AF386359

Atlas of
Skin Pathology

Current Histopathology

Consultant Editor
Professor G. Austin Gresham, TD, ScD, MD, FRC Path.
Professor of Morbid Anatomy and Histology, University of Cambridge

Volume Eleven

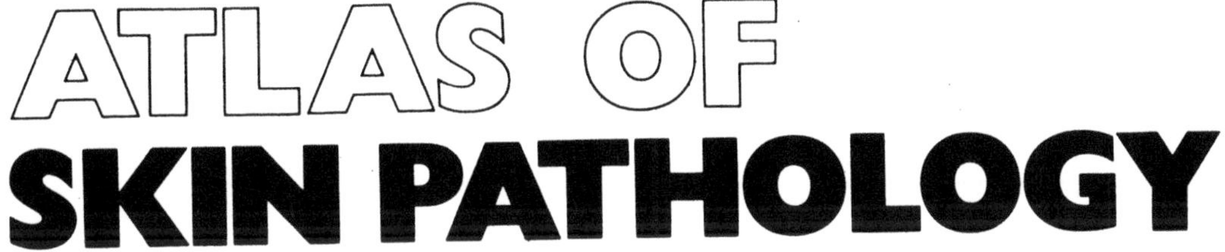

ATLAS OF SKIN PATHOLOGY

BY

R. MARKS
Professor of Dermatology, Department of Medicine

A. KNIGHT
Consultant Dermatologist, Department of Dermatology

P. LAIDLER
Senior Lecturer, Department of Pathology

University of Wales College of Medicine,
Heath Park, Cardiff, Wales
and
University Hospital of Wales,
Heath Park, Cardiff, Wales

SPRINGER-SCIENCE+BUSINESS MEDIA, B.V.

British Library Cataloguing in Publication Data

Marks, R. (Ronald)
    Atlas of skin pathology.—(Current histopathology;
    v. 11)
    1. Skin—Diseases
    I. Title II. Knight, A. III. Laidler, P. IV. Series
    616.5 RL71

    ISBN 978-94-010-8330-0   ISBN 978-94-009-4127-4 (eBook)
    DOI 10.1007/978-94-009-4127-4

Library of Congress Cataloging in Publication Data

Marks, Ronald.
    Atlas of skin pathology.

    (Current histopathology; v. 11)
    Includes bibliographies and index.
    1. Skin—Diseases—Atlases. 2. Histology,
    Pathological—Atlases. I. Knight, A. (Arthur) II.
    Laidler, P. III. Title. IV. Series. [DNLM: 1. Skin
    Diseases—pathology—atlases. W1 CU788JBA v.
    11/WR 17 M346a]
    RL81.M37 1986 616.5'07 86-7233
    ISBN 978-94-010-8330-0

Phototypesetting by Titus Wilson, Kendal.
Colour origination by Tradescanning Ltd., Stockport.

Contents

Consultant Editor's Note

At the present time books on morbid anatomy and histology can be divided into two broad groups: extensive textbooks often written primarily for students and monographs on research topics.

This takes no account of the fact that the vast majority of pathologists are involved in an essentially practical field of general Diagnostic Pathology providing an important service to their clinical colleagues. Many of these pathologists are expected to cover a broad range of disciplines and even those who remain solely within the field of histopathology usually have single and sole responsibility within the hospital for all this work. They may often have no chance for direct discussion on problem cases with colleagues in the same department. In the field of histopathology, no less than in other medical fields, there have been extensive and recent advances, not only in new histochemical techniques but also in the type of specimen provided by new surgical procedures.

There is a great need for the provision of appropriate information for this group. This need has been defined in the following terms.

(1) It should be aimed at the general clinical pathologist or histopathologist with existing practical training, but should also have value for the trainee pathologist.
(2) It should concentrate on the practical aspects of histopathology taking account of the new techniques which should be within the compass of the worker in a unit with reasonable facilities.
(3) New types of material, e.g. those derived from endoscopic biopsy should be covered fully.
(4) There should be an adequate number of illustrations on each subject to demonstrate the variation in appearance that is encountered.
(5) Colour illustrations should be used wherever they aid recognition.

The present concept stemmed from this definition but it was immediately realized that these aims could only be achieved within the compass of a series, of which this volume is one. Since histopathology is, by its very nature, systemized, the individual volumes deal with one system or where this appears more appropriate with a single organ.

This atlas of skin pathology is a valuable addition to the *Current Histopathology* series. It reflects the increasing use of new methods in diagnostic work and illustrates the importance of proper sample preparation and full clinicopathological correlation in achieving diagnostic success. Histochemical reactions of skin are well illustrated here and different enzyme reaction patterns are shown in serial sections. Electron micrographs are included when they assist diagnosis. Careful consultation with clinicians is essential for accurate diagnosis: this information is provided by detailed clinical information accompanying the photomicrographs.

Methods of diagnostic histopathology are frequently changing. New methods are appearing, old ones are being refined and the role of the histopathologist as part of the clinical team is increasingly emphasized. The changing scene is well illustrated by this excellent addition to the series.

G. Austin Gresham
Cambridge

Introduction

Dermatopathology is both exciting and exasperating. Skin has an elegant simplicity in its functions yet a ferocious complexity in its structure. This is one of the paradoxes that underly the pathology of skin disease and may go some way in explaining the multitudinous disorders to which the skin is subject. The ready visibility of the skin may also help explain why straightforward histological examination cannot always provide an answer to a clinicians's question. Quite dramatic appearances may be due to alterations of the relative rates of blood flow, with or without oedema, in the different vascular plexuses or around different structures in the horizontal dimension, neither of which may result in 'much to see' histologically. The inherent sampling error of any histological investigation is of particular importance in dermatopathology. A characteristic disease process may be confined to a particular adnexal structure, a particular stratum of the skin or a particular point in the time course of its evolution.

All these points aside, the skin obeys all the usual 'rules of pathology' and morphological diagnosis with the light microscope is not a separate discipline. In this book we have tried to illustrate the basics of the subject and to emphasize the points in differential diagnosis of the commoner skin disorders. Where possible we have included the various techniques that assist in reaching a diagnosis. We believe that the book should be used 'at the bench' and will also be useful to those who require an uncluttered overview of the subject. With this in mind, we have not given the precise magnification of each of the photomicrographs, but have indicated whether the appearances would be seen down the microscope using a scanning low-power (×2.5–×4) objective (A), a medium-power (×10–×25) (B), a high-power (×40–×100) (C), or a very high-power objective (×100–×250) (D). All the commonly encountered disorders are included but some esoteric diagnoses have been omitted for the sake of clarity. Referencing has been kept to a minimum and should be regarded as a guide to further reading rather than a validation of particular opinions.

We would like to express our thanks to all those colleagues who have helped by providing photographic material for this atlas.

Glossary of Terms. Artefacts. Notes on Techniques

Glossary of Terms

Some special descriptive terms used to describe pathological processes in the skin are defined below. Also included are terms used generally in pathology but which are either used particularly frequently in skin pathology or have acquired a particular significance.

Hyperkeratosis. Thickening of the stratum corneum caused by the accumulation of excess numbers of stratum corneum cells. This occurs in disorders of keratinization because the process of desquamation is disturbed (Figure I.1).

Parakeratosis. The presence of nucleated horn cells in the stratum corneum. Normally the horn cells (corneocytes) are thin lamellae of less than 1 μm thickness. They contain no detectable cytoplasmic contents as these are lost in the granular cell layer. Parakeratosis occurs when the process of keratinization is disturbed such as when the rate of epidermal cell production is increased (as in psoriasis) so that nuclei are not broken down before the stratum corneum is reached and when damage occurs to the upper epidermis (Figure I.2).

Porokeratosis. This is a much more unusual abnormality in which there is a column of parakeratotic cells (cornoid lamella) with hyperkeratosis on either side. It is seen in a number of fairly uncommon disorders (e.g. porokeratosis of Mibelli).

Acanthosis. Thickening of the epidermis due to an increase in the number of epidermal cells. It is usually a consequence of an increased rate of epidermal cell production and is noted in most inflammatory dermatoses. It may occur regularly with regular accentuation of the epidermal rete pegs, when the epidermal thickening is 'psoriasiform', or irregularly as in chronic eczema.

Atrophy. Usually qualified by a term such as 'epidermal' or 'dermal'. Epidermal atrophy signifies decrease in epidermal thickness from the usual four or five cell average to two or three cells thickness with decrease in the usual undulating rete pattern. Dermal atrophy signifies thinning of the dermis. Both epidermal and dermal atrophy occur after use of potent topical corticosteroids and in old age. 'Skin atrophy' implies loss of adnexal elements as well as thinning of epidermal and dermal components.

Hypergranulosis. Thickening of the granular cell layer of the epidermis. Normally the granular cell layer is one to three cell layers thick. Typically the granular cell layer is very thick in lichen planus (Figure I.3).

Hypogranulosis. Absent or deficient granular cell layer. The granular cell layer is often deficient when there is parakeratosis. It is characteristically absent or markedly deficient in autosomal dominant ichthyosis.

Epidermopoiesis. The process of epidermal cell production.

Spongiosis. Epidermal oedema. In spongiosis the epidermal cells retain contact by their desmosomal 'bridges' but are separated by fluid-containing spaces. Typically this occurs in eczema but it is also seen in acute psoriasis and in other inflammatory dermatoses (Figure I.4).

Pseudoepitheliomatous hyperplasia. Massive irregular

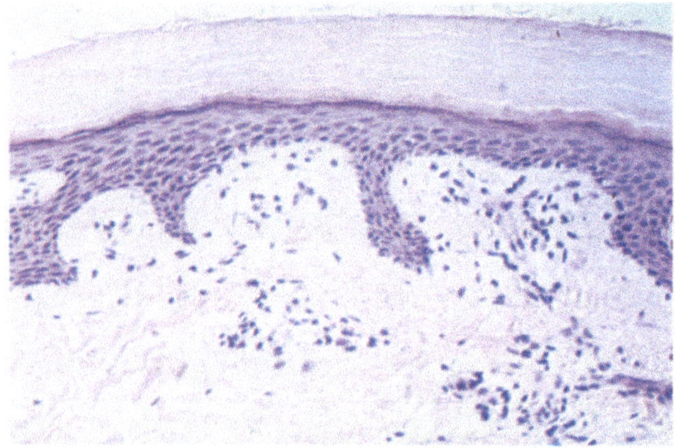

Figure I.1 Hyperkeratosis in skin from patient with lamellar ichthyosis. H & E (B)

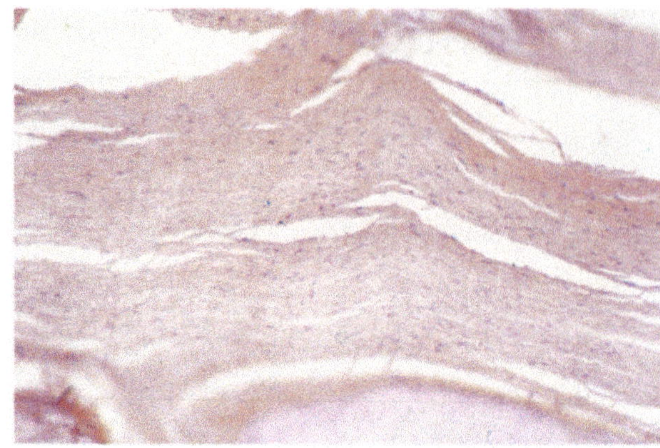

Figure I.2 Parakeratosis. The stratum corneum has retained the nuclei of the epidermis. H & E (C)

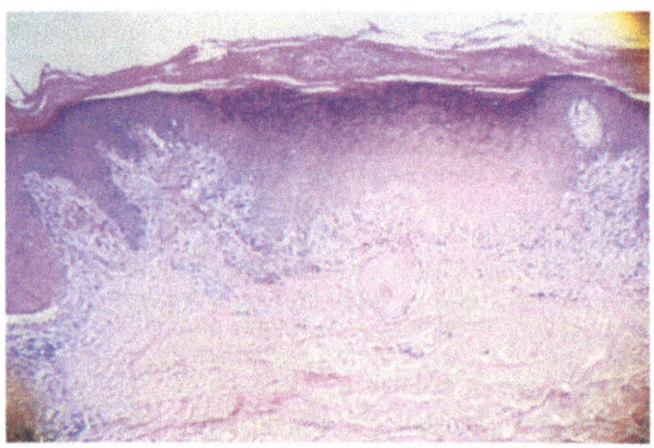

Figure I.3 Hypergranulosis. Marked thickening of the granular cell layer in lichen planus. H & E (A)

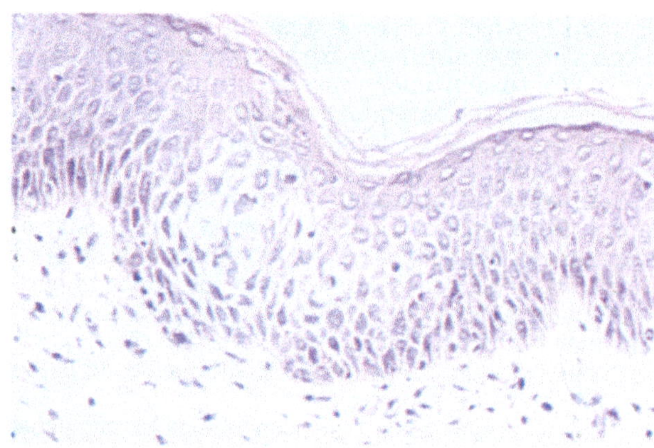

Figure I.4 Spongiosis. The epidermal cells are markedly separated by oedema. H & E (C)

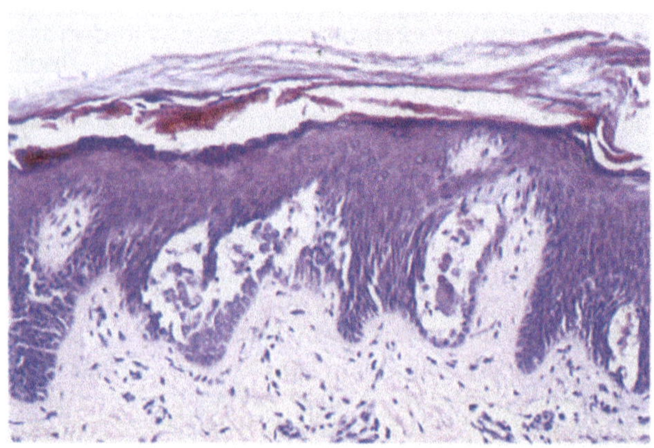

Figure I.5 Acantholysis. Individual epidermal cells can be seen in the suprabasalar cleft within the epidermis. From a patient with pemphigus. H & E (C)

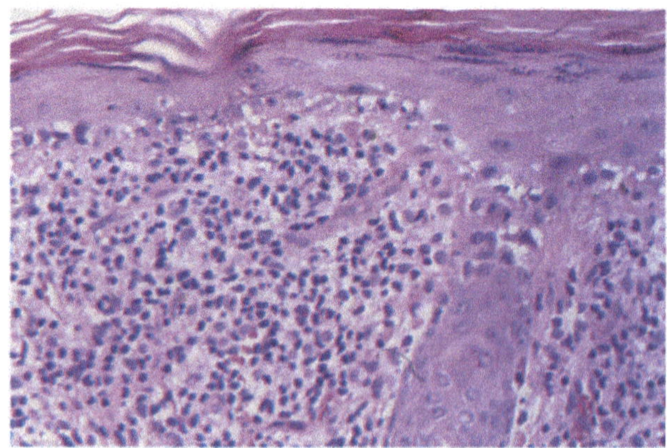

Figure I.6 Basal liquefaction: degenerative change in lichen planus. H & E (C)

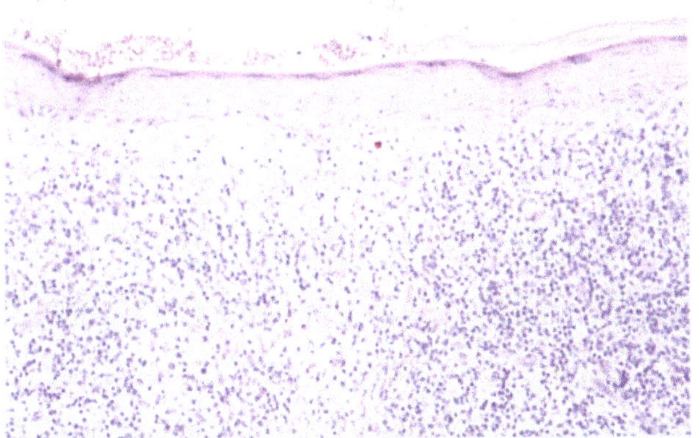

Figure I.7 Colloid bodies: pink globular masses can be seen just beneath the epidermis indicating epidermal cell destruction.   H & E (B)

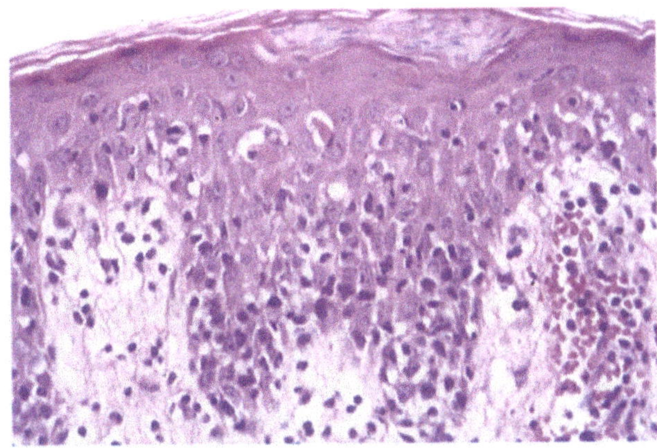

Figure I.8 Exocytosis. Inflammatory cells can be seen to be invading the epidermis. From a patient with pityriasis lichenoides.   H & E (C)

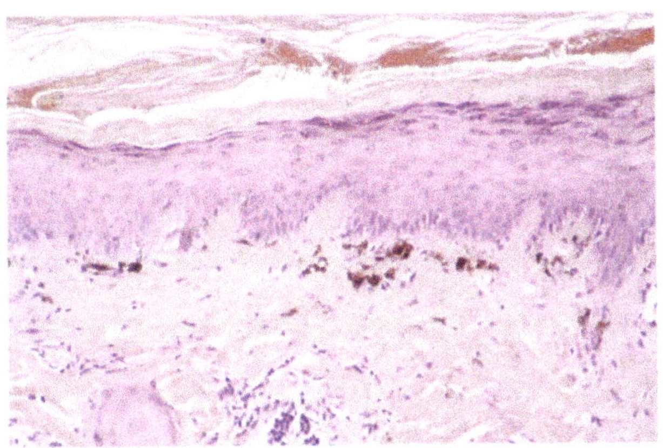

Figure I.9 Pigmentary incontinence. Brown granular pigment is seen beneath the epidermis.   H & E (B)

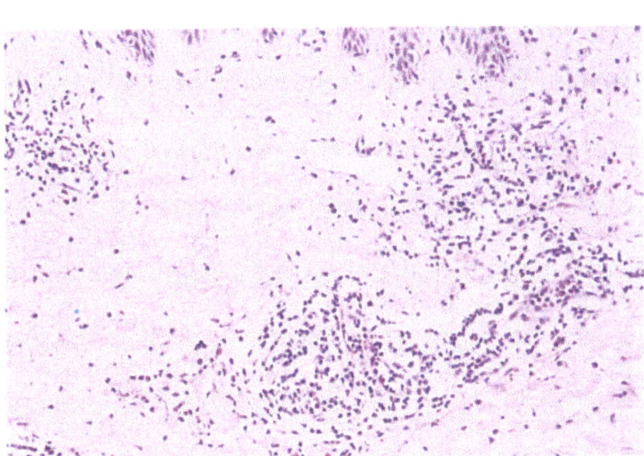

Figure I.10 Leukocytoclastic change. Fragments of polymorphs are seen around the capillary blood vessels.   H & E (C)

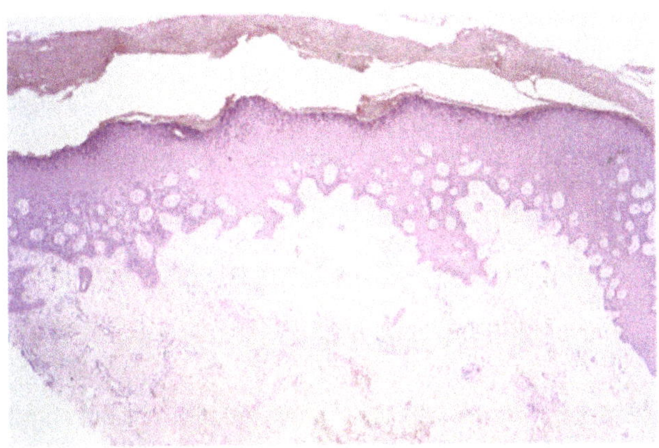

Figure I.11 Oblique cut. The epidermis appears thickened but this is due to an artefact of orientation.   H & E (B)

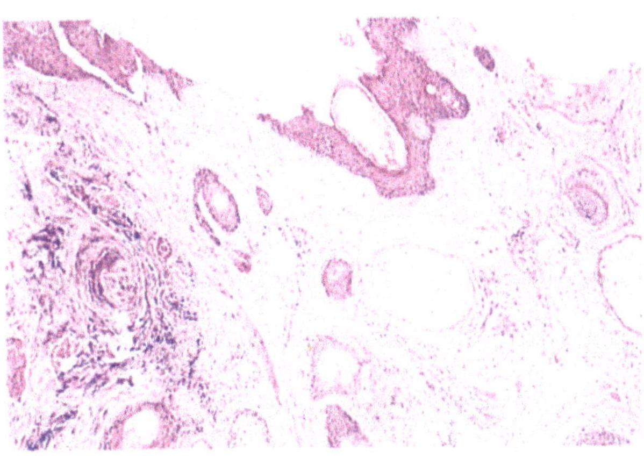

Figure I.12 Crush artefact. The cells appear basophilic and abnormal at the site of crush injury on the left of the figure.   H & E (B)

epidermal thickening (hyperplasia) with some resemblance to squamous cell carcinoma (carcinoma and epithelioma are regarded as synonymous). This degree of epidermal thickening is sometimes seen in the condition known as prurigo nodularis and over the dermal tumour granular cell myoblastoma.

Transepidermal elimination. The process of expulsion of dead or foreign material from the dermis via the epidermis to the exterior by rearrangement of the epidermis so that it engulfs and carries upward the unwanted particles. This process is observed particularly in the condition elastosis perforans serpiginosa but may also be seen in a variety of other conditions, including acne.

Acantholysis. The rounding up of epidermal cells because of dissolution of their desmosomal contacts and their separation one from the other. This condition is classically observed in pemphigus and is the cause of blister formation (Figure I.5).

Dyskeratosis. Abnormal keratinization of epidermal cells in an inappropriate position compared to the surrounding epidermal cells. Malignant dyskeratosis occurs in squamous cell carcinoma and preneoplastic epidermal disorders. Benign dyskeratosis occurs in some disorders of keratinization such as Darier's disease.

Apoptosis. Death and dissolution of epidermal cells within the epidermis. The frequency and significance of this event in normal epidermis is not clear.

Dysplasia. Abnormally growing and differentiating cells with cytological and nuclear abnormalities indicative of neoplastic change.

Liquefactive degenerative change (Hydropic degenerative, vacuolar degeneration). Degenerative change in the basal layer of the epidermis. It is seen typically in lichen planus and lupus erythematosus (Figure I.6).

Colloid body (Civatte body). A homogenous eosinophilic body of approximately the same size as an epidermal cell or larger, and situated either in the basal layer of the epidermis, just below it or occasionally within the body of the epidermis (Figure I.7). Typically colloid bodies are found in lichen planus where they are believed to represent dead epidermal cells.

Exocytosis. Movement of a cell type from its normal location to an abnormal anatomical location. This is a general term but one that is sometimes used to describe the accumulation of inflammatory cells in the epidermis (Figure I.8).

Epidermotropism. The tendency for lymphocytes to accumulate within the epidermis. The term is used to describe the particular situation in mycosis fungoides in which a subset of abnormal T-lymphocytes is particularly 'attracted' to the epidermis and accumulates there in small accumulations known as Pautrier microabscesses.

Pigmentary incontinence. The liberation of melanin pigment from basal epidermal cells due to their damage or destruction. The pigment is liberated into the dermis where it is usually engulfed by phagocytic cells (histiocytes) known as melanophages (Figure I.9). It is a feature of many inflammatory dermatoses including lichen planus and discoid lupus erythematosus.

Papillomatosis. Hypertrophy of the dermal papillae. Typically this is seen in seborrhoeic warts and in some types of naevus cell naevi.

Leukocytoclasia. The destruction of neutrophil polymorphonuclear leukocytes with the liberation of fragments of their nuclei (known as nuclear dust) (Figure I.10). It often accompanies a vasculitis (leukocytoclastic angiitis) and is seen in such disorders as nodular vasculitis, erythema elevatum diutinum and dermatitis herpetiformis.

Vesicle. The accumulation of oedema fluid in small identifiable areas within or beneath the epidermis. Vesicles may arise from accumulation of spongiotic oedema fluid, as in eczema, or from destruction of epidermal cells as in herpes simplex, or from accumulation of oedema fluid within the dermal papillae, as in dermatitis herpetiformis.

Bulla. A bulla is essentially a large vesicle and forms for the same reasons.

Erosion. Loss of protective stratum corneum and epidermis exposing the superficial dermis. The term ulcer usually implies loss of superficial dermis in addition, and persistence.

Lichenoid. This term implies a histological similarity to lichen planus with basal cell destruction, reactive acanthosis and hypergranulosis, and a band-like inflammatory cell infiltrate.

Naevus. A developmental abnormality in which there is a benign hyperplasia of incompletely differentiated tissue elements, often in inappropriate anatomical sites. The term is often used to describe melanocytic naevi ('moles') without the qualifying adjective and the term 'naevus cell' has come to mean the melanocytically derived cells in a melanocytic naevus.

Storiform. Refers to a particular arrangement of tumour cells in a tumour mass where there is an appearance of partial overlapping of successive layers of cells. This arrangement may occur in neurally derived tumours such as neurilemmoma.

Common Artefacts in Skin Pathology

Artefacts due to sectioning. The commonest and often most confusing of artefacts is due to malorientation of the tissue specimen in the wax block. This results in an oblique cut through the tissue, causing some tissue elements to appear in inappropriate sites and others to appear hypertrophied (Figure I.11). If the plane of the section is markedly 'off the vertical plane' the epidermis may seem considerably thickened and may appear to enclose islands of dermis. It is extremely difficult in specimens sectioned in this way to make judgements concerning the deep dermis as often very little of this area of skin is included in the section.

Many skin lesions are small and it is easy to miss the major abnormality in a tissue section. When no abnormality or only minor abnormalities are present it is prudent to obtain futher sections deeper into the block.

When deciding as to the completeness of removal of a tumour it is vital to know the extent to which the tissue has been 'trimmed' before being 'blocked' and to have an adequately orientated section.

Vagaries of the sectioning process can also dislodge fragments of tumour and implant them in unexpected and bizarre anatomical sites. 'Knife carrying over' rarely occurs but the possibility of a fragment of tumour adhering to the microtome blade and being inserted in another section (maybe from a different specimen) has to be borne in mind.

Irregularities in the knife edge often produce odd shatter marks in sections and can produce considerable deformities in sections.

It should be remembered that the trauma of the blade on the tissue specimen often dislodges the stratum corneum so that it is unusual to have the entire thickness of this part of the skin on the section.

Partial blunting of the microtome knife causes uneven thickness of the section. This can give rise to a mistaken impression of the density of cells at one site compared to another.

Artefacts due to surgical techniques. Squeezing the specimen with forceps causes a peculiar artefact with basophilia and alteration of nuclear morphology. It may also cause haemorrhage and destruction of the normal architecture (Figure I.12).

Removal of papillomatous and other exophytic lesions by diathermy or cautery can also give rise to a bizarre appearance with alteration of cellular and nuclear morphology (Figure I.13).

The intracutaneous injection of local anaesthetic does not usually result in any particular artefact but if the injection is made high into the skin it may cause the appearance of oedema and sometimes can cause bleeding.

Artefacts due to preparative and staining techniques. Inadequate fixation (due, for example, to the tissue being removed too quickly from the fixative) may cause the cells to appear swollen or even vacuolated.

Differential shrinkage may cause some parts of the tissue to appear more prominent than they are in life and others to diminish disproportionately.

Brown–black granular deposits are sometimes seen in formalin fixed tissue. These are probably due to a formalin–protein complex which forms under some poorly characterized conditions. They are easily confused by the inexperienced with melanin or blood pigment.

Faulty staining can give rise to several artefacts. These include crystalline stain deposits, uneven staining and inappropriate staining of tissue components.

Wax impregnation can on occasion give rise to an odd 'bubbling' appearance which can cause confusion. Some mounting media crystallize after a few weeks, making proper inspection of the section extremely difficult.

Staining Techniques

Stains are used to demonstrate tissue structure and particular components and deposits. The most usual stain for routine histological sections is haematoxylin and eosin, and this is suitable for virtually all routine purposes. The subject of special stains is complex and for detailed treatment of the subject the reader should consult Drury and Wallington[1]. Table I.1 summarizes the main special stains used for skin and their main uses.

Enzyme Histochemical Techniques

Enzyme histochemical tests identify the presence of particular enzyme activities in tissues. They also enable quantification of the enzyme activity if the tests are performed in a rigorously standardized manner. They depend on reacting slices or sections of the tissue in the presence of the specific substrate for a particular enzyme and revealing the presence of the enzyme activity either by a stable coloured reaction product or by utilizing a product liberated in the reaction to form a stable colour product (Figure I.14). The degree of enzyme activity present is measured either subjectively or accurately with a microdensitometer. The subject is complicated and for detailed treatment the reader should consult reference 2. Table I.2 summarizes the main enzyme histochemical tests of relevance to skin. It should be noted that they are mostly employed for research purposes.

Immunocytochemical Tests

Immunocytochemical tests locate specific biomolecules (or groups of biomolecules) within tissue by using antibodies raised to the specific biomolecules and labelling the antibodies in some way so that they can be visualized (Figure I.15). The subject started off fairly modestly by utilizing the principle to trace the deposition of immunoglobulins and/or complement in tissues with the help of fluorescein isothiocyanate tagged antibodies raised in sheep or rabbits (e.g. in the diagnosis of pemphigus–see page 48). Now with the advent of monoclonal antibodies and new labelling methods the possibilities seem limitless, ranging from the tracing of papilloma virus group antigens in the identification of verruca vulgaris and Bowenoid papulosis of the penis to the identification of components of the dermoepidermal junction in blisters of epidermolysis bullosa for accurate diagnosis. The reader should consult references 3 and 4 for a full

Table I.1 Main special stains used in dermatopathology

Tissue component or substance stained	Stain	Colour change	Notes
Elastic tissue	Weigert	Blue/black	
	Miller	Black	
	Halmi	Magenta	
Collagen	Van Gieson	Red	
Reticulin	Silver stain	Black	
Fat	Oil red O	Red	Most fat is removed in
	Sudan black	Black	processing. For best result
	OTAN technique	Black/brown	unfixed tissue is required.
Glycogen	Periodic acid Schiff	Purple/red	Removed by diastase digestion
Mucosubstances (glycosaminoglycans, proteoglycans)	Alcian blue	Blue	Different substances stained at different pH
	Periodic acid Schiff	Purple/red	Resistant to diastase digestion
	Hale stain	Blue	
Blood pigment (haemosiderin)	Perls' reagent	Blue	
Calcium	Von Kossa	Black	
	Alizarin red S	Red	
	Alkaline methylene blue technique	Blue	On unfixed tissue
Melanin	Fontana (silver)	Black	
	Hamperls	Black	
Epidermal dendritic cells	Gold impregnation techniques	Black	
Nerves	Glees and Marsland silver stain	Black	

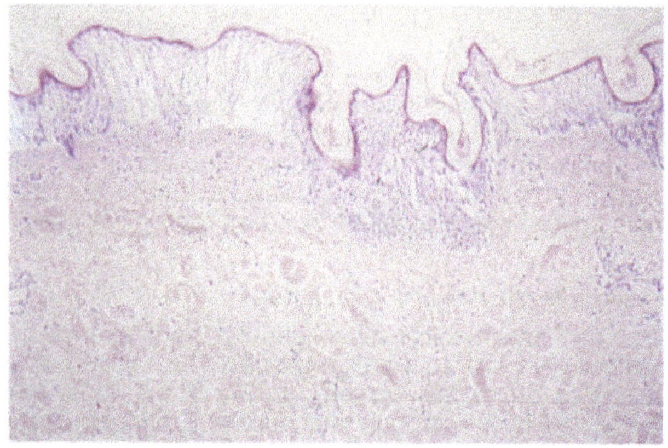

Figure I.13 Burn artefact. The epidermis can be seen vacuolated and degenerate nearby a site of cautery.   H & E (A)

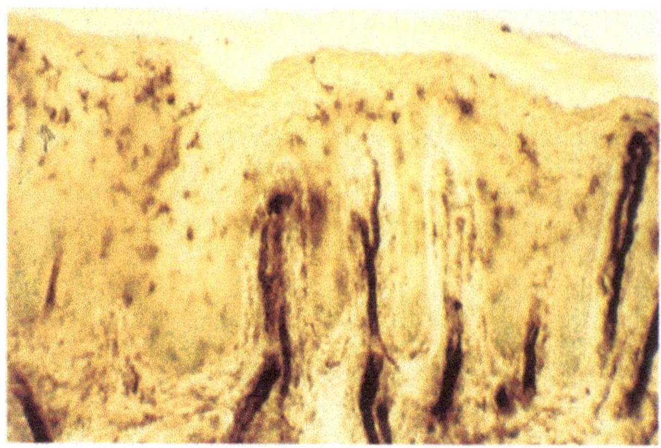

Figure I.14 Adenosine triphosphatase reaction. Histochemical reaction has demonstrated Langerhans cells within the epidermis and both nerves and blood vessels in the dermal papillae.   (B)

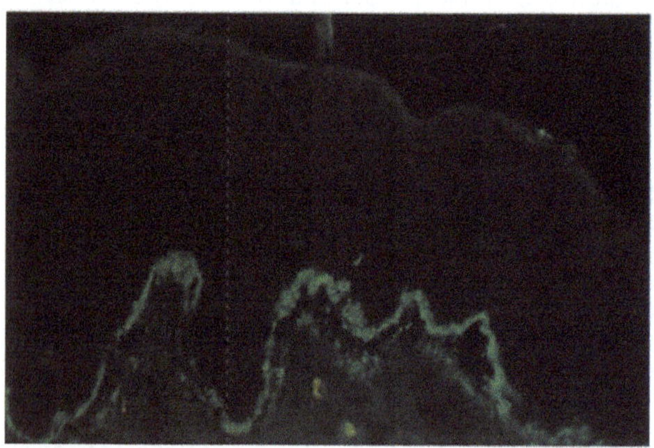

Figure I.15 Immunofluorescence photomicrograph. There is fluorescence subepidermally due to use of an anti-complement antibody and subsequent staining with a fluorescein-tagged reagent. From a patient with pemphigoid. (C)

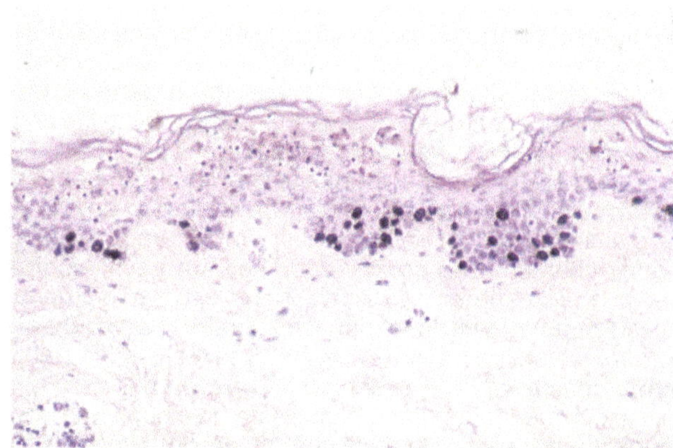

Figure I.16 Autoradiograph after incubation of tissue in the presence of tritiated thymidine. Numerous labelled basal cells in DNA synthesis can be seen. Taken from a piece of skin treated with UV radiation.   (B)

Table I.2 Main enzyme histochemical tests of relevance to dermatopathology

Enzyme histochemical test	Site of reaction	Colour change
Succinic dehydrogenase (and other dehydrogenases of citric acid circle)	Throughout epidermis and epidermal structures. Also in inflammatory cells and endothelium	Blue/black
Lactic dehydrogenase	As above	Blue/black
Glucose-6-phosphate dehydrogenase	Granular cell layer of epidermis	Blue/black
DOPA oxidase (dihydroxyphenylalanine)	Melanocytes	Black/brown
ATPase (adenosine triphosphatase)	Vascular endothelium Nerve fibres	May be black/ brown or red
Non specific esterase	Granular cell layer of epidermis, sweat glands, inflammatory cells	Blue / May be black/brown or red
Acid phosphatase		
Alkaline phosphatase	Endothelium	Black/brown

account of this topic. Some antibodies of use in immunocytochemistry are set out in Table I.3.

Autoradiographic Techniques

Autoradiographic methods enable synthetic reactions to be located and quantified. A radioactively labelled precursor molecule is introduced into the tissue to be studied. In this process the molecule synthesized becomes radioactive and can then be tracked by covering the section with special photographic film. At the site of radioactivity, clumps of photographic silver grains appear. Probably the best-known example of the technique is the demonstration of the sites of premitotic DNA synthesis using the radioactivity labelled precursor tritiated thymidine[5] (Figure I.16).

Table I.3 Main immunocytochemical tests of relevance in dermatopathology

Antibodies directed against:	Diagnostic use
Immunoglobulins and complement components	Pemphigus, pemphigoid, dermatitis herpetiformis
Laminin and type IV collagen	Epidermolysis bullosa, bullous pemphigoid
Lymphocyte subset surface markers	Mycosis fungoides, dermal lymphoma
Intracytoplasmic immunoglobulins (including light chains)	Cutaneous deposits of myeloma
S100 protein	Tumour diagnosis (Schwannoma, granular cell tumour, melanoma)
Factor VIII related antigen and *Ulex europaeus* lectin	Tumour diagnosis (Angiosarcoma, Kaposi's sarcoma)
Carcinoembryonic antigen	Paget's disease, adnexal tumours
Prekeratin	Undifferentiated squamous-cell carcinoma
Neuron-specific enolase	Merkel-cell carcinoma

References

1. Drury, R. A. B. and Wallington, E. A. (1980). *Carleton's Histological Technique*. 5th Ed, (Oxford: Oxford University Press)

2. Chayen, J., Bitensky, L. and Butcher, R. G. (1973). *Practical Histochemistry*. (London: Wiley)

3. Beutner, E. H., Chorzelski, J. P., Bean, S. F. and Jordon, R. E. (1973). *Immunopatholoy of the Skin: Labelled Antibody Studies*. (Stroudsburg: Hutchinson and Ross)

4. Polak, J. M. and Van Noorden, S. (1984). *An Introduction to Immunocytochemistry. Current Techniques and Problems*. (Royal Microscopical Society Microscopy Handbook Ser.) (Oxford: Oxford University Press)

5. Marks, R. (1979). Measurement of epidermal growth activity. In Marks, R. (ed.) *Investigative Techniques in Dermatology*, pp. 127–43. (Oxford: Blackwells Scientific Publications)

Normal Skin

The Epidermis and Stratum Corneum

The prime function of the epidermis is the production of the protective stratum corneum. As conventional histological fixation and sectioning techniques virtually destroy the stratum corneum, this simple truth is not always appreciated (Figure 1.1). The stratum corneum is approximately 15 μm thick over the limbs and trunk and consists of some 15–20 layers of closely interdigitating, flattened corneocytes (each approximately 35 μm in diameter and less than 1 μm thick). Cryostat sectioning and swelling techniques are needed to demonstrate the stratum corneum[1,2]. It must never be forgotten that the skin is a three-dimensional structure and it is sometimes helpful to examine this structure in the horizontal plane using the skin surface biopsy technique[3]. Using this simple method and staining with periodic acid Schiff reagent, it is much easier to identify fungi (Figure 1.2) or other types of microflora than in conventional histological sections[4]. It is also suitable for examination of nucleated horn (parakeratosis).

The epidermis consists of some 3–5 layers of cuboidal or oval basophilic cells (Figure 1.3). The deepest layer is the basal layer. The basal cells and some of the immediately suprabasal epidermal cells form the generative compartment. Cells produced here move upwards to differentiate and eventually become the stratum corneum (keratinization). Mitotic figures are rarely seen in the normal epidermis but cells in the DNA synthesis phase can be identified by presenting the living tissue either *in vivo* or *in vitro* with the radioactively labelled DNA precursor tritiated thymidine, and processing the tissue section by the technique of autoradiography[5] (Figure 1.4). As the epidermal cells move upwards through the epidermis they gradually enlarge and in the granular layer they also become flatter. The differentiated corneocytes (horn cells) are thin (less than 1 μm thick), shield-like structures some 35 μm in diameter. The granular cells are so called because of the accumulation of amorphous, irregular, basophilic granules in their cytoplasm.

Keratin polypeptides are present as tonofilaments in the cytoplasm of basal cells (Figure 1.5) but there is a change in the distribution of the molecular weights of the polypeptides as the keratinocytes become more differentiated so that higher molecular weight species are found higher in the epidermis. The tonofilaments become aggregated into bundles in the granular cell layer under the influence of a histidine-rich protein derived from the granules, known as filaggrin. The tonofilaments are members of the intermediate filament group of cytoplasmic structures and are inserted into the desmosomal plate at the cell periphery.

Keratinocytes are connected to each other by complex lamellated structures known as desmosomes (Figure 1.6). There are also a few tight junctions, but gap junctions are rare. During the process of keratinization a tough, chemically resistant, cross-linked protein wall develops just within the plasma membrane of the granular cell. Small rounded, lamellated bodies develop within the upper part of the Malpighian layer (lamellar bodies, Odland bodies, membrane coating granules). These are expelled into the intercellular space at the junction between the granular cell layer and stratum corneum. It is thought that they 'unfurl' and lay down a layer of glycolipid (ceramide) which is important to the barrier function of the stratum corneum.

During the process of keratinization the keratinocyte nucleus and many of the cytoplasmic organelles disappear. The detail of this process is not as yet fully understood but liberation of lysosomal hydrolases probably plays a role. Certainly esterase and acid phosphatase can be detected by enzyme histochemical techniques in the normal granular cell layer (Figure 1.7).

The dermo-epidermal junction has a particular importance in the pathophysiology of skin disease and an understanding of its structure is important in the interpretation of the morphology in many skin disorders. It is an undulating structure and when seen in the horizontal plane can be seen to be indented by the dermal papillae as a series of fingers poking up into the epidermis. The basal keratinocytes rest on a basal lamina consisting of an electron lucent lamina lucida and an electron-dense lamina densa (Figure 1.8). Hemidesmosomes are specialized structures of the keratinocyte plasma membrane which attach it to the basal lamina and extensions seem to traverse the substance of this structure. This region is complex biochemically, and contains many glycoprotein species, including laminin, entactin and the bullous pemphigoid antigen[6]. At the light-microscope level there is a PAS positive 'basement membrane' between the epidermis and the dermis (Figure 1.9). The dermo-epidermal junction undulates variably, this so-called rete pattern being prominent on the palms and soles and hardly evident on the face. The downward projections of the epidermis are known as epidermal rete pegs and the dermal projections are called dermal papillae.

The Pigmentary System

Melanin pigment is produced by melanocytes in the basal layer of the epidermis. These cells are dendritic and do not possess desmosomes. This fact accounts for their appearance as 'clear cells' (Figure 1.10) which is an artefact due to the effects of fixation. Melanin is produced within cytoplasmic organelles of the melanocyte known as melanosomes. Melanin synthesis can be demonstrated by the DOPA oxidase staining technique in which the substrate dihydroxyphenylalanine is oxidized to melanin pigment (Figure 1.11). When the

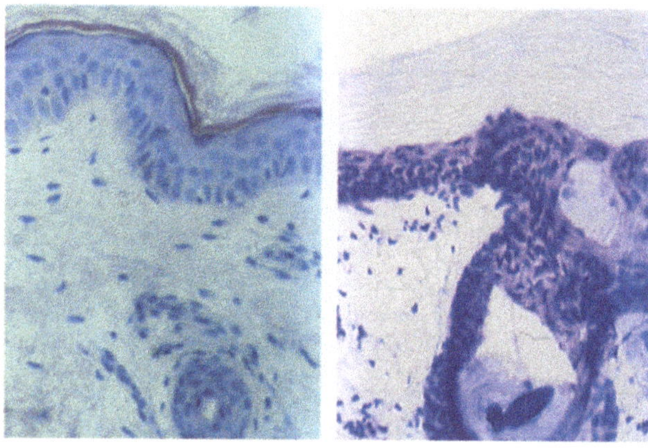

Figure 1.1   Stratum corneum as seen in routinely prepared section (left) and in specially prepared cryostat section (right).   H & E (B)

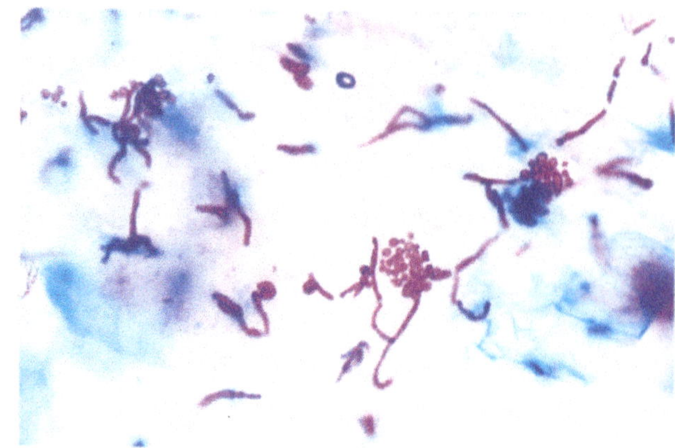

Figure 1.2   Skin surface biopsy stained with periodic acid Schiff reaction to show spores and pseudohyphae of *Pityriasis versicolor*.   PAS (C)

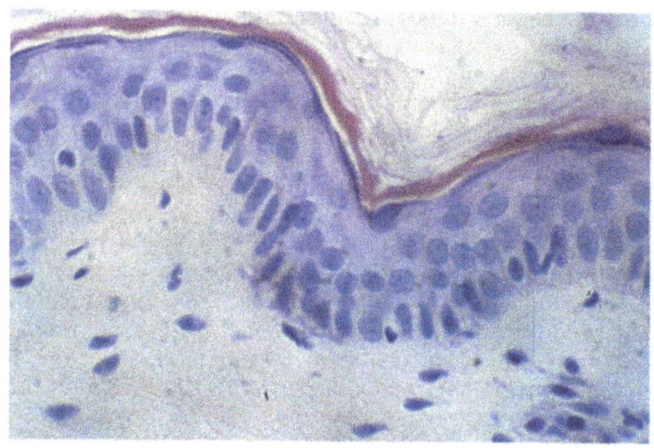

Figure 1.3   Normal epidermis.   H & E (C)

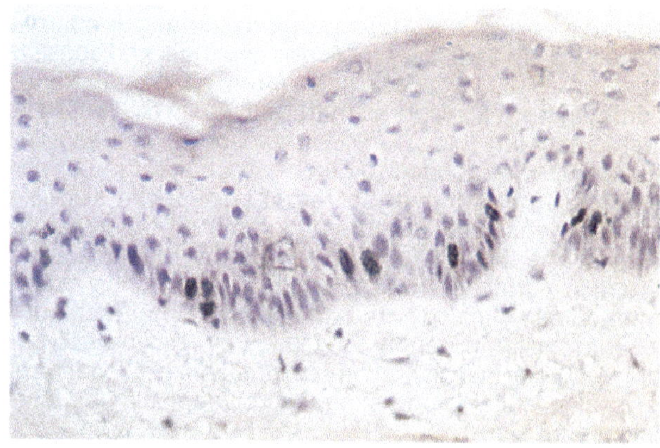

Figure 1.4   Autoradiographically labelled basal epidermal cells in DNA synthesis.   (C)

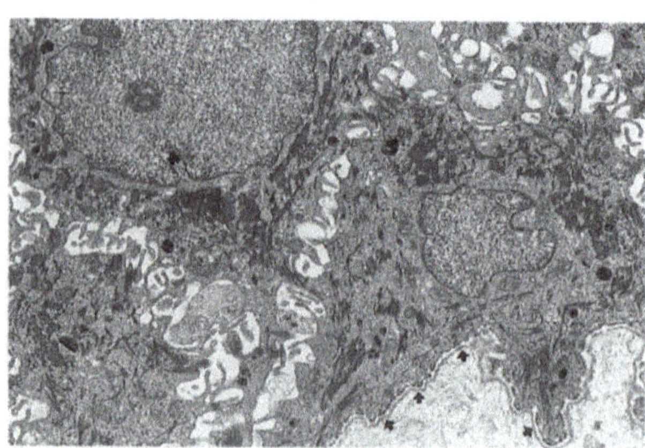

Figure 1.5   Electron micrograph to show keratinocytes in the basal layer of the epidermis supported on basement membrane (arrowed).   × 5300

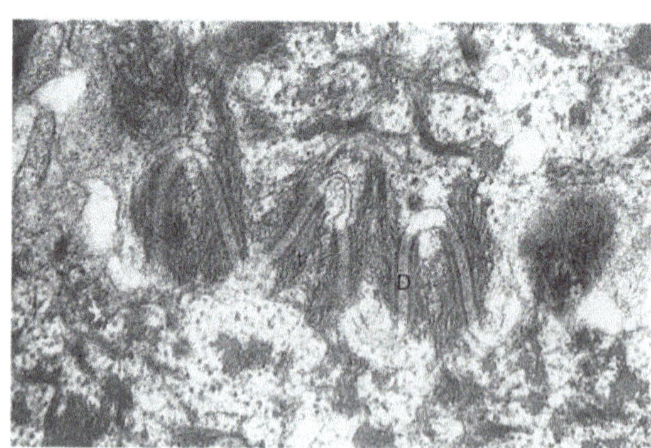

Figure 1.6   Desmosomes (D) between keratinocytes (t = tonofilaments).   × 29 000

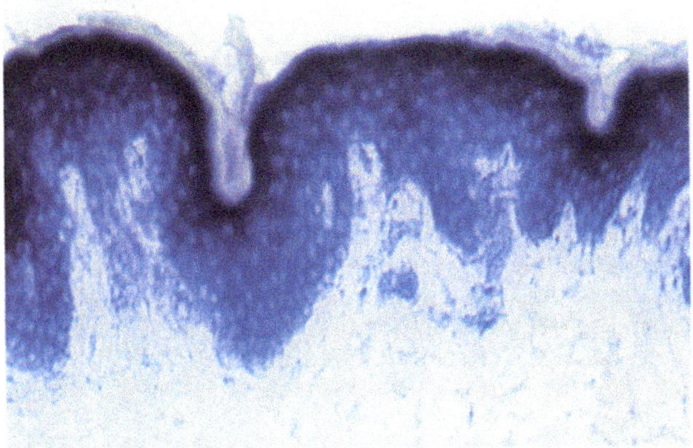

Figure 1.7 Cytochemical reaction to show deposition of Formazan reaction product in epidermis with accentuation in granular cell layer. (C)

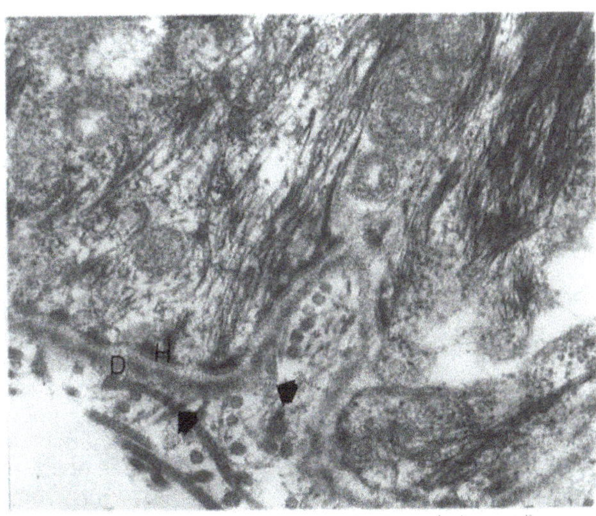

Figure 1.8 Dermo-epidermal junction. Hemidesmosomes (H) on plasma membrane of basal keratinocyte. Fine anchoring filaments appear to cross lamina lucida to the lamina densa (D). On dermal aspect of this there are anchoring fibrils (arrowed). × 40 000

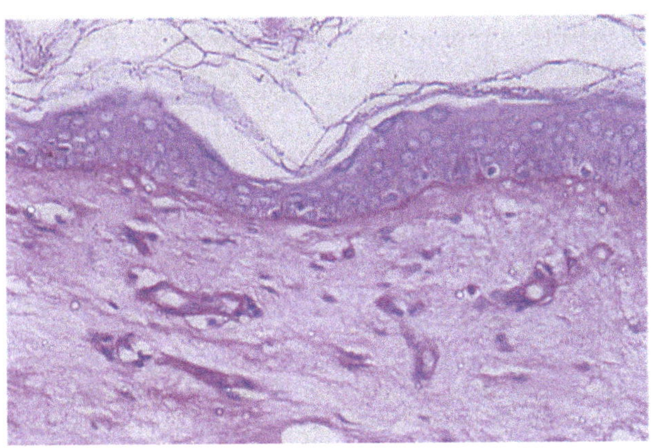

Figure 1.9 Basement membrane demonstrated by periodic acid Schiff reagent. PAS (B)

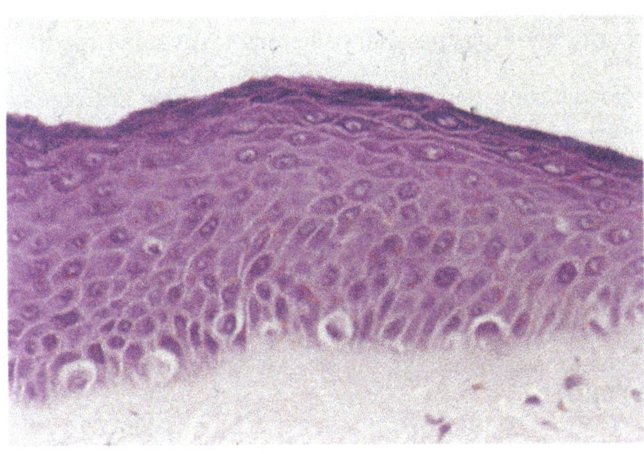

Figure 1.10 Clear cells in basal layer of thickened epidermis. H & E (C)

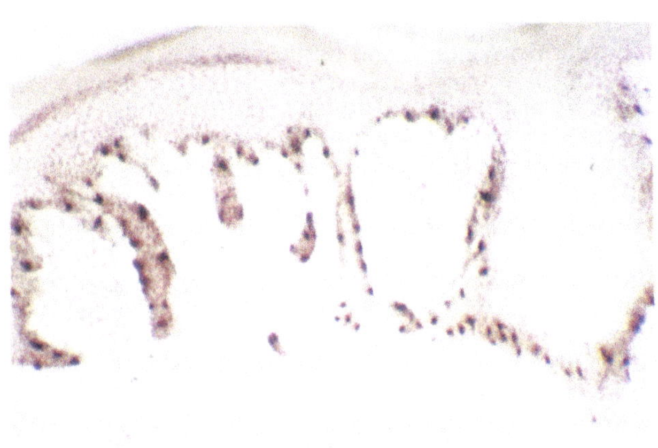

Figure 1.11 Melanocytes demonstrated by dihydroxyphenylalanine (DOPA) reaction in thickened epidermis. (B)

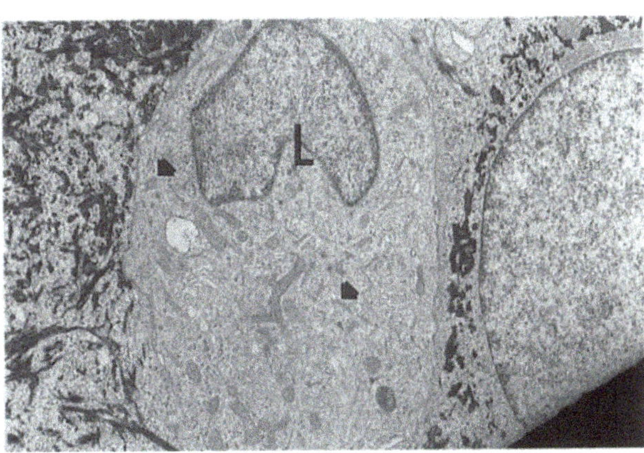

Figure 1.12 Langerhans cell (L) demonstrated between keratinocytes. Rod-like Birbeck granules can be clearly seen (arrowed). × 5300

basal layer of the epidermis is damaged, as, for example, in lichen planus (see page 53), the pigment is shed into the dermis where it is engulfed by macrophages ('melanophages'). Melanocytes account for approximately five per cent of the population of the basal cell layer of the epidermis.

The Langerhans Cell[7]

These dendritic cells appear in light-microscope preparations as 'clear cells' for the same reason as do melanocytes. They are found in the mid epidermal zones and account for some 2–5 per cent of the epidermal population. They are mesenchymal in origin and thought to originate in the bone marrow. Their function is believed to be primarily that of antigen presentation to lymphocytes so that they form an important part of the immune defence system. Ultrastructurally they have a convoluted nucleus and may be identified by the presence of particular structures known as Birbeck granules. These are now thought to represent complex infoldings of the plasma membrane but often appear as tennis racket-shaped structures (Figure 1.12). Langerhans cells may be identified by the adenosine triphosphatase reaction (Figure 1.13), by gold impregnation, or by newer immunolocalization techniques using monoclonal antibodies, e.g. OKT6.

Merkel cells

These are yet another non-keratinocyte cell type found within the epidermis. It is thought that they may have an important neuro-endocrine function, though this has not been fully elucidated. They possess specialized granules which distinguish them ultrastructurally. They may possess desmosomes but do not seem to have tonofilaments.

The Adnexal Structures

Hair follicles and sebaceous glands, eccrine sweat glands and apocrine glands may be regarded as specialized invaginations of the epidermis.

Hair Follicles and Sebaceous Glands

The hair follicles in man have periods of growth (anagen), arrest (catagen) and dormancy (telogen). The relative lengths of these phases of the hair cycle determine the length of the hair. The density of hair follicles is constant and the relative hairiness of individuals depends on the size of the follicle, the length of the anagen phase and the degree of pigmentation of the hair shaft. On the face, chest and upper back, hair follicle structures are well developed but the sebaceous glands are larger than elsewhere and are out of proportion to the size of the hair shaft.

The hair shaft is formed in the hair matrix (Figure 1.14) which is indented by the hair papilla containing blood vessels and tissue that appears to organize the growth of the hair. The hair canal is formed by several layers of specialized epidermal cells – the external root sheath on the outside, the layers of Huxle and Henle, and internal to these, the internal root sheath. The hair shaft itself is covered by cuticular cells. In the middle of the first part of the hair shaft is the hair medulla, and surrounding this, the cortex. All these parts of the hair follicle should be regarded as specialized parts of the epidermis with particular patterns of differentiation[8].

The sebaceous glands drain into the follicular canal at the junction of the upper third and the lower two thirds via a short sebaceous duct. It is a holocrine gland and sebum secretion consists of the breakdown products of mature lipid-laden sebaceous gland cells (sebocytes). Sebocytes are produced by small crescentic basophilic germinative cells at the periphery of the sebaceous gland. As the cells mature they enlarge, become lipidized and vacuolated, and move towards the centre of the sebaceous gland lobule. In the elderly the sebaceous glands of the face often undergo hypertrophy and may form discrete yellowish-orange nodules which may simulate basal cell carcinoma (see page 108).

Eccrine Sweat Glands

These structures are distributed all over the body and are particularly prominent on the palms and soles. The glands drain directly onto the body surface via the eccrine sweat duct which runs from the coiled eccrine sweat gland situated in the deep dermis and pursues a coiled course through the epidermis and stratum corneum (Figure 1.15). The duct is lined by cuboidal cells which are in turn surrounded by myoepithelial cells. Ultrastructurally the lining cells consist of both light and dark cells which probably have different secretory functions. In response to thermal and emotional stimuli the glands produce a watery secretion – eccrine sweat – which contains NaCl and traces of other substances including other electrolytes, urea, proteins and amino acids. The glands are surrounded by a condensation of dermal connective tissue containing a vascular plexus and their autonomic neural supply. The nerves supplying them are sympathetic postganglionic elements but release acetylcholine to stimulate the glands.

Apocrine Sweat Glands

These are located in the axillae, groin, genital, perianal and alveolar skin around the nipple. Rarely they may occur outside these areas. Structurally they are similar to eccrine glands but are larger and drain into the upper parts of the hair follicles of the region concerned. Their lining cells are columnar, rather than cuboidal, and their distal sections can be seen to be in the process of being pinched off to form the apocrine secretion. Both eccrine and apocrine glands contain glycogen granules and may be PAS positive. Apocrine secretion is a thick, viscid lipid containing material whose function is unknown.

The Dermis

The dermis contains the fibrous elements of the skin, interfibrillary amorphous material and connective tissue cells. It also contains the vasculature (blood vessels, lymphatics and vascular plexuses) neural structures (nerves and nerve endings) and the adnexal structures. The dermal collagen supplies most of the mechanical strength and elasticity of the skin and has an important supporting role for the underlying tissues. It extends from the dermo-epidermal junction to the subcutaneous fat and is 0.8 to 2.5 mm in thickness, depending on body site. The fibres have a specific orientation that also depends on body site. The papillary dermis in the immediate subepidermal zone and the upper dermis are much more loosely arranged than the deeper portions of the dermis, which possess broader and more tightly packed collagen bundles (Figure 1.16).

The Fibrous and Amorphous Elements

The fibrous elements consist of collagen and elastin. The collagen fibres form by far the greatest proportion of the visible dermis. They are made of bundles of fibrils which consist of collagen peptides wound around each other arranged in a 'triple helix'. The fibrils can be seen ultrastructurally to be crossbanded every 64 nm (Figure 1.17). Elastic fibres are only visible by special stains. They are arranged in a felt-like band subepidermally and also encircle and bind together the bundles of collagen (Figure 1.18). The elastic network subepidermally has expansions known as elastic globes. Ultrastructurally elastic fibres are broader than collagen and can be seen to consist of an amorphous matrix (elastin) in which are embedded microfibrils. Elastic fibres regenerate extremely slowly after any type of injury and are mostly absent in scarred and inflamed areas.

Reticulin fibres are thin fibrous structures that stain with silver stains in particular and encircle the blood vessels. They probably represent a variety of collagen.

In life the interstices of the dermal fibrous network are filled with an amorphous ground material containing a high proportion of proteoglycan. This is leached out during fixation and processing and is not visible in routine sections.

The Cellular Elements

Interspersed amongst the fibres are spindle or ribbon-shaped fibroblasts. These are the cells that synthesize and secrete all the fibrous elements and the ground substance of the dermis. Ultrastructurally the fibroblasts can be seen to contain abundant endoplasmic reticulum and mitochrondria (Figure 1.19). The normal dermis may also contain a few cells of other types, including mast cells and lymphocytes.

The Dermal Vasculature[9]

The epidermis contains no blood vessels but is nourished and oxygenated by the diffusion of materials from the papillary capillaries in the dermal papillae. These simple capillary loops which derive from the horizontally organized vascular plexuses in the upper and mid dermis can be demonstrated by the alkaline phosphatase or by the adenosine triphosphate histochemical techniques (Figure 1.20). They are little more than thin endothelial tubes resting on a basal lamina. The vessels of the various plexuses in the dermis are thicker and the luminal endothelial cells are surrounded by a layer of perithelial cells. The larger venous channels in the dermis also have a muscular coat and perivascular connective tissue. Arterial vessels tend to be thinner than veins. There are also rich vascular plexuses around the hair follicles and the sweat glands. Arteriovenous shunts occur in the fingertips and the palms and soles. The lymphatic chan-

nels can be recognized by the flatter endothelial cells lining their lumina with nuclei projecting into the lumina and by their angulated or trefoil appearance in histological sections. The presence of red cells in such channels does not necessarily mean that they are not lymphatics, due to the existence of lymphatico-venous channels. Lymphatic valves can occasionally be seen as endothelial tongues crossing the lumen of the vessels.

Dermal Neural Elements

The epidermis contains no identifiable neural structures. Nerve fibres in the dermis can be demonstrated by the adenosine triphosphatase technique or by a silver impregnation technique (e.g. Bodian stain). There is a rich innervation just subepidermally and around the hair follicles. At some sites specialized nerve receptors can be found. The large lamellated (onion skin-like) Vater–Pacini corpuscles are particularly easily seen in palmar and penile skin (Figure 1.21). Meissner corpuscles consist of large clear cells arranged in vertical layers (Figure 1.22).

References

1. Christophers, E. (1970). Eine neue Methode zur Darstellung des Stratum corneum. *Arch. Klin. Exp. Dermatologie*, **237**, 717

2. Mackenzie, I. C. and Linder, J. E. (1973). An examination of cellular organization within the stratum corneum by a silver staining method. *J. Invest. Dermatol.*, **61**, 245

3. Marks, R. and Dawber, R. P. M. (1971). Skin surface biopsy: an improved technique for the examination of the horny layer. *Br. J. Dermatol.*, **84**, 117

4. Marks, R. and Dawber, R. P. R. (1972). In situ microbiology of the stratum corneum. *Arch. Dermatol.*, **105**, 216

5. Marks, R. (1979). Measurement of epidermal growth activity. In Marks, R. (ed.) *Investigative Techniques in Dermatology*. p. 127. (Oxford: Blackwell Scientific Publications)

6. Katz, S. I. (1984). The epidermal basement membrane zone – structure, ontogeny and role in disease. *J. Am. Acad. Dermatol.*, **11**, 1025

7. Hunter, J. A. A. (1983). The Langerhans cell: from gold to glitter. *Clin. Exp. Dermatol.*, **8**, 569

8. Pinkus, H. (1968). Static and dynamic histology and histochemistry of hair growth. In Baccaredda-Bay, A., Moretti, G. and Frey, G. R. (eds.) *Biopathology of Pattern Alopecia*. (Basel: Karger)

9. Pear, R. M. (1983). Vascular supply to the skin: an anatomical and physiological re-appraisal. Parts I and II. *Ann. Plastic Surg.*, **11**, 99–105; 196–205

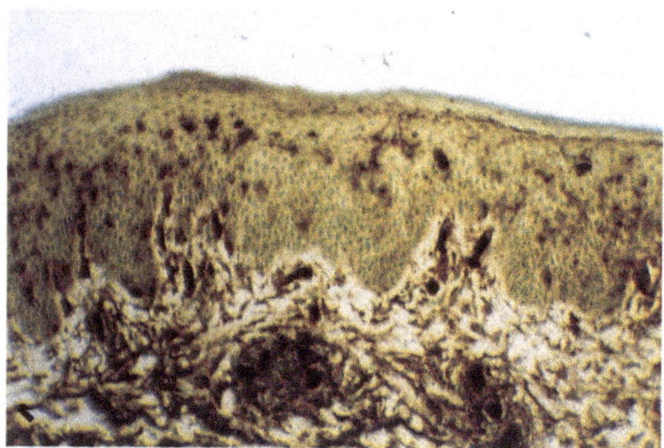

Figure 1.13 Langerhans cells demonstrated by adenosine triphosphatase (ATPase) reaction. (B)

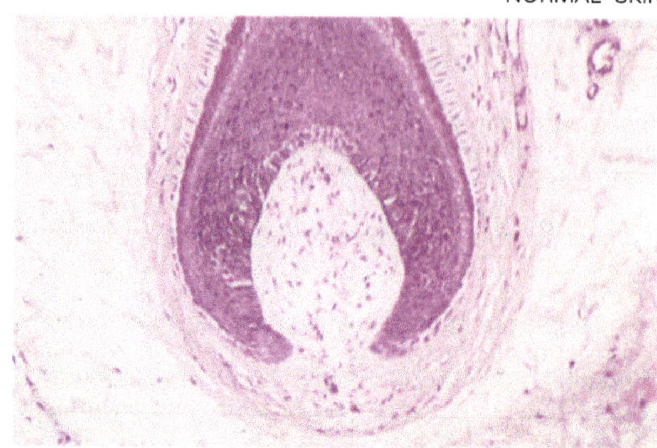

Figure 1.14 Hair papilla and matrix. H & E (B)

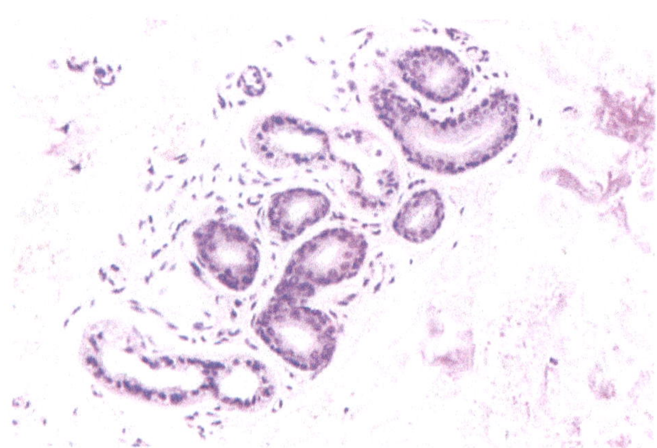

Figure 1.15a Eccrine sweat gland tubules. H & E (B)

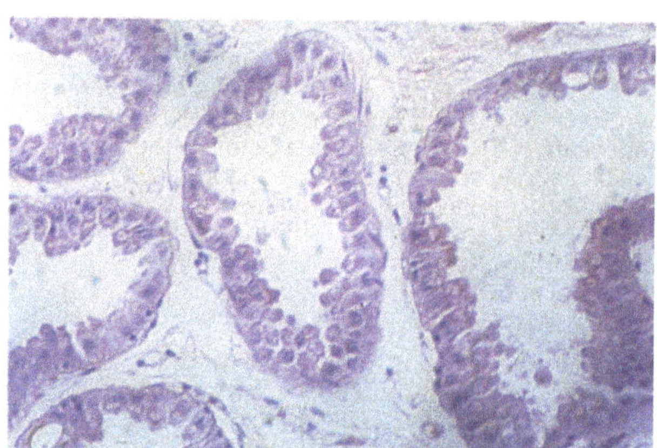

Figure 1.15b Apocrine sweat gland tubules. H & E (C)

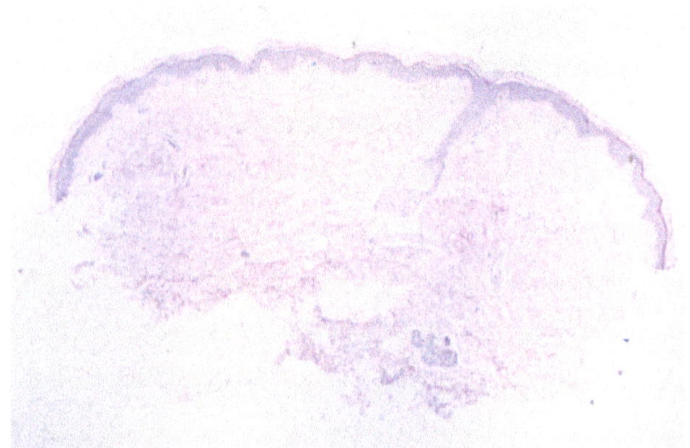

Figure 1.16 Section to show general arrangement of dermis. H & E (A)

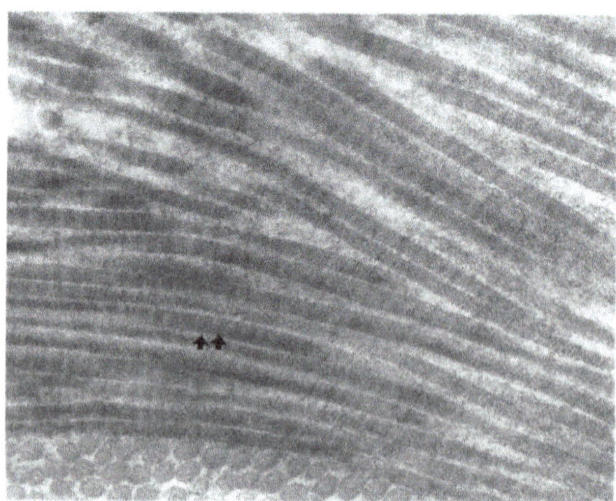

Figure 1.17 Collagen fibres seen in both cross section and longitudinal section. The periodicity can be seen in the longitudinal section (64nm – arrowed). × 35000

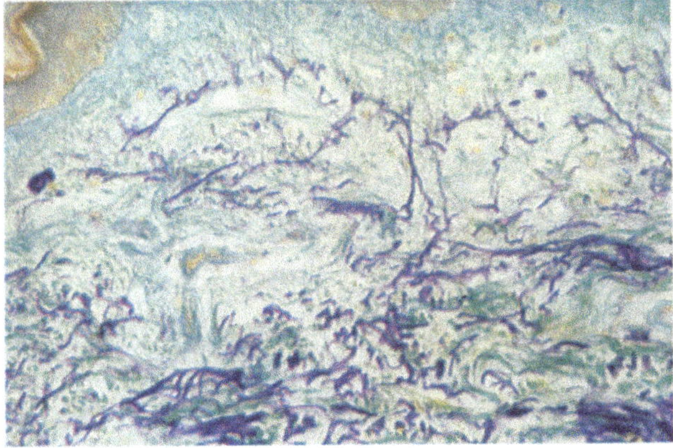

Figure 1.18 Arrangement of elastic fibres demonstrated by Halmi's Trichrome. (B)

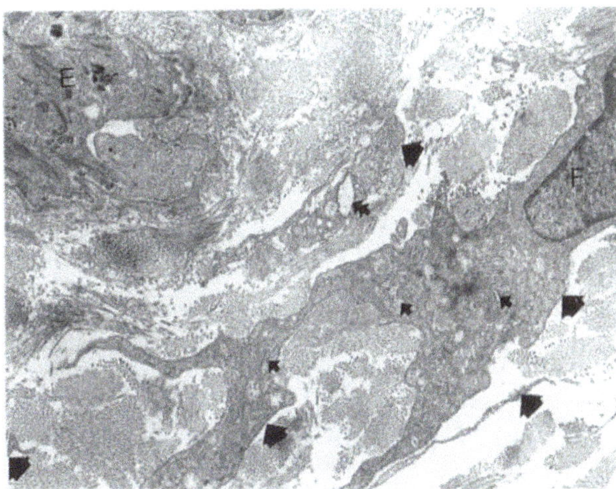

Figure 1.19 Fibroblast nucleus (F) and extensive cytoplasm (large arrows). Endoplasmic reticulum can be seen (small arrows) some of which is dilated (large arrows) (E = epidermis). × 3100

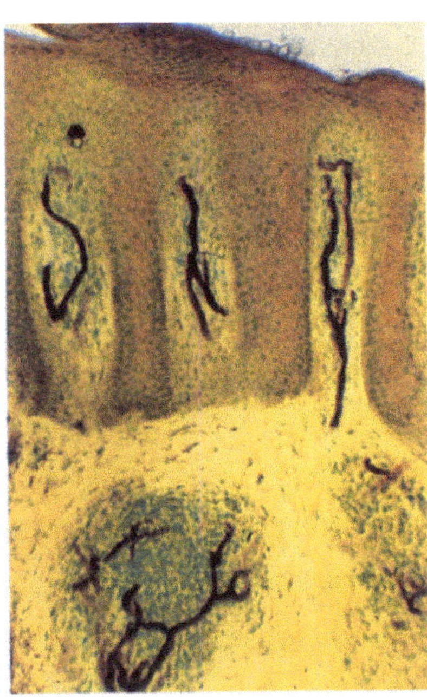

Figure 1.20 Papillary capillaries demonstrated by adenosine triphosphatase stain beneath thickened epidermis. (B)

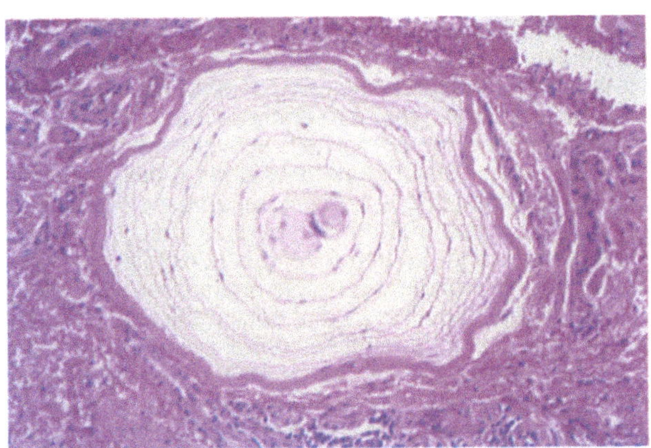

Figure 1.21 Vater–Pacini corpuscles in penile skin. H & E (B)

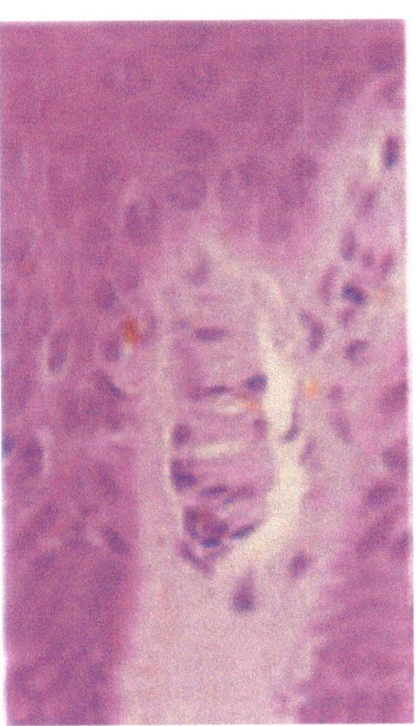

Figure 1.22 Meissner corpuscles. H & E (C)

The sequence of changes that occur in the skin after injury are similar regardless of whether the injury is caused by a knife, by a burn or by a disease process (Figure 2.1). Immediately after injury the extravasated blood clots, due to activation of the clotting cascade, and vasoconstriction occurs. Polymorphonuclear leukocytes accumulate at the site of injury and separate viable from damaged, non-viable tissue components. After some 12 to 24 hours the process of re-epithelialization begins[1]. In the initial stages, epidermal cells actively move over the wounded area. The migrating epidermal cells adopt a spindle- or ribbon-shaped profile, resembling fibroblasts (Figure 2.2). Ultrastructurally they lose their desmosomal apparatus and cell-to-cell contact reverts to primitive interdigitating microvilli. Some 48 hours after wounding, mitotic activity begins at a point behind the leading edge of the sheet of migrating epidermal cells, and on the third and fourth days maturation of the new epidermal cover begins. During the early stages of re-epithelialization the epidermal cells need no specialized dermo-epidermal apparatus, but burrow through the damaged tissue planes, isolating the viable deeper tissues from the superficial necrotic crust, which is eventually sloughed off. Later on, the new epidermis secretes its own junctional apparatus, restoring continuity with the dermis beneath[2].

New blood vessels and the restoration of the capillary network in the damaged skin is a vital step in the repair process. It begins very early in the repair sequence by endothelial buds being generated from the cut capillaries. These ramify in the new tissue, being formed in the subepidermal zone, and recanalize after a few days. Repair of the connective tissue structures takes very much longer and full structural and functional integrity may take many months before the prewounding state is restored. In the early stages, damaged collagen is removed by the action of collagenases, and new collagen is secreted by the fibroblasts that populate the wounded area. The new collagen at first has no particular orientation but the previous orientation is restored after a few weeks by the stresses on the collagenous framework. The original strength of the skin may not be restored for some months. The last components to be restored are the elastic fibres and the neural components. Neither of these components may ever completely regain their prewounding state.

Acute Sunburn

The changes detected will depend on the stage at which the skin is sampled and the dose of ultraviolet radiation received. Amongst the first changes is the development of what are known as sunburn cells in the midepidermis. These are eosinophilic, slightly swollen cells which are either anucleate or have pyknotic nuclei (Figure 2.3).

Enzyme histochemical studies will reveal an increase in hydrolytic enzyme activity (e.g. 'non-specific' esterase activity) in the upper epidermis some 12 hours after irradiation (Figure 2.4). When the exposure has been intense, acute epidermal necrosis occurs. Intraepidermal vesiculation and subepidermal blistering may be observed in less severe injury. After two or three days, epidermal hypertrophy and parakeratosis are noted. Dermal oedema, vascular dilatation and infiltration with a mixture of inflammatory cells accompanies the epidermal changes.

Chronic Solar Damage

All light-exposed skin of Caucasian subjects develops solar damage to a greater or lesser degree. The less pigmented the skin and the greater the degree of sun exposure, the more the damage sustained. The most obvious alteration is in the upper dermis and is known as solar elastotic degeneration or just elastosis, as the damaged connective tissue takes on the staining characteristics of elastic tissue. There is loss of the usual fibrillary structure of the dermal connective tissue and substitution with either irregular strands ('chopped spaghetti appearance') or homogenous material (Figure 2.5). Inexplicably there is always a subepidermal zone some 5 µm or so broad, unaffected by the process. The elastotic change may affect the entire papillary and mid-dermis or if mild, may only involve some areas of the papillary dermis. Interspersed in the abnormal dermis are dilated vascular channels[3].

The relationship between normal elastic tissue and the abnormal, solar-damaged, elastic staining connective tissue has not been satisfactorily characterized. Epidermal atrophy may accompany the elastosis, and focally, areas of dysplasia and frank preneoplastic and neoplastic change occur (see page 111).

Thermal Injury

In severe burns there is loss of tissue and the formation of an eschar of necrotic material at the surface. The burnt area becomes acutely inflamed after a few hours and becomes oedematous and infiltrated with polymorphs and other inflammatory cells. At the margins of the burn, both epidermal and dermal cells take on bizarre shapes and staining reactions (see cautery artefact, page 13). In less severe thermal injury, such as from scalds, subepidermal blisters develop as a result of the intense oedema. When the heating stimulus is less severe and persists over a considerable period of time, such as is seen in erythema ab igne of the legs due to sitting in front of a fire over many years, other changes take place[4]. An elastotic degenerative change is seen in the dermis (Figure 2.6). This differs from that of solar damage in that it extends deeper into the dermis and the elastotic

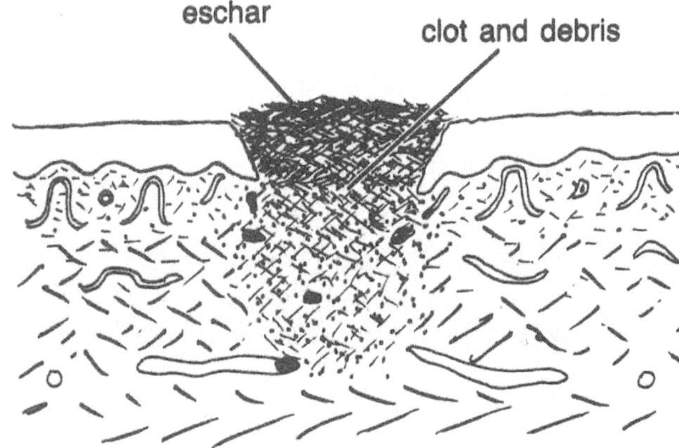

Day 1
Vessel constriction.
Vessel plugged by thrombus, wound cavity filled by thrombus and debris.
Hard eschar forms on surface.
Polymorphs accumulate at wound/eschar interface.
Epidermis just beginning to migrate between eschar and surface.

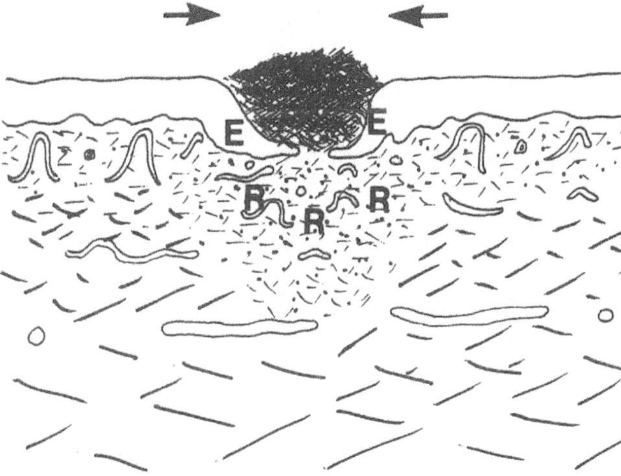

Day 2–5
Epidermal migration (E) onto wound surface below eschar.
Mitosis and maturation occur 1–2 mm back from leading edge.
Thrombus and debris resorbed.
Revascularization (R) of healing area occurs.
Damaged collagen lysed.
Fibroblasts synthesize new collagen.
Wound contraction through activity of myofibroblasts → ←.

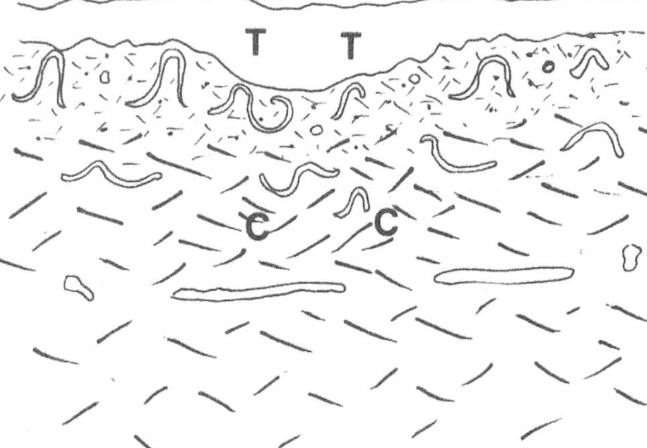

Day 6–42
Post-wounding epidermal thickening (T) persists for some days.
Barrier function restored some 7–10 days after wound closure.
Vascular dilatation may persist for some weeks.
New connective tissue (C) fibres gradually align in direction of stresses.

Figure 2.1 Diagram to illustrate main events in wound healing

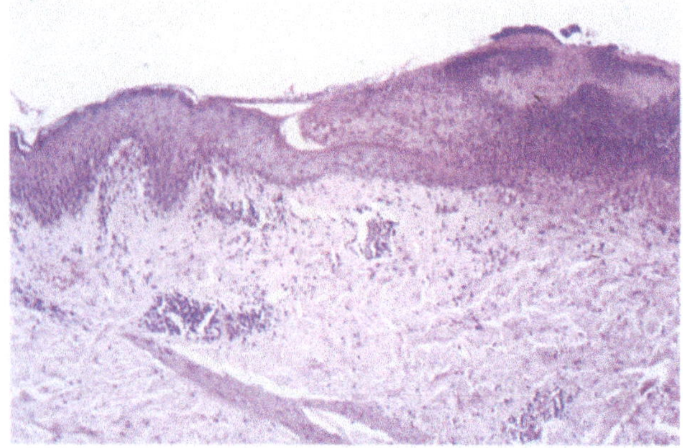

Figure 2.2   Early re-epithelialization of an erosion. A sheet of epithelium is separating slough from viable dermis.   H & E (B)

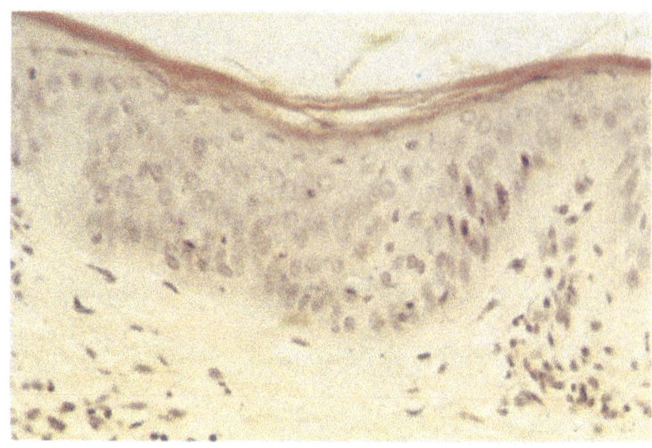

Figure 2.3   There are several eosinophilic cells (sunburn cells) with pyknotic nuclei in the epidermis after UV radiation to the skin.   H & E (C)

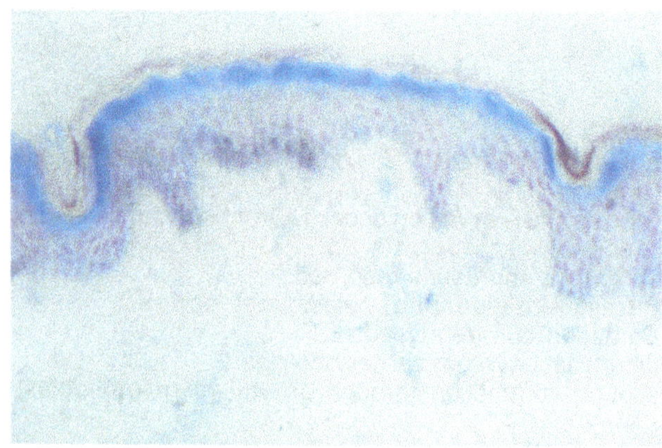

Figure 2.4a   Normal skin to show non-specific esterase reaction in the granular cell layer of the epidermis.   (B)

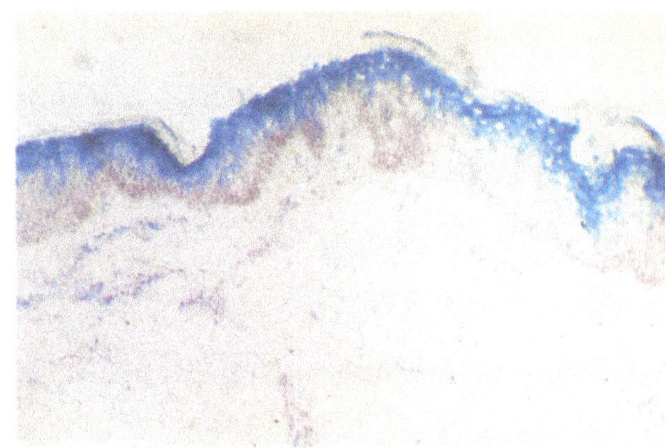

Figure 2.4b   Non-specific esterase reaction in epidermis after UV irradiation.   (B)

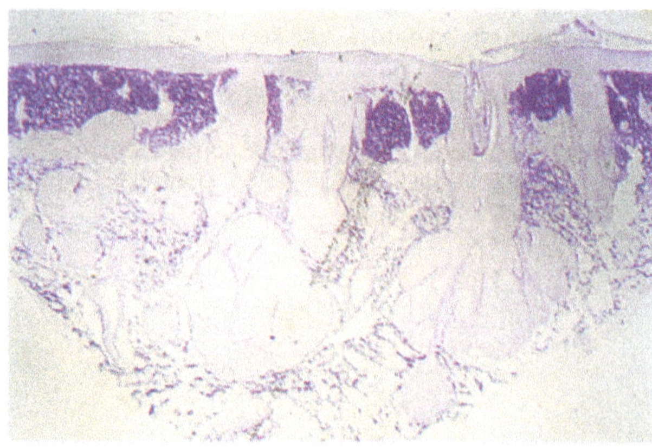

Figure 2.5   Solar elastosis. Solar elastotic degeneration demonstrated by Halmi stain.   (B)

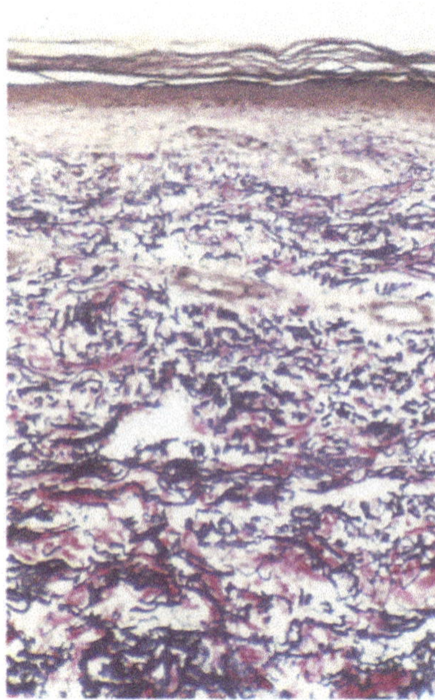

Figure 2.6   Elastotic degenerative change in erythema ab igne demonstrated by orcein stain. The black degenerate material can be seen distributed throughout the dermis.   (B)

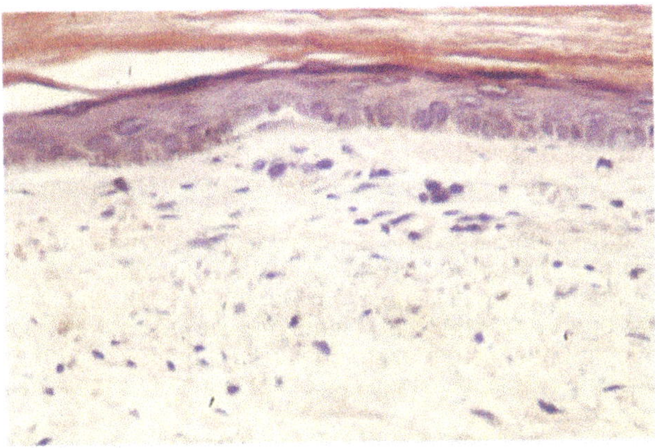

Figure 2.7 Erythema ab igne. There are a number of abnormal appearing cells in the dermis. The epidermal cells show dysplastic change with irregularity in size and arrangement.   H & E (C)

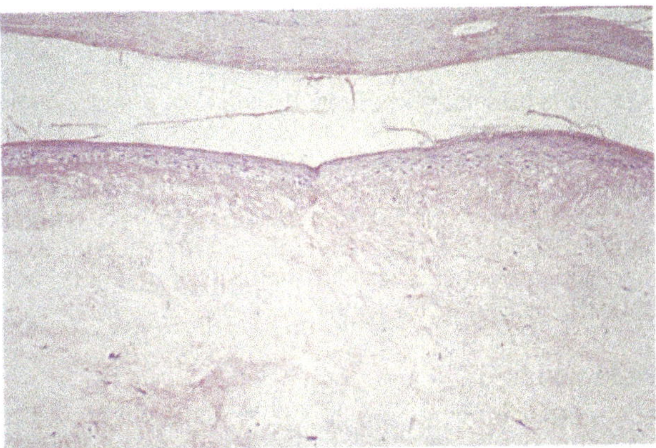

Figure 2.8 Radiation dermatitis at site of radiotherapy some years previously. The upper part of the dermis shows degenerative change and the epidermis is atrophic.   H & E (B)

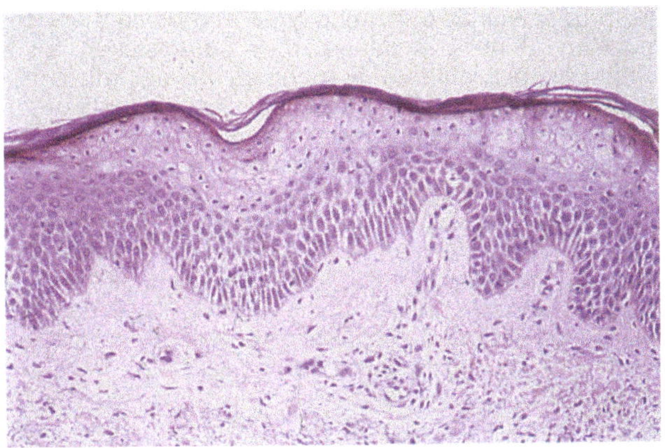

Figure 2.9 Severe chemical injury from dithranol. There is colliquative degenerative change in the upper epidermis.   H & E (C)

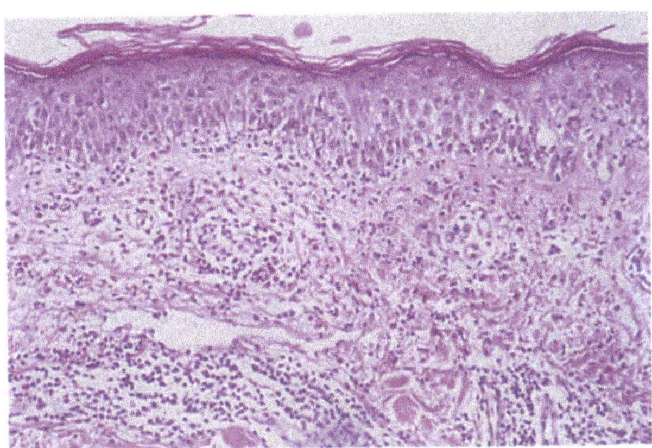

Figure 2.10 Irritant dermatitis after application of sodium lauryl sulphate. The epidermis shows spongiosis and there is a moderately heavy inflammatory cell infiltrate.   H & E (C)

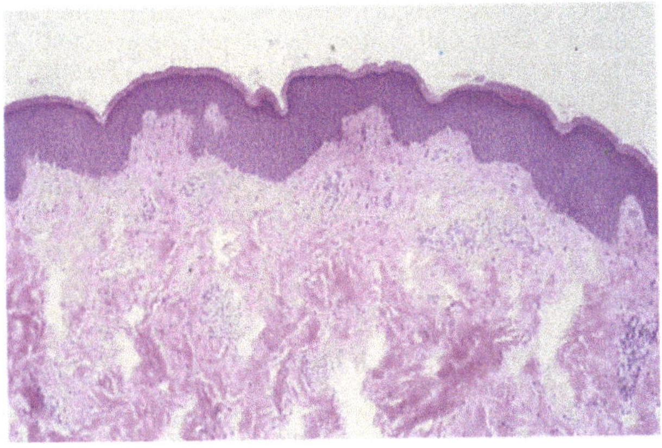

Figure 2.11 Effects of experimentally produced repeated mechanical stimulation showing irregular epidermal hypertrophy.   H & E (B)

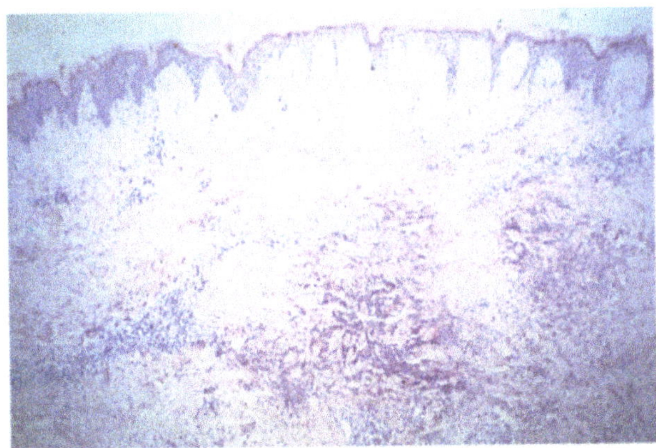

Figure 2.12 Insect bite reaction with upper dermal oedema and accumulation of inflammatory cells in the mid and lower dermis.   H & E (A)

material is less 'homogenized'. In addition, preneoplastic changes may occur in the overlying epidermis. The blood vessel walls are thickened and the endothelial cells may appear bizarre, as indeed may the fibroblasts in the locality (Figure 2.7). Staining for iron pigment reveals heavy deposits of haemosiderin, most of which is in macrophages, accounting for the reticular pigmentation noted clinically.

Radiation Injury

Acute radiation burns are uncommon and are similar to acute thermal burns. Chronic radiation injury is similar to chronic solar and thermal injury in that there is elastotic degenerative change in the dermal collagen. It may be very marked and is responsible for the pronounced telangiectasia observed clinically. In addition to the alterations in the fibrous structure, the cells of the dermis may appear enlarged and bizarre[5]. The epidermis is atrophic and in places abnormal nuclear forms are observed (Figure 2.8). Preneoplastic and neoplastic lesions may develop at the site of injury.

Chemical Injury

The type of damage to the skin is determined by the nature of the chemical agent involved. Corrosive substances such as strong acids and alkalis cause a colliquative necrosis of the epidermis and as much of the dermis as is permeated by the material. Superficial epidermal necrosis may be the only injury if there has been minimal contact (Figure 2.9). Some substances cause a blistering reaction. The vesicant mustard gases are probably the best known chemical agents that can do this but other substances may also be responsible. Cantharidin causes an intraepidermal blister to form as it induces acantholysis (see page 48). Indeed, application of cantharidin has been used to obtain almost pure stratum corneum from the tops of blisters raised *in vivo*. Mildly toxic substances (often called 'irritants') cause an eczematous response (see page 51) which is indistinguishable from eczema due to any other cause (Figure 2.10). If exposure is repeated on several occasions a picture of chronic eczema emerges with epidermal hypertrophy, parakeratosis and a chronic inflammatory cell infiltrate.

Mechanical Injury

Repeated abrasion or friction at the skin surface causes epidermal hypertrophy, hyperkeratosis and sometimes parakeratosis. In addition, lymphocytes and other mononuclear cells accumulate subepidermally (Figure 2.11). Scratching injury may induce patchy deposits of a fibrin-like material just beneath the epidermis. In predisposed subjects the repeated trauma of scratching causes lichenification (see page 51) with massive irregular epidermal hypertrophy, parakeratosis and hyperkeratosis, an inflammatory cell infiltrate, dilation and thickening of small blood vessels, nerve fibre thickening and even fibrosis.

An excoriation is the result of a scratch, usually in response to an itch. It is a linear erosion with partial or complete loss of epidermis at the site of the scratch. Healing rapidly takes place, leaving slight epidermal hypertrophy and inflammation in its wake.

Insect Bites and Stings

A bewildering variety of histological appearances is produced by the ravages of biting and stinging arthropods. Such lesions are frequently misdiagnosed and the possibility of an insect bite should always be remembered. The severity and type of damage induced depends on the type of insect responsible, the degree of success of the 'attack' and the host's inherent or immunological response.

A blistering response is occasionally encountered especially from mosquito bites. The blister is subepidermal and usually rapidly subsides. Rarely, bullous reactions are due to acantholysis – reactions due to blister (Cantharidin) beetles are examples. Tissue necrosis is often present in the early stages and later signs of tissue repair are obvious.

The most frequent difficulty in diagnosis of this category of lesions stems from biopsies of persistent papules or nodules. Many arthropods seem capable of eliciting this sort of response, including the scabies mite[6]. Usually there is a dense infiltrate of a mixture of inflammatory cells (Figure 2.12). The cell types present include lymphocytes, plasma cells, histiocytes, giant cells, neutrophils and eosinophils. The proportions of the various individual cell types are enormously variable and account for the difficulties in diagnosis. Some consist predominantly of lymphocytes, and when the accumulation of cells is dense, may be mistaken for a lymphomatous infiltrate. Sometimes the infiltrate is predominantly perivascular and throughout the depth of the dermis – sometimes giving a lupus erythematosus like picture. Granulomatous inflammation is sometimes observed at the site of an insect bite and in this type there may be remnants of the insect's mouth parts. Eosinophils are often present – sometimes in large numbers – and are helpful in suggesting the diagnosis (Figure 2.13). A dense infiltrate of neutrophils is sometimes seen – on occasion amounting to abscess formation. Neutrophil nuclear fragments ('nuclear dust') may also be present.

Chronic Venous Hypertension (Gravitational Syndrome)

The skin of the lower legs of individuals over the age of 40 presents a distinctive feature regardless as to whether there are clinical changes or not. The small blood vessels show thickened walls and are often increased in number and dilated, giving an undue prominence to the vascular components of the section (Figure 2.14). When there are clinical signs of the gravitational syndrome these vascular features are exaggerated and there are other pathological features superimposed. At times the profusion of vascular elements may be such as to simulate a vascular tumour. The additional presence of inflammation, fibrosis and haemosiderin pigment may lead to a mistaken diagnosis of Kaposi's idiopathic haemorrhagic sarcoma (Figure 2.15), and not unnaturally this situation has been termed 'pseudokaposi's disease'[7].

Often there is marked deposition of haemosiderin pigment within dermal macrophages, and there may also be free red cells extravasated within the dermis. Special stains for fibrin or fibrin immunolocalization procedures reveal that there is a cuff of fibrin around the small blood vessels in the majority of specimens[8] (Figure 2.16). In addition there is a generalized thickening of the dermal connective tissue with fibrosis of the tissues around the site. When severe, deposition of calcium occurs, which can be demonstrated by the appropriate stain.

The degree of dermal inflammatory cell infiltrate is dependent on whether there is eczematous change or ulceration. In these latter instances there is always a pronounced degree of inflammation but there is often an increased number of inflammatory cells even in its absence. The fixed connective tissue cells are also increased in number and enlarged.

The epidermis is variably affected. In longstanding disease epidermal atrophy occurs, but near an ulcer there is often epidermal hypertrophy, occasionally amounting to pseudoepitheliomatous hyperplasia. When an eczematous condition is associated ('varicose eczema') there is spongiosis and parakeratosis as in other forms of eczema.

Ulceration

It is well nigh impossible to determine the aetiological cause of an ulcer from a biopsy specimen as the superimposed secondary changes often swamp the initial provoking disorder. The ulcer base is usually composed of a mixture of tissue debris, fibrin, red cells and polymorphonuclear leukocytes. Below this there are numerous vascular elements and cellular new connective tissue together comprising granulation tissue (Figure 2.17). The edges of the ulcer show epidermal thickening and there may also be tongues of epidermis projecting onto the ulcer itself as evidence of re-epithelialization (Figure 2.18). There is usually considerable oedema and extravasation of red cells within the depths of the ulcer base and a variable amount of inflammation.

When venous hypertension is the cause there are also the changes due to this (see above) but they are less easy to distinguish in the ulcer base. If ischaemia is the cause (such as from large vessel obstruction) the granulation tissue tends to be less prolific and there is less oedema.

Chilblains (Perniosis)

There is usually pronounced telangiectasia and oedema. There may also be a mild inflammatory cell infiltrate and some extravasation of red cells.

Infarction

When blood supply is reduced precipitately to the skin the epidermis is the first tissue to suffer, and depending on the acuity and completeness of the ischaemia is either eroded and crusted, or inflamed and parakeratotic. There is also a variable degree of inflammation, local haemorrhage and oedema.

References

1. Marks, R. (1981). The healing and nonhealing of wounds and ulcers of the skin. In Glyn, L. E. (ed.) *Tissue Repair and Regeneration.* (Amsterdam: Elsevier-North Holland Biomedical)

2. Krawczyk, W. S. and Wilgram, G. F. (1975). The synthesis of keratinosomes during epidermal wound healing. *J. Invest. Dermatol.*, **64**, 263

3. Braverman, I. M. and Fonferko, E. (1982). Studies in cutaneous ageing. I. The elastic fiber network. *J. Invest. Dermatol.*, **78**, 434

4. Shahrad, P. and Marks, R. (1977). The wages of warmth. Changes in erythema ab igne. *Br. J. Dermatol.*, **97**, 179

5. Rubin, P. and Casarett, G. W. (1968). *Clinical Radiation Pathology.* Vol. 1. (Philadelphia: Saunders)

6. Fernandez, N., Torres, A. and Ackerman, A. B. (1977). Pathologic findings in human scabies. *Arch. Dermatol.*, **113**, 320

7. Earhart, R. N., Aeling, J. A., Nuss, D. D. and Mellette, J. R. (1974). Pseudo-Kaposi sarcoma. *Arch. Dermatol.*, **110**, 907

8. Burnand, K., Clemenson, G., Morland, M., Jarrett, P. E. M. and Browse, N. L. (1980). Venous Lipodermatosclerosis: treatment by fibrinolytic enhancement and elastic compression. *Br. Med. J.*, **ii**, 7

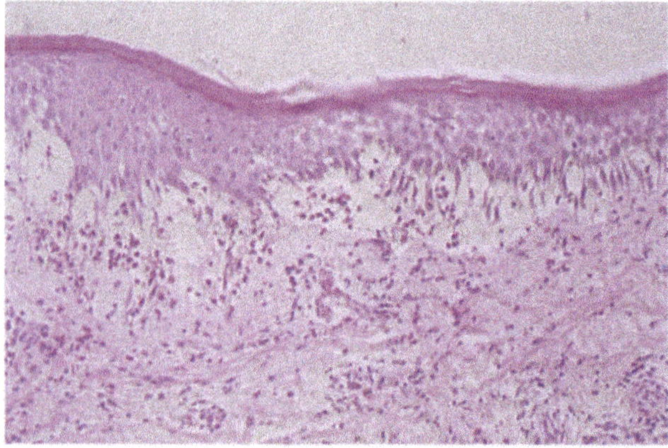

Figure 2.13 Insect bite reaction. There is considerable subepidermal oedema and many eosinophils.   H & E (C)

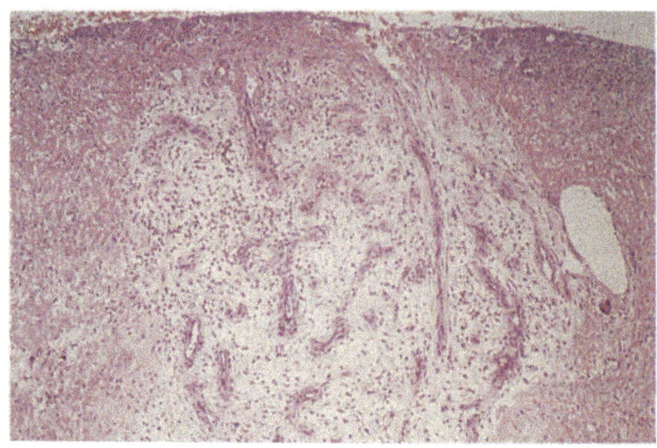

Figure 2.14 Thickened blood vessels of the lower leg in the gravitational syndrome.   H & E (B)

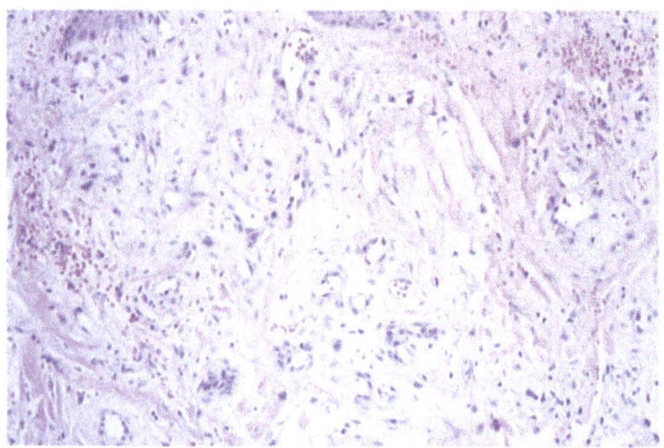

Figure 2.15 Numerous new small blood vessels in the dermis in the gravitational syndrome.   H & E (B)

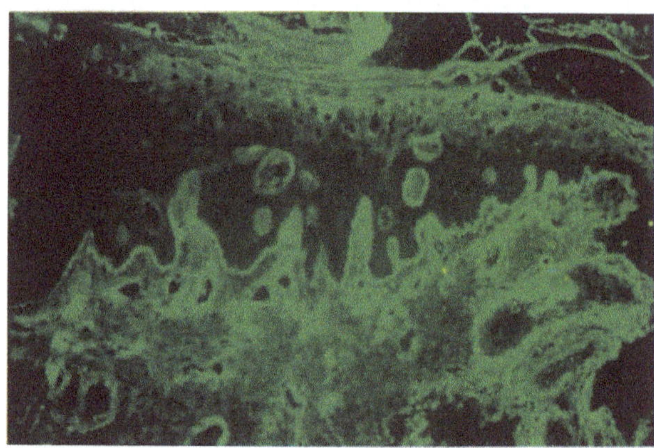

Figure 2.16 Immunofluorescence photomicrograph to show fluorescence around small dermal blood vessels in the gravitational syndrome after staining with anti-human fibrin and fluorescein tagged anti-human globulin.   (B)

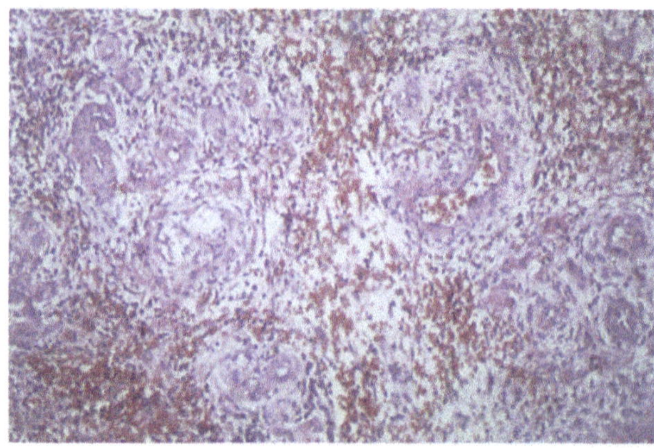

Figure 2.17 Base of gravitational ulcer with numerous small thickened blood vessels, extravasated red cells and accompanying inflammation.   H & E (B)

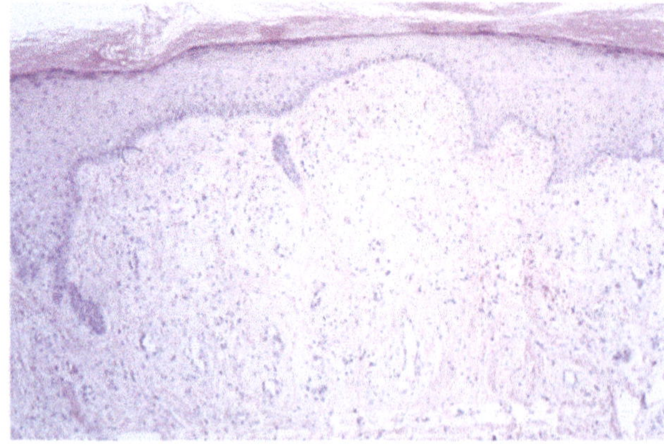

Figure 2.18 Marked epidermal hypertrophy at side of gravitational ulcer.   H & E (B)

Herpes Simplex

This is a common cutaneous infection caused by a virus which is readily identified on electron microscopy. Grouped vesicles are typical and the condition is inflammatory and painful. Regional lymphadenopathy occurs and recurrent attacks of the infection characteristically are seen at the same site. The virus lies dormant between cutaneous infections in the sensory nerve root.

Histopathology

The pathology of the lesions due to Herpes simplex type I is identical to that seen after infection with Herpes virus type II. The characteristic lesion is an epidermal blister (Figure 3.1) with degeneration of epidermal cells and acantholysis. The cells swell and become eosinophilic, the cytoplasm pales, the nuclei shrink and are displaced laterally. This process is termed balloon degeneration (Figures 3.2 and 3.3) and is most prominent in the base of the blister[1]. Epidermal cells burst but the cell walls remain attached to each other forming multilocular vesicles (so called reticular degeneration), which is typical of a viral aetiology. Viral inclusion bodies are seen in the centre of some balloon cells as eosinophilic masses surrounded by a halo. In the upper dermis is a severe inflammatory infiltrate with fibrinoid deposits in the blood vessel walls, neutrophils, extravasated red cells and fragmented neutrophils or nuclear dust.

Herpes zoster and varicella are indistinguishable histologically from herpes simplex. The same inclusion bodies are seen in the three diseases[2].

Varicella. Crops of small superficial vesicles occur over the whole body including the mouth. The histopathological picture resembles herpes simplex but the epidermal damage is much less and the dermal infiltrate is relatively superficial.

Herpes zoster. This is unmistakable clinically because it affects a specific dermatome and is unilateral. The vesicles resemble herpes simplex in type and are also painful because of involvement of the sensory nerve root. The causative virus is varicella which lies dormant in the dorsal root ganglia following a varicella (chicken pox) infection.

Histologically there is a resemblance to herpes simplex though some cases may be very severe resulting in massive epidermal necrosis. The infiltrate extends deep into the subcutis and involves the nerve trunks.

Differential Diagnosis

Erythema multiforme or severe bullous drug eruption may have features suggestive of herpes simplex. The epidermis is oedematous and the cells become necrotic in both conditions. However, in erythema multiforme the dead epidermal cells become pink homogenous blobs and in herpes simplex large balloon cells are the end result. Severe dermal inflammation is seen in both conditions but there are usually more neutrophils in erythema multiforme and eosinophils in drug eruptions.

Viral Wart

The common viral wart requires little clinical description. They may be multiple on the fingers and soles of feet and are extremely common in children and young adults. On the hands they are papular, on the soles they are pushed deeper into the skin, on the face they may be small and flat (plane warts) and on the perianal and genital skin they are often like small polyps.

The viruses of warts belong to the papova group (human papillomavirus group). There are many different antigenic types each being associated with particular clinical types of wart[3,4]. The type responsible for genital warts has been linked with cancer of the cervix and genitalia.

Histopathology

The common wart is an actively growing lesion showing acanthosis, papillomatosis and hyperkeratosis interspersed with parakeratosis. Typically the rete pegs at the lateral margins are elongated and bend inwards giving a claw-like appearance. A characteristic feature of viral warts is vacuolation of the upper Malpighian and granular layers (Figure 3.4). Some of these cells contain large irregular clumps of keratohyaline granules. Others have deeply basophilic round nuclei surrounded by a clear zone (Figure 3.5) and are thought to contain numerous virus particles. The eosinophilic bodies seen in degenerating nuclei do not contain virus particles.

Plane warts in contrast to common warts do not show papillomatosis, only slight elongation of rete ridges and no parakeratosis. There is a more extensive vacuolation of epidermal cells and production of dark basophilic round nuclei. The stratum corneum often has a basket weave appearance.

Genital warts are papillomatous and have many mitotic figures. Occasionally lesions may resemble squamous cell carcinoma but the epithelium has a more orderly arrangement and contains many vacuolated cells and basophilic inclusion bodies. Warts treated with podophyllin show a bizarre cytological picture resembling Bowen's disease.

Differential Diagnosis

Sometimes the typical viral wart features, of vacuolation in the granular cell layer and basophilic inclusion bodies, are absent in typical virus warts. They are then indistinguishable from a simple benign squamous proliferation. Some warts, particularly those in the anogenital region, resemble squamous cell carcinomata. Attention must be paid to the number of mitoses, depth of invasion and degree of dyskeratosis.

Molluscum Contagiosum

This is a common viral infection particularly in children. The virus is a large intra-cytoplasmic virus of the pox group readily identified on electron microscopy. The infection may be contracted in swimming pools or by sexual contact and small pearly dome-shaped papules are seen on the trunk – particularly around the neck and in the groin. The papules have a central umbilication from which cheesy material can be extruded.

Histopathology

The earliest change is oedema in the basal cells of the epidermis. Small granules develop and fuse together resulting in oval eosinophilic bodies. These distend the cell and eventually cause its death and rupture. There is gross proliferation of epidermal cells down into the dermis. The eosinophilic molluscum bodies stream upwards to a central punctum on top of the fully developed papule (Figure 3.6). The molluscum bodies are cytoplasmic masses of virus material. The pathological features of molluscum contagiosum are very easily recognized and the large pink molluscum bodies (Figure 3.7) pouring through the stratum corneum can hardly be mistaken.

Orf

This virus infection is contracted from the mouths of infected lambs and is predominantly seen on the fingers of veterinary surgeons or farmer's wives. A large purple blister-like lesion develops which is painful and lasts 4–6 weeks.

Histopathology

The epidermal ballooning and reticular degeneration resembles herpes simplex. Hovever, the dermis is very oedematous and vascular with a mixed inflammatory infiltrate. A later stage may produce pseudo-epitheliomatous proliferation.

Cellulitis and Erysipelas

It may be difficult to distinguish between cellulitis and erysipelas clinically and both are due to dermal infection with group A streptococci. Erysipelas tends to affect the superficial dermis thus having a more definite border and cellulitis is deep and subcutaneous. In acute infection the patient is ill with a fever and the skin is red and indurated.

Histopathology

There is gross oedema of the dermis with fibrin strands and a very heavy infiltrate of neutrophils around dermal blood vessels as the characteristic features (Figure 3.8). This picture is also shared by Sweet's syndrome (acute febrile neutrophilic dermatosis) which is not due to bacterial infection. Demonstration of gram positive cocci in erysipelas and cellulitis will assist in differential diagnosis but is rarely possible in erysipelas.

Impetigo

A common bacterial infection of the skin caused by *Staphylococcus aureus* predominantly. The skin infection, which may be bullous or consist of superficial crusted erosions, is contagious.

Histopathology

A subcorneal collection of neutrophils is the classical feature of impetigo (Figure 3.9). There is little disturbance of the epidermis. The dermal inflammatory infiltrate varies and may be minimal. Subcorneal pustular dermatosis, candida infection and acute pustular psoriasis may be indistinguishable but a gram stain will reveal the presence of cocci in impetigo. Acantholysis is a feature of subcorneal pustular dermatosis and the budding spores of a candida infection will be visible with PAS staining.

Boils and Carbuncles

A staphylococcal folliculitis is the basis for boils and furuncles. Inflammatory products are found within and around the hair follicle. A boil is a raised red painful inflammation of one follicle and a carbuncle involves multiple follicles. Discharge of pus through the orifices is normal.

Histopathology

In a staphylococcal folliculitis neutrophils accumulate in large numbers resulting in abscess formation (Figure 3.10). The connective tissue surrounding the follicle is infiltrated with neutrophils and becomes necrotic. Below or around the follicle an abscess develops which destroys the follicle and contains readily demonstrable staphylococci. This pus is finally evacuated. Acne vulgaris causes an inflammatory reaction much less than a staphylococci infection. A foreign body granuloma may result from rupture of the follicle in acne vulgaris. The presence of hair or stratum corneum gives a clue to the aetiology.

Syphilis

The causative organism is the motile *Treponema pallidum* which is widely distributed in the body well before any inflammation becomes apparent. The primary cell histologically is the plasma cell and syphilis should be considered when plasma cells are seen in moderate or large numbers.

Primary Syphilis

The chancre is a firm indurated lesion usually on the genitalia, on the lips or in the anorectal region.

Histopathology. The epidermis is thickened, oedematous, covered by parakeratotic scale and invaded by inflammatory cells. Lymphocytes and plasma cells infiltrate the dermis in large numbers. The endothelial cells of blood vessels are swollen and increased in number. Silver stains reveal treponemas in the epidermis particularly.

Secondary Syphilis

During this phase the patient may have a fever with influenza-like symptoms, lymphadenopathy and a rash which is very variable. In most cases it is non-itchy, macular, erythematous on the face, trunk, limbs and invariably the palms and soles. However, the clinical manifestations are very variable and many other types of rash have been described.

Histopathology. A range of pathological reactions are seen in secondary syphilis[5]. There may simply be a non-specific perivascular lymphocytic infiltrate. However, plasma cells are present in large numbers in roughly three-quarters of cases and are a very useful diagnostic feature. The blood vessels throughout the dermis show endothelial thickening in half the cases (Figure 3.11). The epidermis may be oedematous, acanthotic and invaded with round cells. Pallor of the nuclei leads to a washed-out appearance of the epidermis. In the papulosquamous variety of secondary syphilis the epidermal rete pegs are elongated as in psoriasis (Figure 3.12) and even microabscesses appear. Treponemas are difficult to demonstrate in secondary syphilis.

Differential diagnoses of secondary syphilis include a drug eruption, pityriasis lichenoides chronica, psoriasis and a reticulosis. The presence of plasma cells however should always alert one to syphilis.

Tertiary Syphilis

Various dermatological entities may be produced by tertiary syphilis. The gumma is only one and others include nodules, ulcerated nodules, plaques and tumours.

Histopathology. A tuberculoid granuloma is frequently seen in cutaneous tertiary syphilis. Differentiation may be possible by noting several points. The lupus vulgaris granuloma is higher in the dermis and more organized in appearance than that of tertiary syphilis. Plasma cells are rare in lupus vulgaris and common in syphilis. Necrosis is not seen commonly in lupus vulgaris but is present in syphilis. Fibrosis is a constant feature in tertiary syphilis and is best demonstrated by absence of elastic fibres in and around the granuloma. The acid orcein–Giemsa stain is useful colouring elastic fibres black. The absence of eosinophils points against a fungal granuloma.

Tuberculosis

Mycobacterium tuberculosis evokes different responses in the skin depending upon the site of inoculation, the dose of organisms and the immunity of the patient.

Primary Tuberculosis

In primary tuberculosis a primary complex of the local lesion and satellite lymphadenopathy develops – similar to that in the lung. Initially the histological changes are non-specific but later an epithelioid and lymphocytic response develops. When the skin is involved ulceration is usual and acid-fast bacilli are demonstrable. Finally the lesion may lead to death of the patient or immunity develops and it becomes lupus vulgaris.

Lupus Vulgaris

Lupus vulgaris is cutaneous tuberculosis in a patient with considerable immunity to *M. tuberculosis*. Clinically brownish-red plaques develop on the face or neck and gradually extend. Some areas ulcerate but most become chronically inflamed and heal with scarring.

Histopathology. The typical tuberculoid granuloma consists of a collection of epithelioid cells[6] surrounded by a dense lymphocytic and plasma cell infiltrate (Figures 3.13 and 3.14). In the central area of epithelioid cells are giant cells some of which have the peripherally arranged nuclei of the Langhans type (Figure 3.15). Central caseation necrosis is not a prominent feature. The granuloma is usually in the upper dermis but may completely fill the dermis and the subcutis. The overlying epidermis may erode and ulcerate centrally but may be thickened and papillomatous at the edges. Acid-fast bacilli are present in such few numbers that they are difficult to demonstrate.

Differential diagnosis includes other infections with a tuberculoid pattern: syphilis, leprosy, atypical mycobacterial infections and some deep fungus infections. Some foreign bodies produce a similar picture including zirconium, beryllium, suture materials, talc and starch. In addition the granulomatous forms of rosacea may be difficult to differentiate.

Tuberculosis Verrucosa Cutis

This is a cutaneous exogenous infection with *M. tuberculosis* in a person with a high degree of immunity. Clinically the lesion is a warty growth on a finger of a pathologist handling cadavers or on the buttocks of a child from a country with a high incidence of pulmonary tuberculosis.

Histopathology. The epidermis is thickened, papillomatous and may show pseudoepitheliomatous hyperplasia. There is an acute inflammatory infiltrate in the upper dermis with abscess formation. In the mid and deep dermis a tuberculoid granuloma develops with significant central necrosis. Acid-fast bacilli may be demonstrable. The picture resembles a swimming-pool granuloma (*M. marinum*) and sporotrichosis.

Scrofuloderma

This is a cutaneous infection as a result of direct extension from an infected lymph node or bone. Initially a bluish-red painless swelling it rapidly ulcerates.

Histopathology. The central area shows non-specific changes but a biopsy from the edge should reveal tuberculoid features and central necrosis. Acid-fast bacilli will be readily demonstrated.

Leprosy

Mycobacterium leprae affects the skin and cutaneous nerves. The clinical form of the disease depends upon the patient's immunity against the organism. Tuberculoid leprosy occurs in persons with a high degree of immunity and few organisms are found. Lepromatous leprosy occurs in persons with poor immunity to *M. leprae* and numerous bacilli are present. Between these extremes are borderline tuberculoid and borderline lepromatous leprosy. The tuberculoid type has depigmented hypoaesthetic skin lesions and thickening of peripheral nerves. Lepromatous leprosy which is teaming with organisms is symmetrical on the face with skin thickening and mucosal involvement.

Histopathology

The organism primarily involves the nerves and is phagocytosed by Schwann cells. If cellular immunity is low tissue macrophages take up the bacilli and become filled with organisms (foamy macrophages) (Figure 3.16). If the cellular immunity is high the bacilli are destroyed by histiocytes which form epithelioid tubercles.

Lepromatous Leprosy

An extensive upper dermal infiltrate is separated from a flattened epidermis by a Grenz zone of normal collagen[7]. Foamy macrophages predominate resembling xanthoma cells. These are full of acid-fast bacilli and are called Lepra cells. Skin appendages are destroyed and the infiltrate extends into the fat. The cutaneous nerves also contain bacilli but are better preserved than in tuberculoid leprosy.

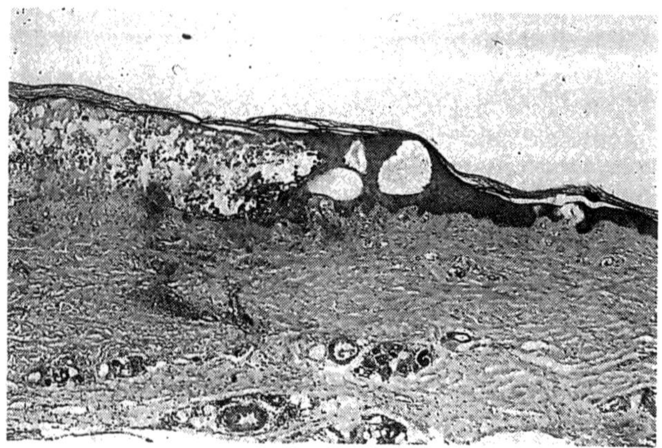

Figure 3.1 Herpes simplex. Blistered epidermis with gross cell destruction and reticular degeneration. H & E (A)

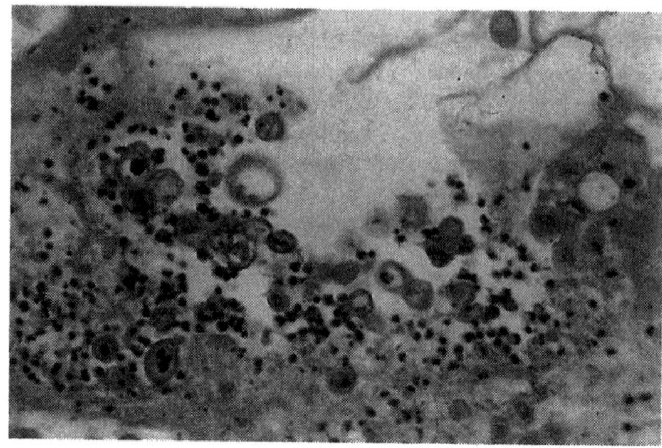

Figure 3.2 Herpes simplex. Epidermal cell destruction with some balloon cells. Lymphocytic infiltrate and some reticular degeneration. H & E (C)

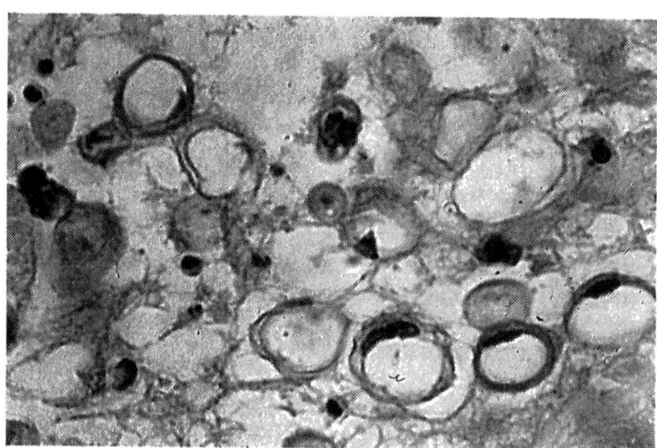

Figure 3.3 Herpes simplex. Balloon cells. H & E (D)

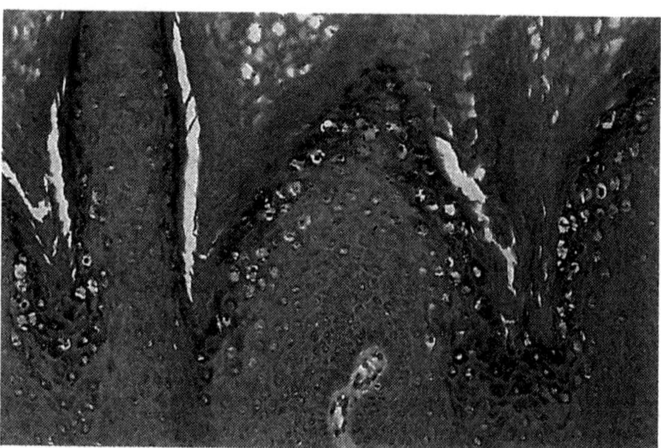

Figure 3.4 Virus wart. Gross hyperkeratosis and acanthosis. Very prominent vacuolated granular cell layer. H & E (B)

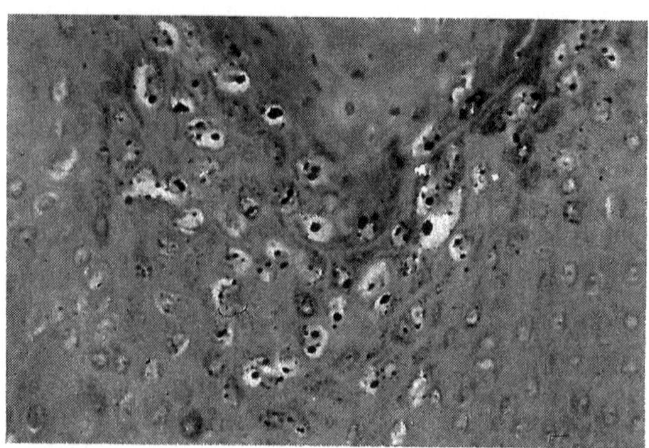

Figure 3.5 Virus wart. Vacuolated granular cell layer with basophilic round nuclei and a surrounding halo. These are thought to contain viral particles. H & E (C)

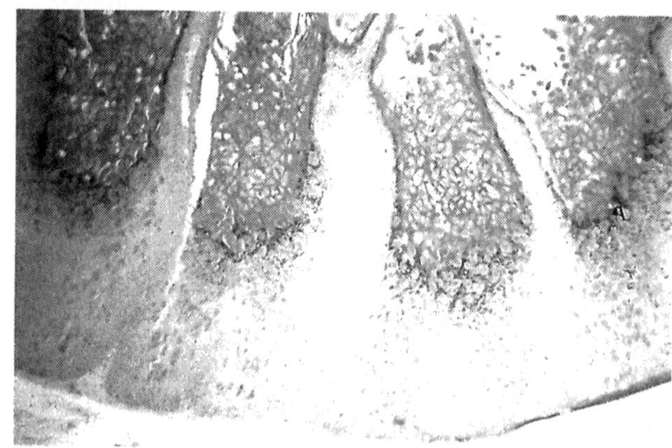

Figure 3.6 Molluscum contagiosum. Masses of eosinophilic molluscum bodies streaming upwards to a central punctum. H & E (B)

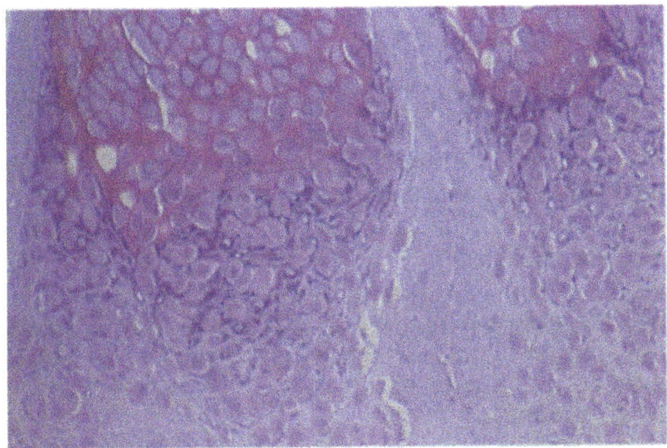

Figure 3.7 Molluscum contagiosum. Large pink molluscum bodies in the epidermis. H & E (C)

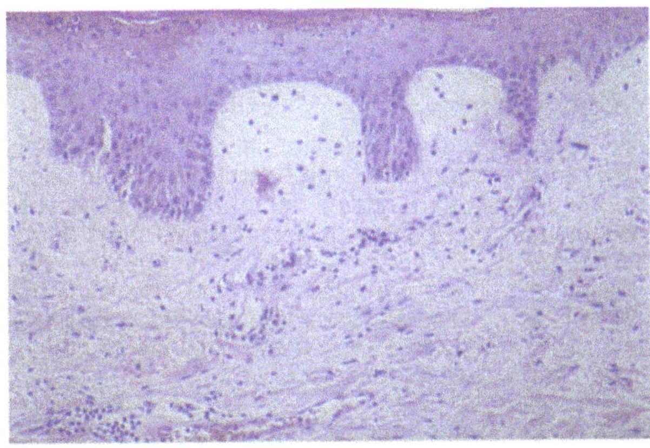

Figure 3.8 Erysipelas. Papillary oedema and neutrophils in upper dermis. H & E (C)

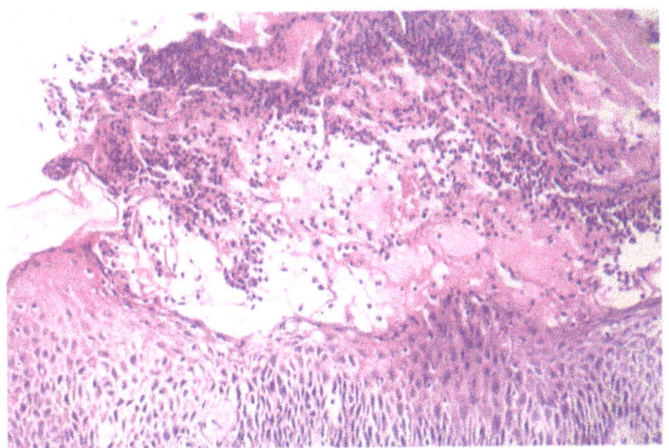

Figure 3.9 Impetigo. Subcorneal collection of neutrophils and some oedema within the epidermis. H & E (B)

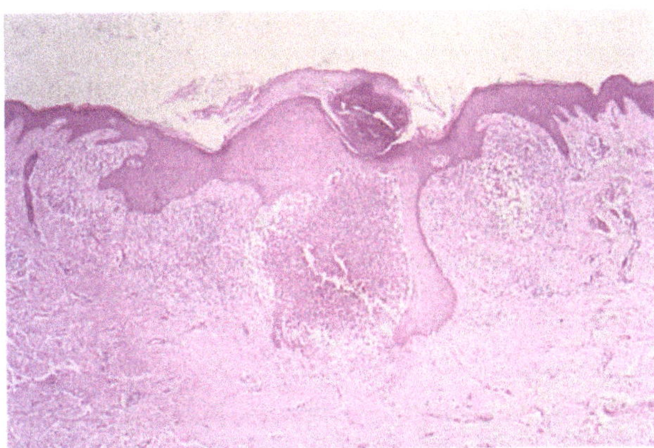

Figure 3.10 Folliculitis. Ruptured hair follicle filled with a neutrophil abscess. H & E (B)

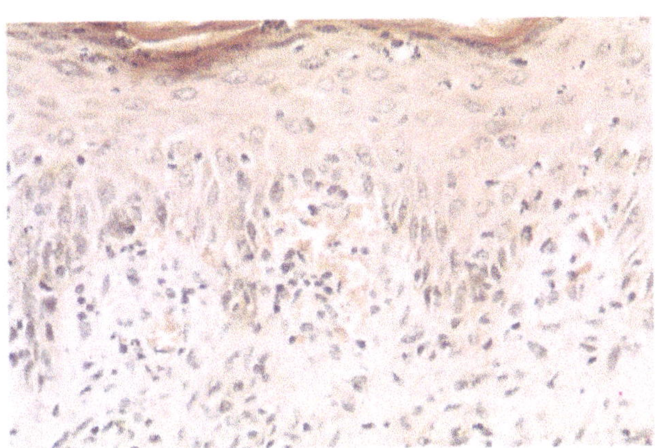

Figure 3.11 Secondary syphilis. Superficial blood vessels thickened with an increased number of large endothelial cells. Lymphocytic perivascular infiltrate invading the epidermis. Only an occasional plasma cell visible. H & E (C)

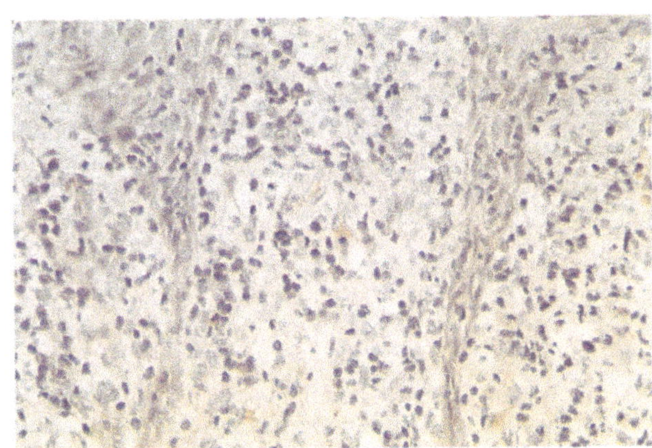

Figure 3.12 Secondary syphilis. Elongated, rather pale epidermal rete pegs. Invasion of epidermis with lymphocytes. Large numbers of lymphocytes and plasma cells throughout the upper dermis. Thickening of capillary blood vessels. H & E (C)

Tuberculoid Leprosy

The recognition of cutaneous nerve involvement is important and requires a large deep biopsy. Epithelioid cell granulomata form around necrosing dermal nerves. The granulomata may be indistinguishable from sarcoidosis (Figures 3.17 and 3.18) and acid-fast bacilli within the necrotic nerves are difficult to find. However the tuberculoid granulomata are more elongated because they follow nerves and silver stains may identify nerve tissue within the necrotic areas.

Atypical Mycobacterial Infections

Mycobacterium marinum

This is the most common of the atypical mycobacteria to cause cutaneous infections. It is responsible for swimming-pool and tropical fish-tank granulomata. In both cases the organism gains entry through a break in the skin. Red papules or nodules appear on the fingers, elbows or knees and subcutaneous nodules may develop along the lymphatic vessels in a 'sporotrichoid' pattern.

Histopathology. Early lesions show a non-specific inflammatory infiltrate with neutrophils, lymphocytes and epithelioid cells. After a few months multinucleate giant cells and epithelioid cell granulomata are present. Typical tuberculoid granulomata are seen only after 6 months[8]. Necrosis within the granulomata is infrequent and the epidermis becomes papillomatous and hyperkeratotic. Acid-fast organisms can be identified in early lesions. Differentiation from tuberculosis verrucosa cutis or lupus vulgaris is not possible and it is necessary to culture the organism.

Buruli Ulcer

Caused by *Mycobacterium ulcerans*, Buruli ulcer occurs in widely distributed tropical countries. The endemic areas cluster around water courses or swamps. Following minor trauma, often on a limb, a painless subcutaneous nodule breaks down to form a necrotic shallow ulcer which extends rapidly.

Histopathology. Acute necrosis of the dermis and subcutis is the earliest feature. Clusters of acid-fast bacilli are easily seen in necrotic material. The subcutaneous fat becomes necrotic and may calcify. There is little inflammatory reaction and rarely any granulomatous reaction.

Superficial Fungus Infections

These include dermatophyte (ringworm), pityriasis versicolor and candida infections. Generally a fungus does not invade living tissue but may still evoke an inflammatory response. The organism is found in stratum corneum, hair and nails only. The exceptions are *Trichophyton rubrum* and *Candida* which rarely invade tissue to produce granulomata.

Dermatophytes

Dermatophytes of the *Trichophyton* species produce inflammatory ringed eczematous looking lesions. The infection is common between the toes and in the groin, but may also occur in the scalp and elsewhere on the body.

Histopathology. There is an eczematous reaction in the epidermis which is frequently patchy. The characteristic hyphal filaments are difficult to see on H and E staining, they are best seen with PAS[9]. Although they can be seen anywhere in the stratum corneum (Figure 3.20),

the follicular openings are more likely to be affected. In some dermatophyte infections there is invasion of the hair (Figure 3.19) and this should be sought in scalp biopsies where there is inflammation and hair loss[10].

Pityriasis Versicolor

This is a common superficial fungus infection caused by the *Pityrosporon* species. Clinically the rash is on the upper trunk. On dark skin small slightly scaly depigmented round patches are seen and on pale skin the patches appear brown.

Histopathology. There is little or no reaction in the dermis or epidermis. The stratum corneum may be a little thickened and characteristic small filaments and grouped spores are readily seen in PAS sections.

Acute Candidiasis

Organisms may be found on human skin and do not necessarily cause an infection. *Candida albicans* is the common yeast organism associated with human infection. Moist flexures become inflamed and the margin is lined by small superficial pustules.

Histopathology. The primary lesion is a subcorneal pustule resembling impetigo. There may be some spongiform change in the epidermis and the differentiation from pustular psoriasis is difficult without special stains to demonstrate the small hyphal filaments and budding spores. The organism is only found in the stratum corneum.

Chronic Muco-cutaneous Candidiasis

This is caused by a defect in cell-mediated immunity resulting in widespread lesions on the skin, particularly hands, feet, periorally, and mucous membranes. Various immune deficiencies give rise to this disorder which may be lethal in infancy, non-lethal in early life or acquired in later life. Candidal granulomata are characteristic of chronic mucocutaneous candidiasis and the organism does invade viable skin[11].

Histopathology. The pathological features are those of acute candidiasis with granulomata. A feature of the latter is gross papillomatosis and hyperkeratosis with a dense dermal infiltrate of lymphocytes, neutrophils, plasma cells and multinucleate giant cells. *Candida albicans* is found in the stratum corneum and rarely in the viable epidermis and dermis.

Deep Mycoses

North American Blastomycosis

This is caused by *Blastomyces dermatitidis* and occurs as a primary cutaneous inoculation, pulmonary and systemic blastomycosis. The primary cutaneous form is rare and is seen only following a laboratory or autopsy room infection.

Histopathology. Initially in the primary cutaneous inoculation blastomycosis there is a non-specific inflammatory infiltrate and large numbers of budding organisms. Verrucous lesions have considerable downward proliferation of the epidermis and intraepidermal abscesses. Multinucleate giant cells are scattered within a mixed inflammatory infiltrate and organisms are difficult to find even with PAS staining. The verrucous type of blastomycosis must be differentiated from tuberculous verrucosa cutis which has fewer neutrophils and no fungal spores.

Actinomycosis

Actinomycosis is caused by *Actinomyces israeli*, a gram-positive bacterium formerly thought to be a fungus. It may be found as a saprophyte in tonsillar crypts and may produce an area of woody skin over the mandible or maxilla with discharging sinuses. Characteristic yellow sulphur granules, which are clumps or organisms, are in the purulent discharge. Pulmonary and intestinal infections occur.

Histopathology. Granulation tissue containing abscesses leading to sinuses is seen in the indurated skin. The diagnosis is made by finding the 'sulphur granules' within the abscesses. On H and E sections they are clumps of filamentous bacteria staining a basophilic colour and having a lobulated appearance. At the edge is a radiating fringe of eosinophilic clubs. The granules are surrounded by neutrophils. The size of the granules vary from 25 µm to 3500 µm. *Actinomyces israeli* bacterial filaments can be seen with the Gram stain in the centre of the granules. They are identical to Nocardial filaments except that they are not acid fast (Figure 3.21).

Sporotrichosis

Sporotrichosis is caused by *Sporothrix schenckii*. The primary cutaneous inoculation of the fungus is through a prick in the skin from a thorn or splinter of wood. It occurs in North and South America and in the mining areas of South Africa. A painless red nodule appears at the puncture site and a line of other nodules develop along the draining lymphatics.

Histopathology. An ulcerated primary lesion of sporotrichosis shows no diagnostic feature but simply a non-specific inflammatory infiltrate. The epidermis may be hyperplastic and intraepidermal abscesses do occur. The lymphatic nodules develop granulomata within the inflammatory infiltrate. A central suppurative zone composed of neutrophils is surrounded by a tuberculoid zone and at the periphery lymphocytes and plasma cells[12]. A PAS stain is necessary to recognize the oval spores of *Sporothrix schenckii* within the granulomata. Infections with *Mycobacterium marinum* have the same histological appearance as the cutaneous nodules of sporotrichosis.

Phycomycosis (Mucormycosis)

Infection of the skin with these fungi is uncommon. Primary cutaneous inoculation phycomycosis occurs only in severely debilitated diabetics or immunosuppressed patients. There is a chronic subcutaneous phycomycosis in tropical areas affecting otherwise healthy individuals. Typically hard well-defined indurated areas enlarge painlessly on the face.

Histopathology. Very large long non-septal hyphae (Figure 3.22) are seen in non-specific areas of necrosis or granulation tissue. Ring-shaped structures represent cross-sections of hyphae. PAS staining allows easier identification.

Leishmaniasis

Cutaneous Leishmaniasis

This occurs around the Mediterranean coast and is caused by *Leishmania tropica*. It is transmitted by the bite of the sand fly. The average incubation period is 2 months. The wet or early ulcerative type starts like a boil then breaks down to a superficial ulcer. Healing occurs in 2–6 months. The dry type has a longer incubation period, heals more slowly over 12 months and is plaque-like.

Histopathology. The dermis is filled with large histiocytes containing large numbers of organisms[13] (Leishman–Donovan bodies) (Figure 3.23). These are protozoa and are round or oval 2–4 µm in diameter with a large peripherally placed nucleus. They are visible with H and E stain but are best seen with Giemsa stain. The epidermis is initially acanthotic and later ulcerates. Late recurrences are indistinguishable from lupus vulgaris.

American Cutaneous and Mucocutaneous Leishmaniasis

This occurs in Central and South America and is caused by *L. brasiliensis*. Mucous membranes are involved either by direct spread from cutaneous inoculation or as a secondary feature. The pathological changes are similar to cutaneous leishmaniasis except that gross epidermal proliferation results in a warty appearance of the primary lesion.

Scabies

Scabies is an infestation by human *Sarcoptes scabeii* mite. It is an intensely itchy condition and is readily transmitted by body contact. There is no characteristic pathological pattern. The picture may resemble an insect bite reaction (see page 28) and the burrowing female mite within the stratum corneum is rarely seen. Serial sections of a burrow may reveal the female acarus and possibly some eggs[14] (Figure 3.24).

Cutaneous Amoebiasis

The causative organism is *Entamoeba histolytica* which occurs as a motile form in the large bowel and may encyst outside the body. Cutaneous infection results from contamination of a wound with the organism or by extension from the liver or gut to the skin.

Histopathology. The resulting granuloma is not diagnostic. Fresh, non-necrotic, material suspended in saline may reveal motile trophozoites.

References

1. McSorley, J., Shapiro, L., Brownstein, M. H. *et al.* (1974). Herpes simplex and varicella-zoster: comparative histopathology of 77 cases. *Int. J. Dermatol.*, **13**, 69
2. Blank, H. and Haines, H. (1976). Viral diseases of the skin, 1975. A 25 year perspective. *J. Invest. Dermatol.*, **67**, 169
3. Gross, G., Pfister, H., Hagedorn, M. *et al.* (1982). Correlation between human papillomavirus (H.P.V.) type and histology of warts. *J. Invest. Dermatol.*, **78**, 160
4. Orth, G., Jablonska, S., Breitbard, F. *et al.* (1978). The human papilloma viruses. *Bull. Cancer*, **65**, 151
5. Abell, E., Marks, R. and Wilson-Jones, E. (1975). Secondary syphilis. A clinico-pathological review. *Br. J. Dermatol.*, **93**, 53
6. Montgomery, H. (1937). Histopathology of the various types of cutaneous tuberculosis. *Arch. Dermatol. Syph.*, **35**, 698
7. Ridley, D.S. (1974). Histological classification and the immunological spectrum of leprosy. *Bull. WHO*, **51**, 451
8. Jolly, H. W. Jr. and Seabury, J. H. (1972). Infections with *Mycobacterium marinum*. *Arch. Dermatol.*, **106**, 32
9. Birt, A. R. and Wilt, J. C. (1954). Mycology, bacteriology and histopathology of suppurative ringworm. *Arch. Dermatol.*, **69**, 441
10. Graham, J. H., Johnson, W. C., Burgoon, C. F. *et al.* (1964). Tinea capitis. *Arch. Dermatol.*, **89**, 528

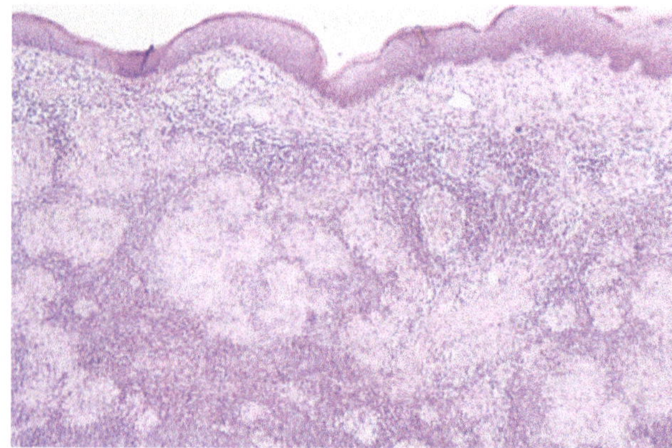

Figure 3.13 Lupus vulgaris. Tuberculoid granulomata throughout the dermis. Note the granulomata are surrounded by a dense lymphocytic infiltrate. H & E (B)

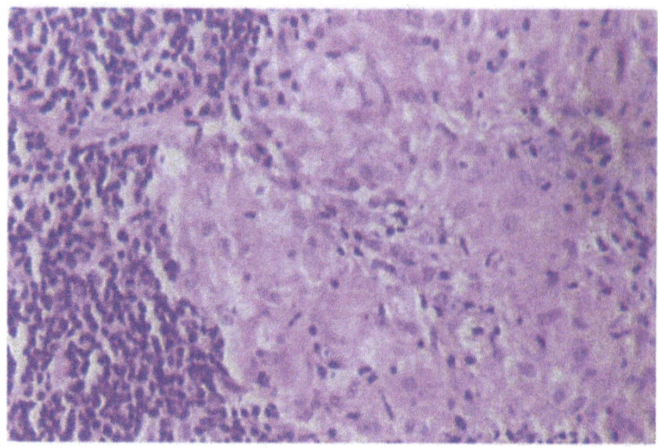

Figure 3.14 Lupus vulgaris. Epithelioid cells surrounded by a dense lymphocytic infiltrate. H & E (C)

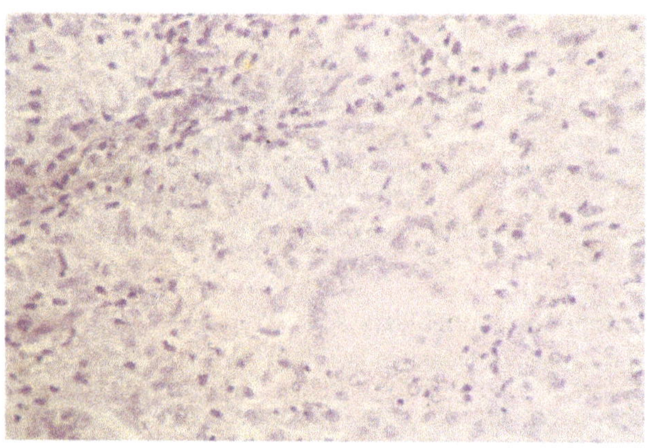

Figure 3.15 Lupus vulgaris. Large Langhans giant cell within an epithelioid granuloma. H & E (C)

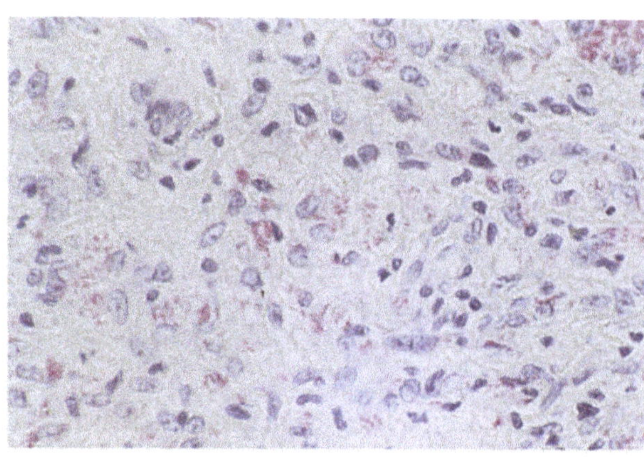

Figure 3.16 Lepromatous leprosy. Foamy lepra cells full of acid-fast bacilli. Z.N. stain (C)

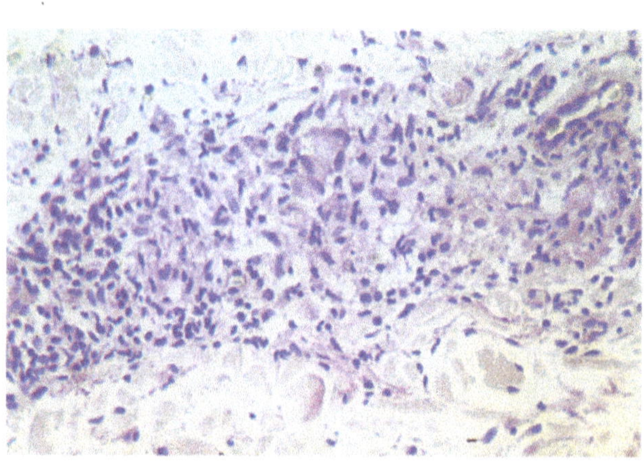

Figure 3.17 Tuberculoid leprosy. Epithelioid cell granuloma with very little surrounding lymphocytic infiltrate. The granuloma resembles sarcoidosis but is based on a nerve. H & E (C)

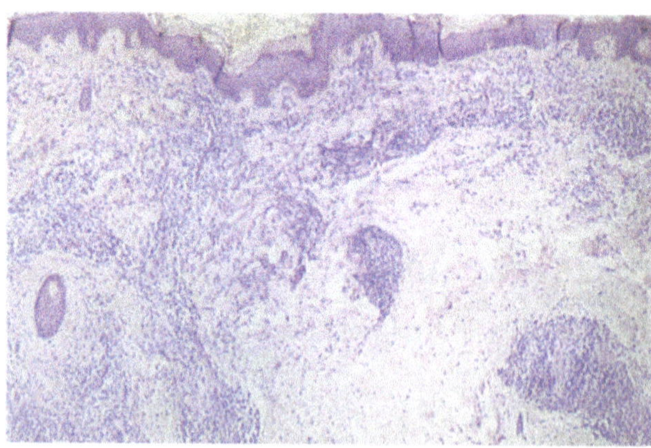

Figure 3.18 Tuberculoid leprosy. Epithelioid cell granulomata in mid dermis with little surrounding lymphocytic infiltrate. The granulomata resemble sarcoidosis but are around cutaneous nerves. H & E (B)

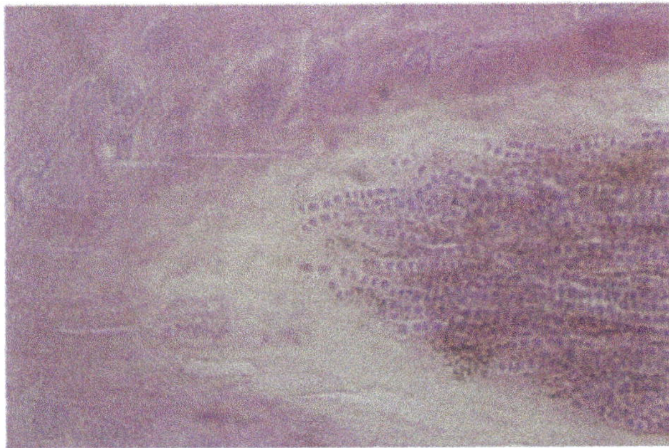

Figure 3.19 Dermatophyte infection of hair. Note the hyphal filaments almost reaching the hair matrix.   H & E (D)

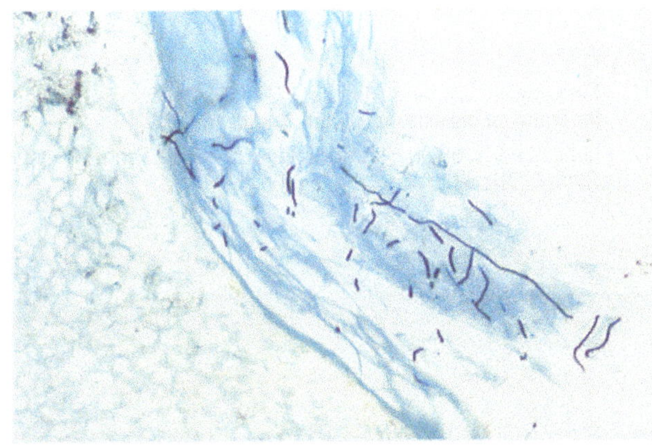

Figure 3.20 Dermatophyte infection. Note hyphae limited to stratum corneum and stained black. Grocott's silver stain.   (D)

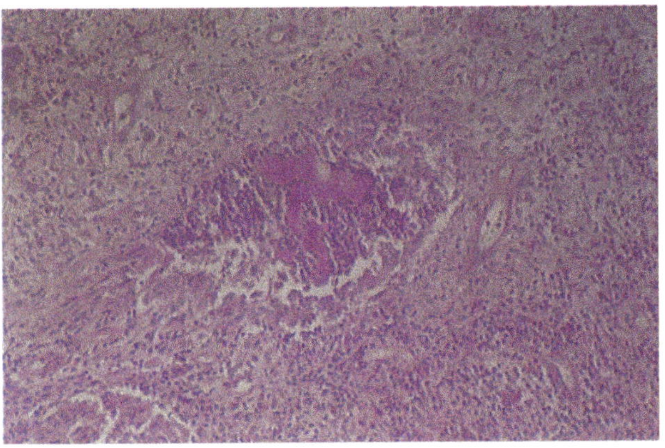

Figure 3.21 Nocardiasis. Clumps of organisms (granules) surrounded by neutrophils. This picture is very similar to that seen in Actinomycosis.   H & E (C)

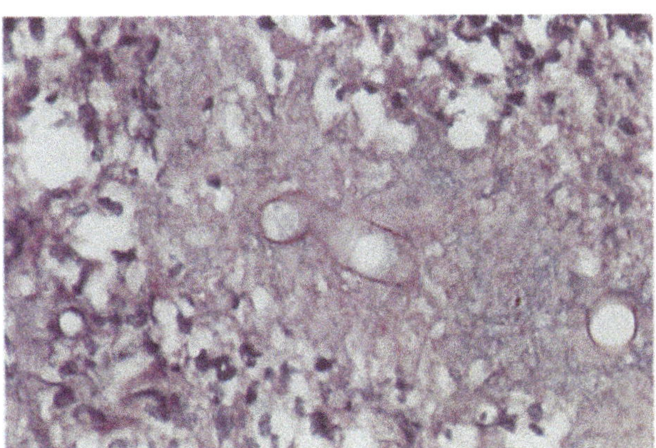

Figure 3.22 Mucormycosis. Subcutaneous inflammation and necrosis. In the centre is a large ring-shaped section of a hypha. Surrounding inflammatory cells include eosinophils.   PAS (C)

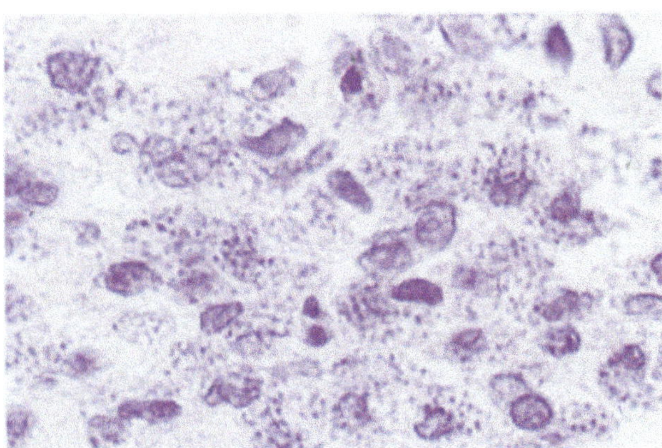

Figure 3.23 Leishmaniasis. Large histiocytes filled with Leishman–Donovan bodies.   Giemsa stain (D)

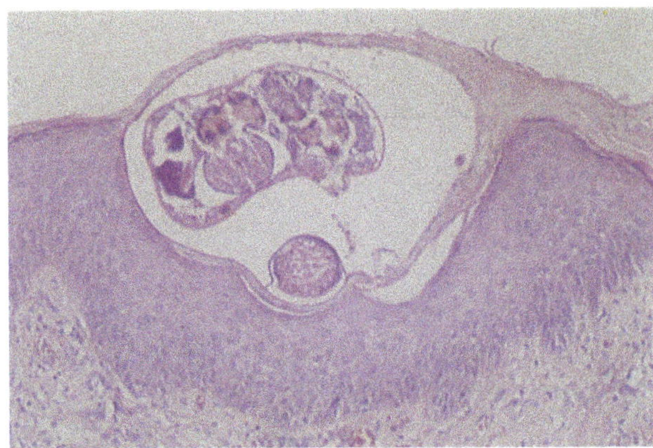

Figure 3.24 *Sarcoptes scabeii*. A female acarus and egg in a burrow situated within the stratum corneum.   H & E (C)

11. Kirkpatrick, C. H. and Montes, L. F. (1974). Chronic mucocu-
     taneous candidiasis. *J. Cutan. Pathol.*, **1**, 211

12. Lurie, H. I. (1963). Histopathology of sporotrichosis. *Arch.
     Pathol.*, **75**, 421

13. Kurban, A. K., Malak, J. A., Farah, F. *et al.* (1966). Histopathol-
     ogy of cutaneous leishmaniasis. *Arch. Dermatol.*, **93**, 396

14. Fernandez, N., Torres, A. and Ackerman, A. B. (1977). Patho-
     logic findings in human scabies. *Arch. Dermatol.*, **113**, 320

Disorders of Keratinization

This term is used to describe disorders in which there is a primary fault in the process of epidermal differentiation and (or) desquamation. It includes the ichthyotic disorders and a number of other quite uncommon disorders in which there is scaling and hyperkeratosis.

The Ichthyotic Disorders

These are disorders characterized by persistent generalized scaling without inflammation. The commonest is known as *autosomal dominant ichthyosis* in which the scaling is generally mild and spares the flexures. Histologically the only distinguishing feature is the absence or deficiency of granular cell layer (Figure 4.1). A similar but less common disorder is *X-linked ichthyosis*. This is inherited as a sex-linked characteristic so that it is manifest in boys only, but carried by the female. This resembles autosomal dominant ichthyosis but is more severe, involving the flexures and the sides of the neck. Interestingly it differs from the dominant condition histologically in that the granular layer is exaggerated rather than deficient (Figure 4.2). In recent years it has been found that patients with sex-linked ichthyosis have steroid sulphatase deficiency and a consequent accumulation of cholesterol sulphate in the stratum corneum. Although abnormalities in lipid metabolism have been identified in autosomal dominant ichthyosis these are non-specific and do not inform concerning the underlying fault[1]. It has been suggested that lipids are involved in normal desquamation but conclusive evidence on the mechanism(s) of involvement is not yet available[2].

Refsum's Syndrome (Ataxia Heredopathia Neuritiformis)

This rare disorder of keratinization seems to be due to a deficiency in alpha hydroxylation of branched-chain fatty acids, although which particular enzyme is involved is not clear. In particular, dietary phytanic acid cannot be metabolized so that abnormal phytanates accumulate in tissues[3]. It is a recessively inherited multisystem disorder characterized by retinitis pigmentosa, nerve deafness, peripheral neuropathy and ichthyosis. Histologically the epidermis is slightly thickened with mild hypergranulosis. A particular feature that distinguishes the disorder is the presence of lipid vacuoles in the basal layer of the epidermis[4] (Figure 4.3). These are visible throughout the epidermis ultrastructurally[5] (Figure 4.4). Cell kinetic studies in which autoradiographic labelling indices were determined after exposure to tritiated thymidine showed that unlike other types of phenotypically similar ichthyosis vulgaris the ichthyosis in Refsum's disease is 'hyperproliferative' (Figure 4.5).

Epidermolytic Hyperkeratosis (also known as bullous ichthyosiform erythroderma)

This is a rare dominantly inherited disorder in which there is generalized scaling and hyperkeratosis as well as a background of erythema. In addition there is a tendency to blistering with trauma that seems to improve with age. Even more rarely the disorder only occurs at localized sites either as a form of verrucous naevus or as a type of palmoplantar keratoderma[6].

Histopathology. The epidermis is irregularly thickened. The most typical feature is a degenerative change in the mid and upper epidermis, in which vacuoles appear in the epidermal cells, which become disrupted. This change is generalized and consistent and of unknown cause. It is most prominent in the granular cell layer whose granules are more irregular and larger than normal (Figure 4.6). The epidermis shows an increased rate of cell production – presumably to keep pace with the cell destruction in the upper layers. The metabolic basis for this disorder is not understood.

Non-bullous Ichthyosiform Erythroderma (NBIE)

This disorder is recessively inherited in contrast to the dominantly inherited bullous type. In infancy generalized erythema is usual but this is less prominent in older subjects. The scaling is fine and bran-like and there is little hyperkeratosis. The pathology demonstrates a psoriasiform hyperplasia of the epidermis (Figure 4.7). There is marked parakeratosis but no epidermal invasion by polymorph neutrophils and neither tortuousity or dilatation of papillary capillaries nor suprapapillary plate thinning. Autoradiographic cell kinetic studies with tritiated thymidine have demonstrated a high labelling index in the disease – similar to that in psoriasis[7]. Abnormalities in the lipid content of the stratum corneum have been described[8].

Lamellar Ichthyosis

This is another rare, recessively inherited form of ichthyosis. The clinical hallmark of the disorder is thick scaling and hyperkeratosis, giving an almost reptilian appearance. This is mirrored in the histological appearance which usually shows inconspicuous epidermal thickening overall but hypergranulosis and pronounced hyperkeratosis (Figure 4.8).

Tylosis (Hyperkeratosis Palmaris et Plantaris)

There are several disorders which are characterized clinically by marked thickening and (or) scaling of the skin of all or parts of the palms and soles. The mode of inheritance varies with the particular phenotypic expression of the condition. Histologically the picture is not

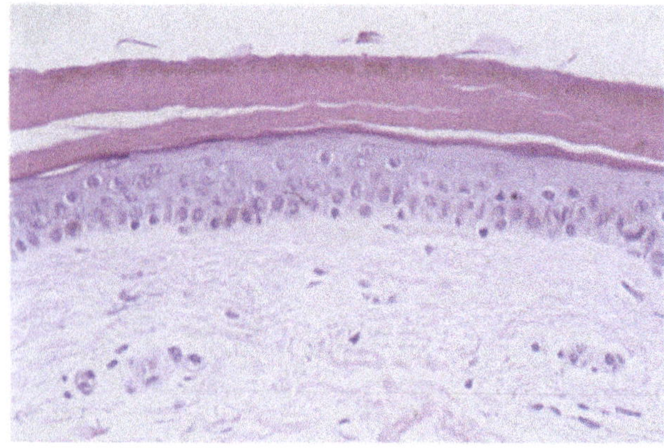

Figure 4.1 Autosomal dominant ichthyosis. The granular cell layer is barely present. H & E (C)

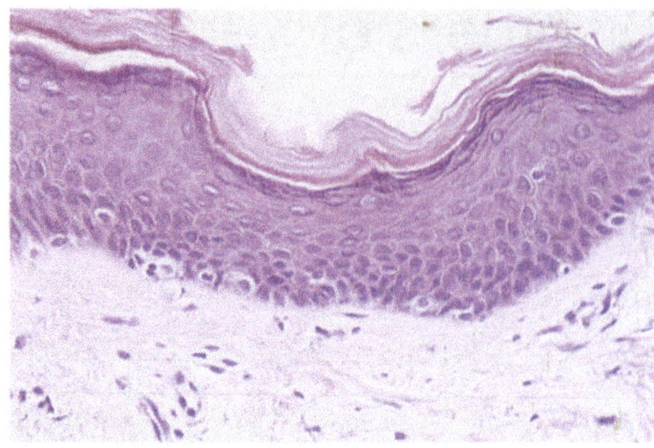

Figure 4.2 Sex-linked ichthyosis. There is accentuation of the granular cell layer. H & E (C)

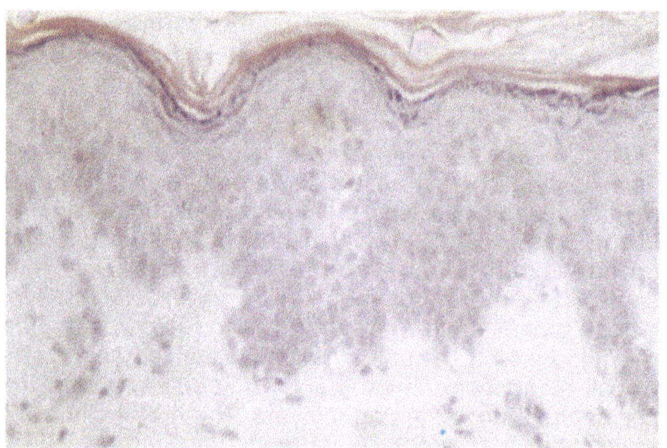

Figure 4.3 Refsum's syndrome. Note the vacuolated cells in the basal layer as well as epidermal thickening. H & E (C)

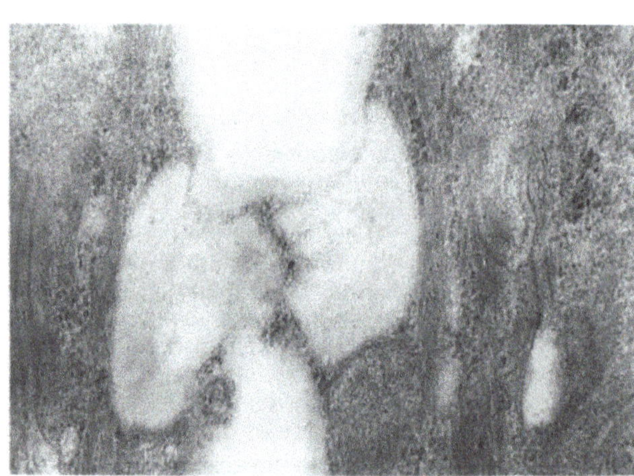

Figure 4.4 Electron micrograph to show lipid droplets in cytoplasm of keratinocytes from patient with Refsum's syndrome. × 30 000

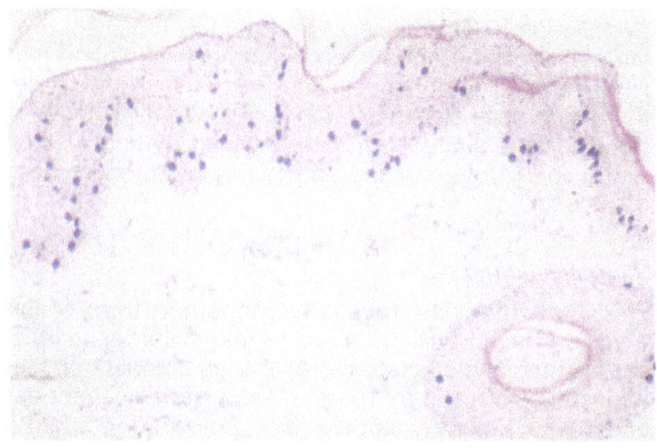

Figure 4.5 Autoradiograph from patient with Refsum's syndrome showing many basal keratinocytes labelled after injection of tritiated thymidine before biopsy. (B)

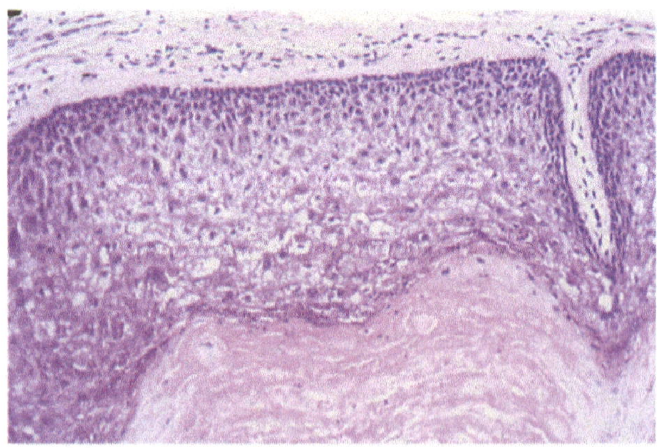

Figure 4.6 Epidermolytic hyperkeratosis (bullous ichthyosiform erythroderma) showing reticulate degenerative change in upper epidermis. H & E (C)

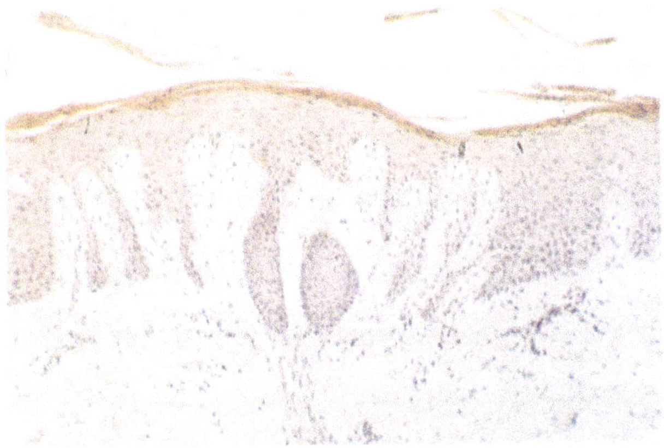

Figure 4.7 Non-bullous ichthyosiform erythroderma. There is epidermal thickening and parakeratosis.   H & E (C)

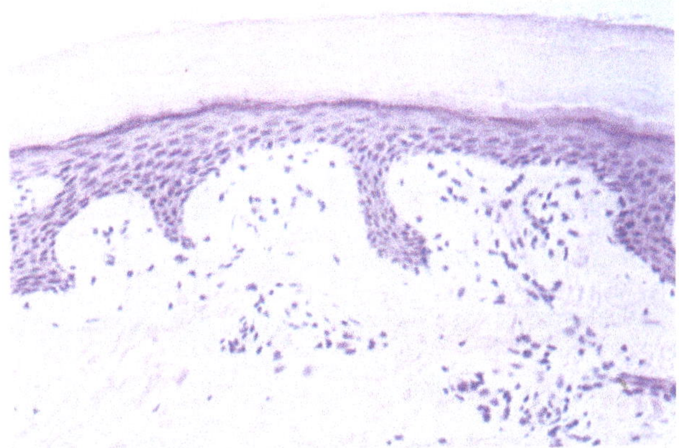

Figure 4.8 Lamellar ichthyosis. There is slight hypergranulosis and marked compact hyperkeratosis.   H & E (C)

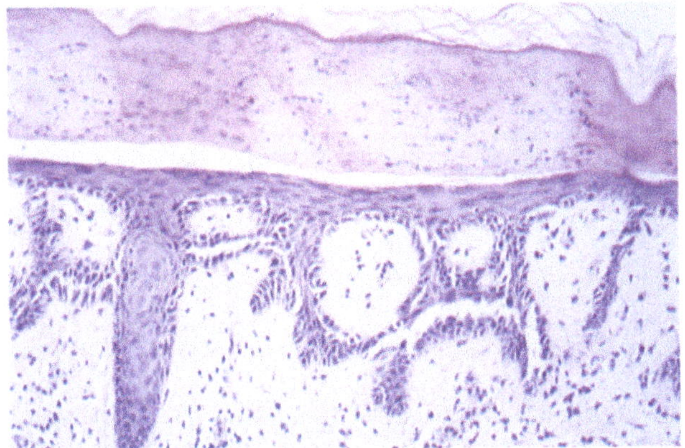

Figure 4.9 Darier's disease. Note the suprabasal cleft.   H & E (C)

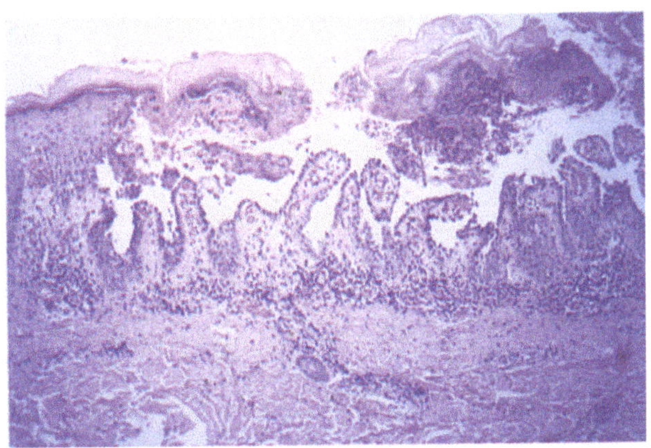

Figure 4.10 Darier's disease. Villous arrangement and suprabasilar clefting.   H & E (B)

distinctive, showing only uniform epidermal thickening and hyperkeratosis.

Other Disorders of Keratinization

Darier's Disease (Keratosis follicularis)

Darier's disease is included in this section for convenience as a disorder of keratinization as it is a genodermatosis that results in scaling, crusting and hyperkeratotic areas and is marked by histological changes in the differentiating part of the epidermis. However, it may be more correctly categorized as a disease of epidermal cohesion. The face, scalp, shoulders and chest are preferentially involved although any area can be affected. Horny papules and scaling occur in the affected sites. Episodes of crusting and exudation on the affected areas develop. Small pits on the palms and linear fissures in the finger nails are also characteristic. The disorder may be transmitted as a dominant characteristic but many cases have no family history and are presumably 'new mutations'.

Histopathology.   The most characteristic feature of the disorder is suprabasilar clefting within the epidermis. Epidermal cells that have become rounded and lost contact with their neighbours (acantholytic cells) may be

found within the cleft (Figure 4.9). The bottom of the cleft, i.e. the basal layer, may show irregular villous-like hypertrophy. In the epidermis above the cleft individual swollen dyskeratotic cells (corps ronds) are found, while small dark and dense bodies known as 'grains' are also seen sometimes (Figure 4.10). Ultrastructurally the cells show abnormalities of the tonofilament desmosomal plate complex[9]. Unlike pemphigus there are no characteristic immunofluorescent findings. For differential diagnosis of suprabasilar clefting, see Chapter 5.

Chronic Benign Familial Pemphigus (Hailey-Hailey disease)

This uncommon disorder has some similarity to Darier's disease but is considered in Chapter 5.

References

1. Dykes, P. J. and Marks, R. (1978). Lipid synthesis in ichthyotic conditions. In Marks, R. and Dykes, P. J. (eds.) *The Ichthyoses.* pp. 31–36. (Lancaster: MTP)

2. Elias, P. M. (1983). Epidermal lipids, barrier function and desquamation. *J. Invest. Dermatol.,* **80** (Suppl.), 44s

3. Davies, M. G., Reynolds, D. J., Marks, R. and Dykes, P. J. (1978). The epidermis in Refsum's disease (Heredopathia atactic polyneuritiformis). In Marks, R and Dykes P. J. (eds.) *The Ichthyoses.* pp. 51–64. (Lancaster: MTP)

4. Davies, M. G., Marks, R., Dykes, P. J. and Reynolds, D. (1977). Epidermal abnormalities in Refsum's disease. *Br. J. Dermatol.*, **97**, 401

5. Blanchet-Bardon, C., Anton-Lamprecht, I., Puissant, A. and Schnyder, U. W. (1978). Ultastructural features of ichthyotic skin in Refsum's syndrome. In Marks, R. and Dykes, P. J. (eds.) *The Ichthyoses*. pp. 65–70. (Lancaster: MTP)

6. Klaus, S., Weinstein, G. D. and Frost, P. (1970). Localised epidermolytic hyperkeratosis: A form of keratoderma of the palms and soles. *Arch. Dermatol.*, **101**, 272

7. Hazell, M. and Marks, R. (1985). Clinical, histologic and cell kinetic discriminants between lamellar ichthyosis and nonbullous congenital icthyosiform erythroderma. *Arch. Dermatol.*, **121**, 489

8. Williams, M. L. and Elias, P. M. (1985). Heterogeneity in autosomal recessive ichthyosis: Clinical and biochemical differentiation of lamellar ichthyosis and nonbullous congenital icthyosiform erythroderma. *Arch. Dermatol.*, **121**, 477

9. Gottlieb, S. K. and Lutzner, M. A. (1973). Darier's disease: an electron microscopic study. *Arch. Dermatol.*, **107**, 225

The skin can develop vesicles and bullae as a result of diverse causes through mechanisms affecting different levels of the epidermis and dermis[1]. Histological diagnosis of bullous skin disorders requires attention to several key points. These include:

(1) The presence or absence of an inflammatory cell infiltrate, its predominant cell type and the distribution of the inflammatory cells within the dermis.
(2) The type of changes in the epidermis (spongiosis, acantholysis, balloon degeneration, individual cell death or widespread necrosis, pustule formation, and the presence or absence of exocytosis).
(3) The level of separation or clefting which may be subcorneal, in the prickle cell layer, suprabasally or subepidermally in the papillary dermis.

For light microscopy to yield this information, it is essential to take a biopsy before the blisters are fully formed. Established blisters or 'old' lesions are often unhelpful because the important details are lost as blister formation evolves. Indeed the appearances may be quite misleading in some cases of subepidermal blistering disease as the level of separation becomes located intraepidermally following regeneration of new epidermis from the margin of the lesions or from hair follicles. Accordingly, there are occasions when a firm histological diagnosis cannot be made by light microscopy.

Immunofluorescence and electron microscopy have made the diagnosis of bullous disease more precise. For example, immunofluorescence microscopy may distinguish the pemphigus group of disorders from other acantholytic disorders such as Hailey–Hailey disease and transient acantholytic dermatosis. It also allows ready differentiation between bullous pemphigoid, dermatitis herpetiformis and herpes gestationis, conditions which on routine light microscopy sometimes show overlapping features.

Electron microscopy, by defining the precise site of clefting, is most useful in the diagnosis of epidermolysis bullosa: a term applied to a heterogenous group of genetically determined skin disorders, whose common feature is blistering after trivial injury.

Blisters may also be a component of several skin disorders such as viral and bacterial infections, eczema and disorders of keratinization but these diseases are discussed elsewhere. This chapter discusses only those diseases in which blisters are the outstanding clinical feature and includes pemphigus and its variants, bullous pemphigoid, dermatitis herpetiformis and epidermolysis bullosa. Porphyria cutanea tarda, although a blistering disease, is described along with other forms of prophyria in Chapter 12.

Congenital Disorders

Epidermolysis Bullosa

Epidermolysis bullosa is the term applied to a variety of congenital disorders which have the common feature of an abnormal susceptibility to blistering of the skin as a result of trivial trauma. The various forms of epidermolysis bullosa are defined by the level of clefting within the basal layer of the epidermis and the dermo-epidermal

Table 5.1 Epidermolysis Bullosa

Type	Inheritance	Level of Separation (precisely identifiable only in electron-micrographs)
Epidermal		
Hands and feet	Dominant	Intra-epidermal
Simplex	Dominant	Basal epithelial cells
Junctional		
Letalis	Recessive	Between epithelial basal cells and epithelial basement membrane
Dermal		
Dystrophica	Dominant or recessive	Between epidermal basement membrane and dermis
Acquisita	—	Dermo-epidermal junction between basement membrane and dermis

junction[2] (see Table 5.1). The simplex type shows degeneration of the basal epithelial cells and a suprabasal bulla. In the letalis type the separation is in the basement membrane of the epidermis and the condition is recessively inherited. There is cleavage in the upper dermis in the dystrophica type which may show dominant or recessive patterns of inheritance. The deeper the level of clefting within the skin, the more susceptible to scarring is the resultant blister.

Histological examination of a blister in epidermolysis bullosa shows the characteristic combination of a subepidermal bulla without an inflammatory infiltrate (Figure 5.1). Other than in epidermolysis bullosa this combination is only seen in bullous prophyria cutanea tarda and in the latter condition there is usually a characteristic PAS-positive deposit around dermal capillaries and 'festooning' of dermal papillae so that they protrude into the cleft. It is not possible to distinguish between some of the forms of epidermolysis bullosa with the light microscope. With the electron microscope, however, the precise site of clefting can be identified[3] (see Table 5.1 and Figures 5.A, 5.B). Letalis-type epidermolysis occurs on the outer surface of the basement membrane due to abnormality of the desmosomes in this region. Ultrastructural examination of dystrophic epidermolysis shows an intact junction between epidermis and base-

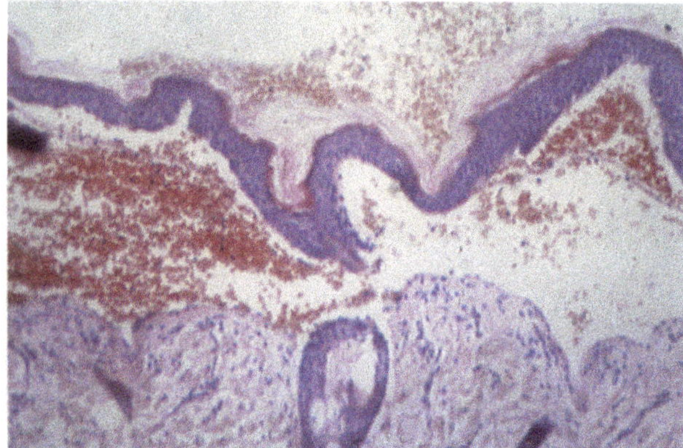

Figure 5.1   Epidermolysis bullosa. Dystrophic recessive type, dermo-epidermal separation. The dermis is oedematous with sparse infiltrate. Accurate localization of the split demands electron microscopy.   H & E (B)

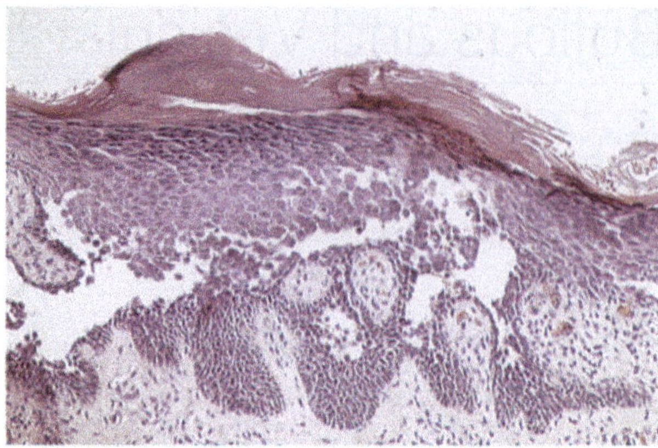

Figure 5.2   Hailey–Hailey disease. Separation of epidermal cells both singly and in clumps. The separation is above the basal layer and there is some 'delapidated brick wall' appearance.   H & E (B)

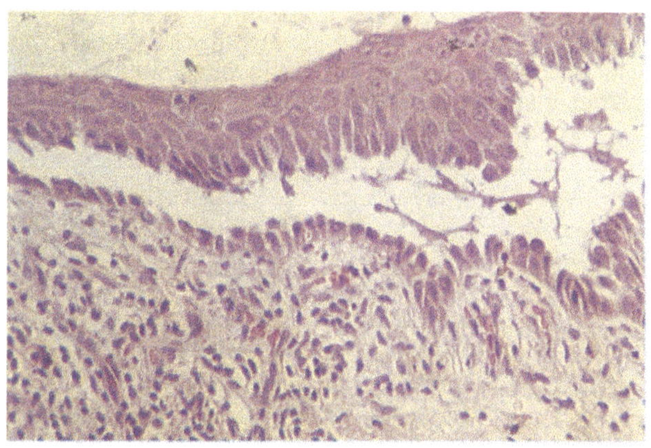

Figure 5.3   Pemphigus vulgaris. Suprabasal cleft, acantholytic cells in roof of blister. Basal cells form the base of the blister. Dermal infiltrate of lymphocytes and some eosinophils.   H & E (B)

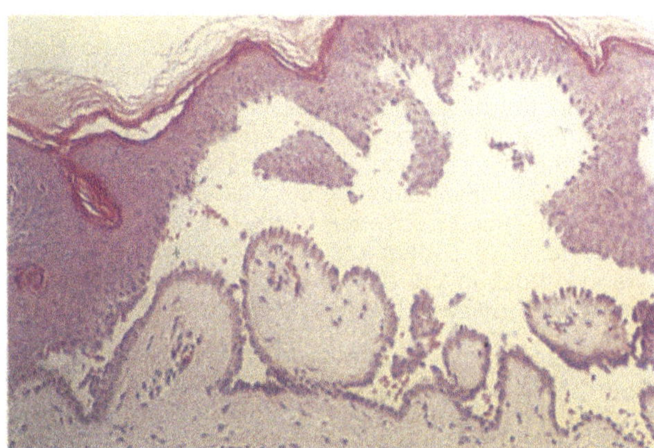

Figure 5.4   Pemphigus vulgaris. Suprabasal cleft (floor of blister lined by basal cells) and floor of blister interrupted by upward 'villous' projections. Acantholytic cells in blister.   H & E (B)

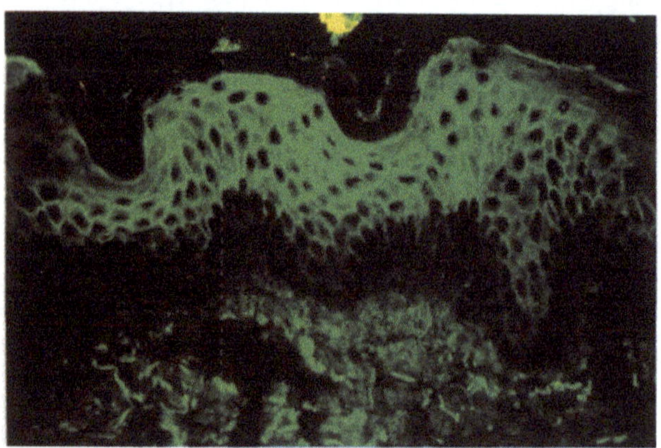

Figure 5.5   Pemphigus vulgaris. Immunofluorescence of perilesional skin using anti-IgG. There is fluorescence of the periphery of epidermal cells (intercellular fluorescence). Also positive with anti-C3.   (B)

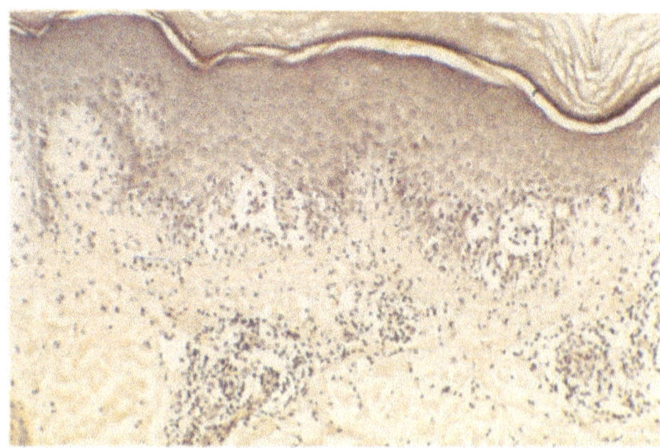

Figure 5.6   Erythema multiforme. Upper dermal oedema with some intra-epidermal vesicles and exocytosis. Mainly perivascular dermal mononuclear cell infiltrate.   H & E (B)

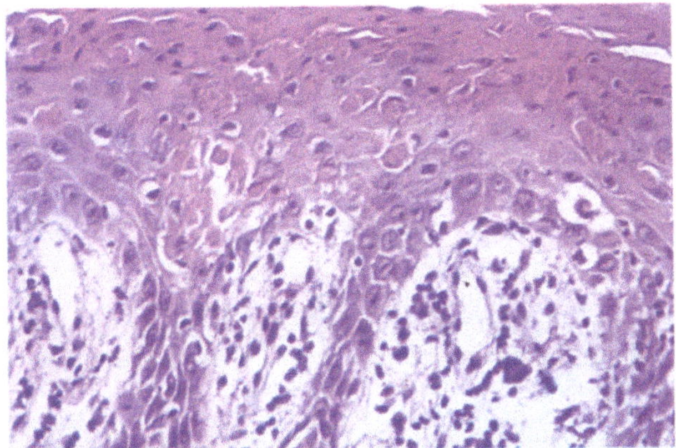

Figure 5.7 Erythema multiforme. Epidermal oedema and individual epidermal cells showing eosinophilic necrosis. H & E (D)

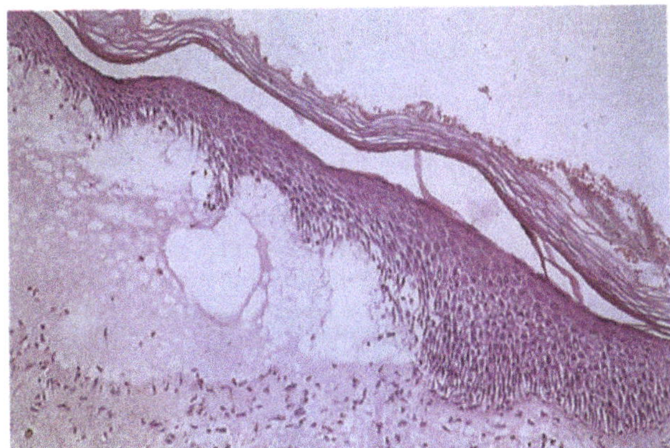

Figure 5.8 Bullous pemphigoid. Subepidermal blister with intact epidermis forming the roof. Flattened dermis with an infiltrate of eosinophils and neutrophils. H & E (B)

Figure 5.9 Bullous pemphigoid. Direct immunofluorescence of perilesional skin using anti-IgG. A smooth narrow band is present along the dermoepidermal junction. Also positive with anti-C3. (B)

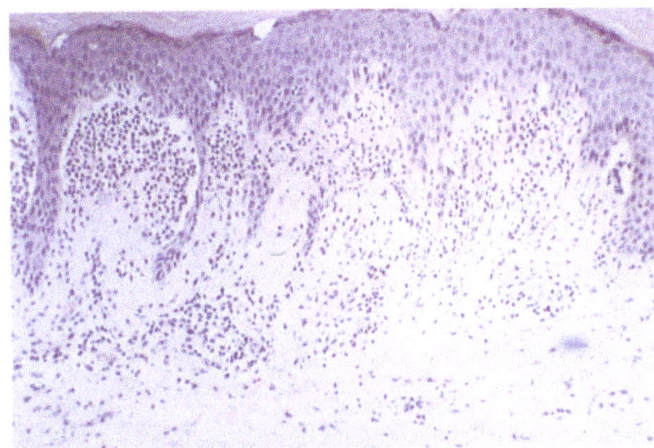

Figure 5.10 Dermatitis herpetiformis. Pre-bullous skin showing early dermoepidermal separation and papillary collections of neutrophils. H & E (B)

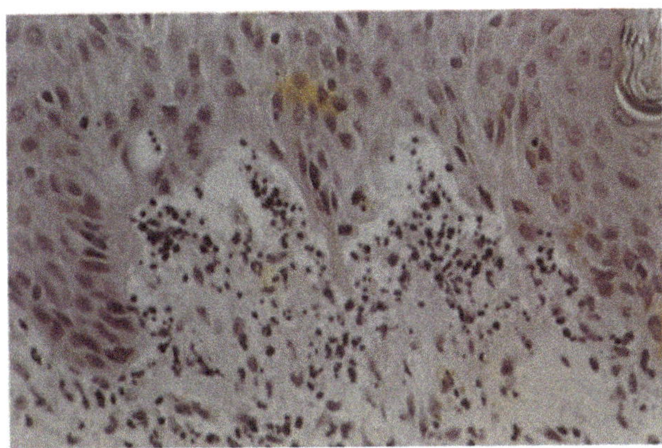

Figure 5.11 Dermatitis herpetiformis. Dermo-epidermal separation in the papillae which are full of neutrophils and nuclear dust. H & E (C)

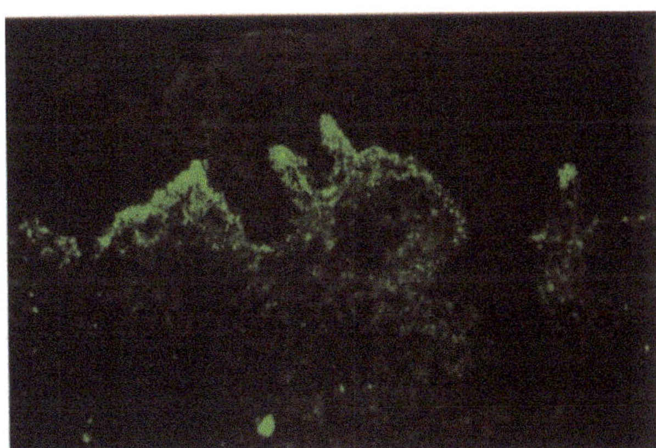

Figure 5.12 Dermatitis herpetiformis. Direct immunofluorescence of normal uninvolved skin using anti-IgA. There is a speckled fluorescence concentrated in the dermal papillae. (B)

ment membrane, with clefting of the upper dermis and abnormalities of the anchoring fibrils. Immunofluorescence staining may also help in diagnosis. Antibodies labelled with fluorescein can be used to demonstrate type IV collagen and laminin, the latter being found in the lamina lucida of the basement membrane. In junctional epidermolysis bullosa both type IV collagen and laminin are found in the base of the bulla. In dystrophic epidermolysis bullosa these substances are demonstrable in the *roof* of the blister. Immunofluorescence is also useful in the diagnosis of epidermolysis bullosa

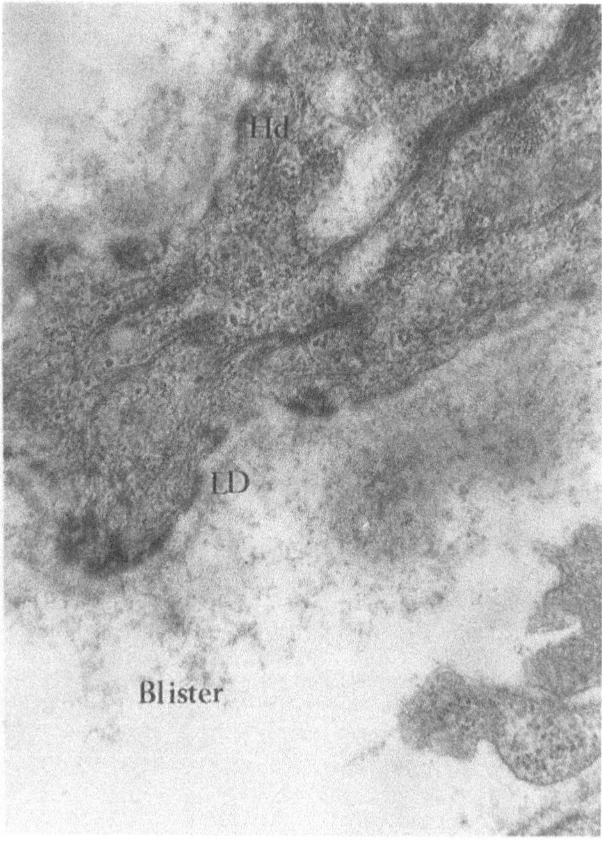

Figure 5.A Epidermolysis bullosa dystrophic recessive type. There are no anchoring fibrils on the dermal side of the lamina densa (LD). Hd is hemidesmosome. × 8650

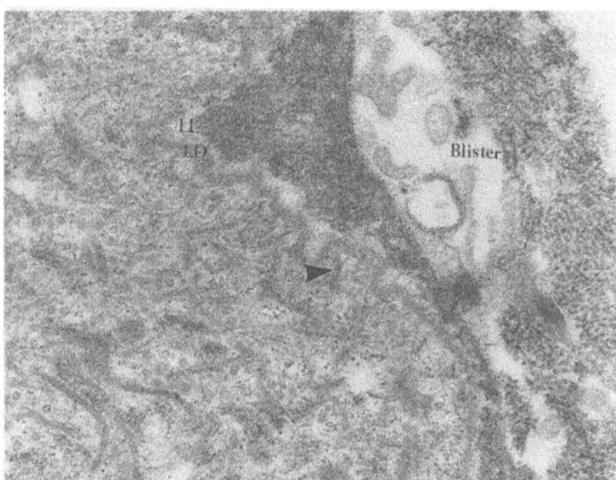

Figure 5.B Epidermolysis bullosa simplex. Note presence of anchoring fibrils arrowed. The blister contains remnants of epidermal cells which show little sign of attachment to lamina densa (LD). LL is lamina lucida. × 12 600

acquisita, in which linear deposits of immunoglobulins and complement are seen along the dermo-epidermal junction throughout the skin.

Chronic Familial Benign Pemphigus

Familial benign pemphigus (Hailey–Hailey) has some histological features in common with Darier's disease (Chapter 4), but clinically they are quite different. Hailey–Hailey is autosomal dominant in inheritance and presents as a vesicular exudative and crusted disorder affecting the axillae, groins and back of the neck. The hyperkeratosis, which is such a feature of Darier's disease, is barely apparent clinically in Hailey–Hailey.

In histological sections, the clefts in Hailey–Hailey are suprabasal as in Darier's disease, but the acantholysis is much more extensive and is characteristic in appearance[4]. Thus the desmosomes between adjacent cells appear to be still loosely attached so that the affected keratinocytes become separated but not completely free-floating. Their appearance is rather similar to bricks separated by copious mortar (Figure 5.2). There is also acanthosis and papillomatosis. Although corps ronds and grains may be seen in the skin in Hailey–Hailey disease, they are infrequent and often absent.

Although the clinical differences between Darier's disease and Hailey–Hailey are usually clear, this is not always the case in pemphigus vulgaris. This disorder may resemble Hailey–Hailey disease, although Hailey–Hailey does not occur on mucous membranes or affect large areas of the trunk, face or limbs. In histological sections, it is the widespread distribution of the rather peculiar type of acantholysis which distinguishes Hailey–Hailey best from pemphigus vulgaris. Immunofluorescence studies of frozen sections are negative in Hailey–Hailey disease and this negative finding is useful in cases in which the histological appearances are equivocal.

Incontinentia Pigmenti

The syndrome of incontinentia pigmenti is most commonly seen in female infants and children. It is a disease which passes through various stages, each with rather characteristic appearances. The earliest manifestations, occurring in the first few days of life, are small vesicles described as eosinophilic spongiosis. The vesicles are intraepidermal, rather small in size and circular in outline. Characteristically, they are separated by bands of intact keratinocytes. The eosinophil polymorph infiltrate is moderate to marked in degree. As the lesions mature, the vesicles disappear leaving only a vacuolated basal layer with acanthosis of the overlying epidermis and large amounts of melanin in the underlying dermis. This persists through the third stage of the disease when the epidermal changes regress. Clinically, the vesicles disappear and the affected sites develop warty lesions which gradually atrophy leaving a bizarre pattern of pigmentation over the skin of the trunk. Although eosinophilic spongiosis is a good indicator of vesicular incontinentia pigmenti, it must be remembered that similar changes are also seen in allergic dermatitis and arthropod-bite reactions.

Acquired Disorders

Pemphigus

The blisters of pemphigus are usually flaccid, and are easily disrupted. Bullae may occupy large areas of the skin and include the mucosa of the oral cavity. Two histological types of pemphigus are seen; suprabasal, exemplified by pemphigus vulgaris and superficial, of which pemphigus foliaceus is the main example.

Pemphigus Vulgaris

In this condition the cleft develops suprabasally (Figure 5.3). Acantholysis is the characteristic feature which helps to distinguish pemphigus vulgaris from bullous pemphigoid. Only small numbers of inflammatory cells (including eosinophils) are seen at the base of the blister, except in the variant called pemphigus vegetans in which very large numbers of eosinophils produce an intraepidermal pustule. In typical pemphigus vulgaris dermal papillae are covered by a single layer of epidermal cells (the so-called 'villi') (Figure 5.4) and the suprabasal cleft extends down into the hair follicles.

When the biopsy is of an early lesion, the appearances in pemphigus vulgaris are usually characteristic. Nonetheless, immunofluorescence staining using an indirect method is useful in confirming the diagnosis[5]. Intercellular staining is seen at the periphery of keratinocytes using fluorescein-labelled antibodies to IgG and C3 (Figure 5.5). Electron microscopy has shown that the acantholysis in pemphigus vulgaris is primarily due to the dissolution of intercellular cement[6]. This finding may explain the susceptibility of the oral mucosa to pemphigus, in that mucosal cells have fewer desmosomes than those in the epidermis. When desmosomes separate they do so in the plane of the attachment plates, so that tufted tonofilaments remain adherent to the isolated cell surface. Immunoperoxidase methods applied to electron microscopy have shown that the IgG antibodies are located in this intercellular cement in cases of pemphigus vulgaris.

Pemphigus Foliaceus

Although other features, including the results of immunofluorescence staining, are the same as in pemphigus vulgaris, the clefting in pemphigus foliaceus is subcorneal or between granular cells. This plane of cleavage is immediately beneath the granular layer and so dyskeratosis is characteristically superficial. Shrunken, basophilic epidermal cells are seen in the granular zone.

Erythema Multiforme

This is a relapsing condition, idiopathic but sometimes precipitated by viral infections or drugs and characterized by erythematous plaques, macules or papules. Blisters and erosions occur on these erythematous areas and the mucosae are often affected. Individual lesions usually heal after about a month but may subsequently relapse. The severity and extent of the changes seen in erythema multiforme may also be very variable with the most severe manifestations being seen in Stevens–Johnson disease.

The characteristic histopathological changes of bullous erythema multiforme are subepidermal blistering and adjacent basal vacuolation (Figure 5.6). In lesions which are clinically more severe, the abnormalities are principally within the epidermis and consist of focal necrosis of keratinocytes (Figure 5.7) associated with the typical subepidermal clefting and vacuolation of the basal layers[7]. A superficial perivascular inflammatory-cell infiltrate is seen in the upper part of the dermis and the dermal papillae show well-marked oedema. Drug-induced erythema multiforme tends to show less epidermal involvement and a more prominent superficial perivascular dermatitis with acute inflammatory cells also being seen at the dermo-epidermal junction.

Table 5.2 Subepidermal Blistering Diseases

	Epidermal cell death	Dermal infiltrate	Immuno-fluorescence
Erythema multiforme	++	mixed	negative
Bullous pemphigoid	−	eosinophils	linear BM IgG and C3
Porphyria cutanea tarda	−	very scanty	Not diagnostic
Dermatitis herpetiformis	−	neutrophils	IgA normal skin

Erythema multiforme should be readily distinguished from other subepidermal blistering diseases because of the epidermal cell death. In addition the very severe upper dermal oedema in erythema multiforme is absent in bullous pemphigoid, porphyria cutanea tarda and dermatitis herpetiformis.

Toxic Epidermal Necrolysis

Clinically toxic epidermal necrolysis is characterized by sheets of epidermis separating and appearing to slide over the base like scalded skin. The condition has two types – the adult and infantile forms – which have a different aetiology despite their clinical similarity[8]. The adult type is caused by a drug reaction and the infantile variety by a staphylococcal bacterial toxin. In both forms epidermal cell necrosis is the major feature. The necrosis in the infantile type is limited to the upper epidermis though the lower epidermal cells are frequently distorted and shrunken. In the adult type necrosis occurs in the whole epidermis. Little dermal inflammation is present in either variety.

Bullous Pemphigoid

This blistering skin disease commonly affects the elderly and is characterized by tense bullae affecting the skin surfaces. The blisters are often several centimetres in diameter and have blood-stained contents. The disorder spontaneously regresses after some months even without steroid therapy. Unlike pemphigus vulgaris, lesions are only rarely seen in the mouth. Some lesions may present as urticarial patches without blistering, when appearances may resemble those of erythema multiforme.

The level of cleavage in early lesions is subepidermal (Figure 5.8), but it is quite characteristic of bullous pemphigoid that there are prominent epidermal regenerative changes at the base of the lesion so that the cleft may appear to be intraepidermal or even subcorneal as the bullae mature. Even in regenerating bullae there is no acantholysis, and this is a useful feature in distinguishing between bullous pemphigoid and pemphigus vulgaris[9]. The degree of dermal inflammatory infiltrate seen in bullous pemphigoid varies considerably from one lesion to another. In lesions taken from erythematous skin the predominant cell is the eosinophil polymorph. The infiltrate is usually of less intensity than that seen in dermatitis herpetiformis, in which the predominant acute inflammatory cell is usually the neutrophil. Direct immunofluorescence testing of frozen sections from perilesional skin shows a positive binding in virtually every case for antibodies to IgG and C3 in a linear distribution along the basement membrane zone (Figure 5.9). In the rare cases which are negative for immunoglobulins, a similar distribution of staining for C3 can be seen. Immunoperoxidase localization of IgG in ultrastructural studies of the skin in cases of bullous pemphigoid have shown that the antibody is located in the lamina lucida above the basement membrane of the epidermis[10]. Consequently, type IV collagen is adherent to the base of the ulcer, and this can be demonstrated in immunofluorescence studies.

Cicatricial Pemphigoid (Benign Mucous Membrane Pemphigoid)

This condition is similar to bullous pemphigoid except that the lesions commonly affect the mucous membranes, including the conjunctiva, as well as the skin. The disorder is much more limited in extent than bullous pemphigoid and is chronic and recurrent, resulting in scarring of the affected areas[11]. Immunofluorescence findings may be similar to those of bullous pemphigoid but are much more variable. In many cases, the only immunoglobulin found is IgA, and some cases show positive staining with only C3[12]. Unlike bullous pemphigoid, circulating antibodies are demonstrable in only a small proportion of cases of cicatricial pemphigoid. The histological appearances differ in that the predominant inflammatory cell is neutrophil rather than eosinophil in type, although the clefting is still subepidermal in location.

Dermatitis Herpetiformis

Dermatitis herpetiformis is a vesicular rather than a bullous skin disease. The vesicles often arise on erythematous or urticarial patches. In contrast to bullous pemphigoid the lesions are usually symmetrical, occur on the extensor surfaces and are seen at all ages. Vesicles are not seen in the mouth. Most cases of dermatitis herpetiformis are associated with gluten-sensitive enteropathy.

The characteristic microscopic feature of dermatitis herpetiformis is the presence of microabscesses, composed of neutrophil polymorphs, at the tips of the dermal papillae (Figure 5.10). The early vesicles are formed by subepidermal clefting over these microabscesses and the fully formed bulla is the result of coalescence of these vesicles. Fully mature bullae may contain significant numbers of eosinophils. In most cases there is evidence of leukocytoclasis (Figure 5.11) with many neutrophil fragments around the vessels of the upper and mid dermis. Immunofluorescence staining shows a characteristic granular deposit of IgA (Figure 5.12) at the dermo-epidermal junction in the dermal papillae of non-vesicular skin[13]. It is the granular deposit type of dermatitis herpetiformis which is associated with gluten-sensitive enteropathy[14]. Once a clinically apparent bulla appears, the IgA is usually lost from the basement membrane. In about 15 per cent of cases the immune deposit is linear. Patients with this pattern of IgA deposition (so-called 'linear IgA dermatosis') tend not to have a gluten enteropathy and may not respond to dapsone therapy as readily as the majority.

Herpes Gestationis

This condition shows many of the clinical and histological features of bullous pemphigoid but it occurs in pregnancy or the puerperium, and is characterized by immunofluorescence staining for fractions of complement such as C3 and C1q without the presence of immunoglobulins[15].

References

1. Jordon, R. E. and Provost, T. (1981). Vesiculo-bullous skin diseases. In Good, R. A. and Day, S. B. (eds): *Comprehensive Immunology, 7, Immunodermatology*, pp. 361-376. (New York: Plenum)

2. Pearson, R. W. (1962). Studies on the pathogenesis of epidermolysis bullosa. *J. Invest. Dermatol.*, **39**, 551

3. Anton-Lamprectt, I. (1978). Electron microscopy in the early diagnosis of genetic disorders of the skin. *Dermatologica*, **157**, 65

4. Palmer, D. D. and Perry, H. O. (1962). Benign familial chronic pemphigus. *Arch. Dermatol.*, **86**, 493

5. Beutner, E. H. and Jordon, R. E. (1964). Demonstration of skin antibodies in sera of pemphigus vulgaris patients by indirect immunofluorescent staining. *Proc. Soc. Exp. Biol. Med.*, **117**, 505

6. Lever, W. F. (1979). Pemphigus and pemphigoid. A review of the advances made since 1964. *J. Am. Acad. Dermatol.*, **1**, 2

7. Bedi, T. R. and Pinkus, H. (1976). Histopathological spectrum of erythema multiforme. *Br. J. Dermatol.*, **95**, 243

8. Lyell, A. (1979). Toxic epidermal necrolysis (the scalded skin syndrome). A re-appraisal. *Br. J. Dermatol.*, **100**, 67

9. MacVicar, D. N., Graham, J. H. and Burgoon, C. F. (1963). Dermatitis herpetiformis, erythema multiforme and bullous pemphigoid: a comparative histopathological and histochemical study. *J. Invest. Dermatol.*, **41**, 289

10. Sams, W. M. Jr and Gammon, W. R. (1982). Mechanism of lesion production in pemphigus and pemphigoid. *J. Am. Acad. Dermatol.*, **6**, 431

11. Person, J. R. and Rogers, R. S. (1977). III: Bullous and cicatricial pemphigoid: clinical, histopathogenic and immunopathologic correlations. *Mayo Clin. Proc.*, **52**, 54

12. Michel, B., Bean, S. F. Chorzelski, T. *et al.* (1977). Cicatricial pemphigoid of Brunsting-Perry. Immunofluorescent studies. *Arch. Dermatol.*, **113**, 1403

13. Chorzelski, T. P., Beutner, E. H., Jablonska *et al.* (1971). Immunofluorescence studies in the diagnosis of dermatitis herpetiformis and its differentiation from bullous pemphigoid. *J. Invest. Dermatol.*, **56**, 373

14. Katz, S. I. and Strober, W. (1978). The pathogenesis of dermatitis herpetiformis. *J. Invest. Dermatol.*, **70**, 63

15. Carruthers, J. A. (1978). Herpes gestationis. A re-appraisal, *Clin. Exp. Dermatol.*, **3**, 199

Eczema

The terms eczema and dermatitis are synonymous. The various types of eczema cannot be readily distinguished histologically. Histological classification therefore resolves simply into (a) acute, (b) chronic and (c) lichenification. In acute eczema the skin is red, swollen and may blister. Chronic eczema tends to be rather dry and scaly and lichenification is a reactive thickening partially due to scratching.

Histological Findings

Acute eczema. Oedema fluid appears between and within the epidermal cells (Figure 6.1). The cells separate from each other and the bridges between are stretched (Figure 6.2). This oedematous appearance is known as spongiosis[1]. Rupture of the intercellular connections and of epidermal cells leads to focally exaggerated spongiosis and vesicle formation. In severe cases reticular degeneration results when vesicles are separated by thin septa derived from the remnants of ruptured epidermal cells. Mononuclear cells may migrate into the epidermis and are also seen in large numbers around the upper dermal blood vessels. Other cell types observed including polymorphs and eosinophils are also occasionally seen. The vessels are dilated and surrounded by oedema. Parakeratotic areas are present (Figure 6.3) in the stratum corneum and there may be coagulated plasma and some neutrophils particularly in older lesions.

Chronic eczema. Vesicles are usually absent but there may be some degree of spongiosis. However, occasionally changes of acute eczema are superimposed on the chronic changes described below. Acanthosis and elongation of the rete ridges mimic psoriasis. Patches of parakeratosis will be seen between layers of normal thickened stratum corneum. Very few inflammatory cells are seen within the epidermis and there are no collections of inflammatory cells in the stratum corneum. The inflammatory cell infiltrate which varies in intensity is around the upper dermal blood vessels. There may be thickening of the blood vessel walls and an increase in number of capillaries and fibrosis in the upper dermis. Occasionally an eosinophilic amorphous material is present immediately beneath the epidermis. This is thought to represent fibrin deposition from the trauma of scratching.

Lichenification. The epidermis is irregularly hyperplastic and often more thickened than in psoriasis. Areas of acanthosis, hypergranulosis and hyperkeratosis adjoin areas of parakeratosis (Figure 6.4). The rate of epidermal cell production is increased and the transit time decreased[2] (Figure 6.6). There is some degree of papillomatosis resulting from elongation of the dermal papillae. There may be fibrosis and loss of elastic fibres in the dermal papillae as a result of repeated inflammation and mechanical injury and the consequent repair. The

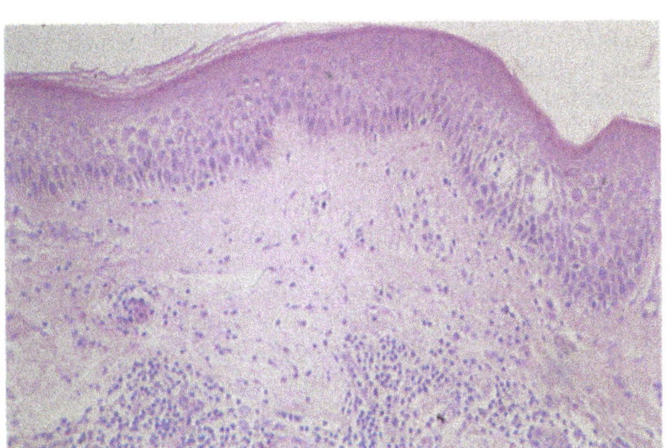

Figure 6.1 Eczema. Two focal areas of spongiosis. Mid dermal perivascular mononuclear cell infiltrate. H & E (B)

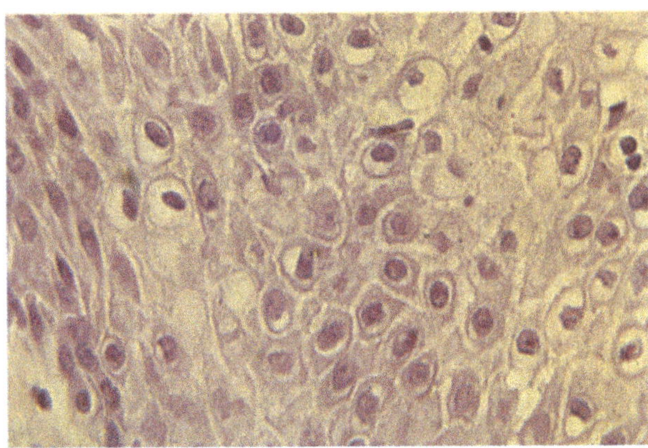

Figure 6.2 Eczema. Oedema of epidermal cells and between the cells the intercellular bridges are stretched. H & E (C)

papillary capillaries may be thick walled and the sebaceous glands tend to shrink. In nodular prurigo the epidermal hyperplasia is exaggerated[3] and there are superimposed changes due to mechanical injury.

Differential Diagnosis of Eczema

These include psoriasis, dermatophyte infection, pityriasis rosea, pityriasis lichenoides chronica and pre-mycosis fungoides.

Chronic psoriasis may appear similar to lichenified eczema particularly if the typical Munro abscess of neutrophils in the stratum corneum is absent[4]. The epidermis in lichenification is irregularly thickened without the regular bulbous enlargement of rete pegs and without the thinning over the dermal papillae which is so characteristic of psoriasis.

Dermatophytes produce an eczematous reaction and the hyphal filaments will not be visible with an H & E section but show well with PAS staining. The hyphae are present only in the horny layer particularly in the orifices of hair follicles.

Pityriasis rosea also produces an eczematous type of reaction with spongiosis. Vesicles are almost always found despite the lesions being clinically dry and scaly.

Focal areas of lymphocytic epidermal invasion are characteristic of pityriasis lichenoides chronica. Spongiosis is not normally present but some epidermal oedema is normal. Focal epidermal cell death may be evident (see page 64). The parakeratotic scale is not layered between orthokeratotic horn as it is in eczema.

Parapsoriasis of the benign type and also early pre-mycosis fungoides may be indistinguishable from chronic eczema. Mild parakeratosis and a banal lymphocytic perivascular infiltrate may be the only findings. Only in the later stages of pre-mycosis fungoides do the characteristic mycosis fungoides cells make their appearance in the dermis amongst the lymphocytes and histiocytes and begin to invade the epidermis.

Actinic Reticuloid

This is a rare eczematous type of reaction in elderly persons thought to be triggered by sun exposure. The epidermis is thickened and there is a deep dense lymphocytic dermal infiltrate which simulates mycosis fungoides and invades the epidermis (Figure 6.5).

Psoriasis

Psoriasis is a common inherited skin disease of unknown cause with a variable clinical pattern. The classical chronic type consists of thick dark red plaques covered in a silvery scale on the elbows, knees and scalp. Under certain circumstances the skin becomes less scaly and more red and sore. The whole skin may become red resulting in an erythroderma and a rare clinical type is a generalized superficial pustulation of the skin. The pathological features vary according to the clinical pattern.

Pathodynamics

The two most important features are an increased rate of epidermal cell production and the migration of neutrophils into the epidermis and stratum corneum[5]. These two features are always present to varying degrees.

Histopathological Features

Chronic plaque-type psoriasis. This shows a thickened abnormal stratum corneum characterized by patchy para-keratosis due to rapid bursts of epidermal cell activity. The parakeratotic horn lies in horizontal layers and within this remnants of migrated neutrophils are seen (Figure 6.7). The neutrophil collections (Munro abscesses) are an important diagnostic hallmark of psoriasis[6]. They may be distinguished quite easily from the parakeratotic horn as clusters of small dark round bodies while the parakeratotic horn is arranged longitudinally around the collections. A PAS stain may be helpful in identification of neutrophils within the epidermis. The epidermis is thickened and there is elongation of the rete pegs with bulbous enlargement of the rete peg tips (Figure 6.8). Above the dermal papillae the epidermis is thinned. This gives a characteristic clubbed appearance to the epidermal pegs. Mitotic figures are seen in the suprabasal epidermis as well as in the basal layer reflecting the increased rate of epidermal cell production. The granular cell layer is absent. The dermal papillae contain dilated and tortuous capillaries. There is a moderate amount of inflammatory cell infiltrate comprising mainly lymphocytes particularly around the upper dermal blood vessels. Within the vascular lumina neutrophils may be seen. They are rarely present in the dermis though they are often seen migrating through the epidermis.

Erythrodermic psoriasis. This is a form of psoriasis without the thickening of the stratum corneum and elongation of the rete pegs. The epidermis is oedematous and contains many mitotic figures (Figure 6.9). Neutrophils migrate in large numbers through the epidermis to form micro-abscesses in the stratum corneum which are larger and more numerous than in the chronic scaly form of psoriasis. The upper dermal blood vessels are engorged and cuffed with a moderate amount of inflammatory cell infiltrate.

Widespread pustular psoriasis. This is an extension of erythrodermic psoriasis with superficial sheeted pustulation[7]. Biopsy is difficult as the skin may fragment. The neutrophils form a layer of pus in the stratum corneum and thus give an appearance like impetigo –though without the micro-cocci. There may be many mitotic figures in the epidermis. Oedema is a constant feature in the epidermis and upper dermis (Figure 6.10). The upper dermal blood vessels are engorged and cuffed with lymphocytes, histiocytes and a few neutrophils.

Subcorneal pustular dermatosis. This is a very rare disease having pathological features very similar to those of acute pustular psoriasis. There is a subcorneal collection of neutrophils and acantholysis is also a feature (Figure 6.11). It must be differentiated from acute psoriasis and impetigo.

Palmar plantar pustular psoriasis. This is a variant of psoriasis in which clinical pustules appear in localized areas on the palms and soles. There is a massive migration of neutrophils into the epidermis in focal areas only[8]. The affected epidermis is oedematous and the final result is a form of spongiotic pustule (Kogoj spongiosis) (Figure 6.12). A true intraepidermal pustule may result. The pustulation remains intact due to the thickness of the overlying stratum corneum. At a later stage of the process large collections of desiccated polymorphs are visible within the stratum corneum.

Pityriasis rubra pilaris. This is an uncommon inflammatory skin disorder of unknown cause. In the early erythrodermic phase it resembles psoriasis with widespread erythema and scaling, though at some sites a characteristic plugging of follicles with horny spines may be seen. As in psoriasis there is a high rate of epidermal

Table 6.1 Differential diagnosis of chronic psoriasis

	Psoriasis	Pityriasis lichenoides chronica	Pityriasis rubra pilaris	Lichenification	Hypertrophic lichen planus
Parakeratosis	+	+	+	+	−
Munro abscess	+	−	−	−	−
Prominent granular cell layer	−	−	+	+	+
Neutrophils in epidermis	+	−	+	−	−
Follicular plugging	−	−	+	−	+

cell production. The parakeratosis tends to be continuous rather than intermittent as seen in psoriasis and the parakeratotic horn cells tend to be thicker. There is sebaceous gland atrophy and some proliferation of the erector pili muscles. In the later stages horny plugs fill the follicular openings and the epidermis is evenly thickened though the papillae and ridges are accentuated. The granular layer may be prominent and in some instances appears vacuolated (Figure 6.13).

Differential Diagnosis of Psoriasis

Conditions to be differentiated histologically are: pityriasis rubra pilaris, subcorneal pustular dermatosis, impetigo, Bowen's disease, lichenification, pityriasis lichenoides chronica, hypertrophic lichen planus and a psoriasiform naevus.

Table 6.2 Differential diagnosis of acute pustular psoriasis

	Psoriasis	Impetigo	Subcorneal pustular dermatosis
Micrococci	−	+	−
Acantholysis	−	+−	+
Mitoses increased	+	−	−

Psoriasis may be difficult to differentiate from pityriasis rubra pilaris (PRP) but with a prominent granular cell layer and follicular plugging in PRP it should be possible (Table 6.1). Subcorneal pustular dermatosis resembles pustular acute psoriasis and differentiation may not be possible but acantholysis favours the former (Table 6.2). Impetigo is similar to both these conditions but a Gram stain will show the micrococci in the subcorneal pus. Bowen's disease resembles acute psoriasis but only because both conditions show numerous mitotic figures (Figure 6.14). However, in Bowen's disease many mitoses will be abnormal, many individual cells will be keratinized early and total loss of polarity of the epidermal cells is characteristic. There is elongation of rete ridges and acanthosis in lichenification but no neutrophils will be seen in the stratum corneum. The granular cell layer is often prominent in lichenification and reduced in chronic psoriasis. Pityriasis lichenoides chronica (PLC) should not be mistaken for psoriasis. There is migration of lymphocytes into the epidermis in PLC and neutrophils in psoriasis. The parakeratotic scale of PLC is not layered between normal stratum corneum but comes off as a whole. The epidermis in PLC is not much thickened and does not react to the invading lymphocytes. Also the lymphocytic epidermal invasion is very focal. Hypertrophic lichen planus shares with chronic psoriasis epidermal thickening but is irregular

and more extensive in the former. Psoriasis typically has a reduced granular layer and hypertrophic lichen planus shows hypergranulosis. Parakeratosis is not a feature of lichen planus. A psoriasiform naevus is either present at birth or develops in early childhood. It is often linear and clinically resembles psoriatic skin. Histologically however there is usually much less parakeratosis, no Munro micro-abscesses and a prominent granular cell layer − though the epidermal rete pegs may be prominent.

Lichen Planus

A common disorder of unknown cause with small mauve or dark red shiny papules predominantly on the wrists, ankles and sacral area and feathery white lesions on the buccal mucosa.

Histology

Histologically the main features are: (a) hyperkeratosis; (b) hypergranulosis; (c) irregular epidermal acanthosis; (d) erosion of the basal layer; and (e) a band-like infiltrate hugging the epidermis[9] (Figure 6.15).

The stratum corneum is thickened and there is no parakeratosis – an important diagnostic feature. Thickening of the granular layer is irregular and the cells appear larger than usual and contain large coarse granules. The thickening of the epidermis affects the rete ridges as well as the stratum malpighium. The rete ridges may be pointed giving a saw-tooth effect and the papillae between are domed.

There is erosion of many basal cells but in places smaller spindle-shaped basophilic epidermal cells are evident. The border between the epidermis and dermis is clouded by a dense cellular infiltrate beneath and between the basal cells. Colloid bodies will be visible in the lower epidermis and upper dermis. These are round and pink and are found where basal cells are damaged. These bodies have no nucleus and tend to be clumped together.

The infiltrate predominantly consists of lymphocytes with a few histiocytes. It hugs the lower epidermis and there is no deep component. Melanophages are seen in the upper dermis as the pigment is liberated from the basal layer. There may be discrete areas of dermo-epidermal separation – the so-called Max-Joseph clefts (Figure 6.16).

Pathodynamics

It is likely that the epidermal cell destruction results from an immune reaction. The thickening and hypergranulosis results from the usual reaction of the epidermis to injury subsequent to migration of epidermal cells into the injured area.

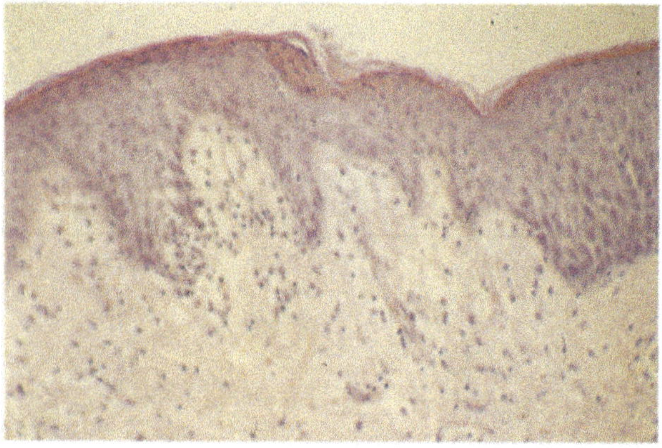

Figure 6.3 Eczema. Parakeratosis. Mild oedema in epidermis and gross oedema in upper dermis. H & E (B)

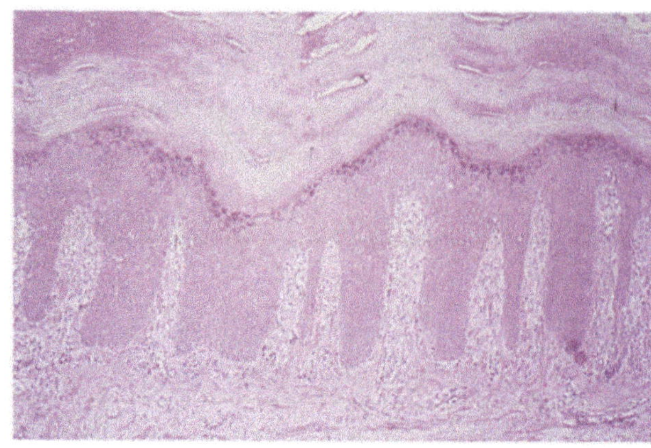

Figure 6.4 Lichenification. Hyperkeratosis. Elongated, psoriasiform rete pegs but with prominent granular cell layer. H & E (B)

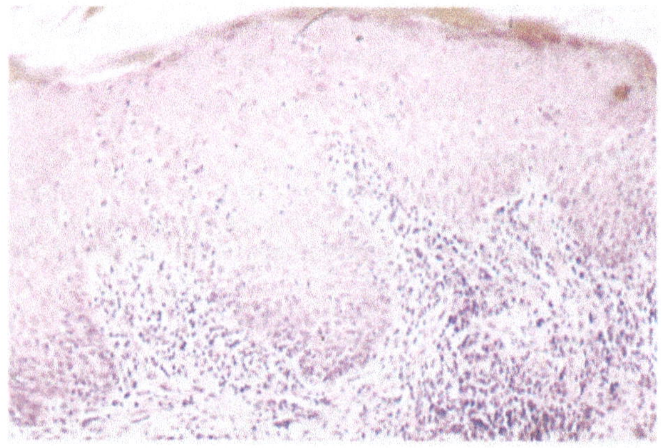

Figure 6.5 Actinic reticuloid. Acanthotic epidermis and a dense lymphocytic dermal infiltrate which may be confused with mycosis fungoides. Invasion of the epidermis with lymphocytes. H & E (B)

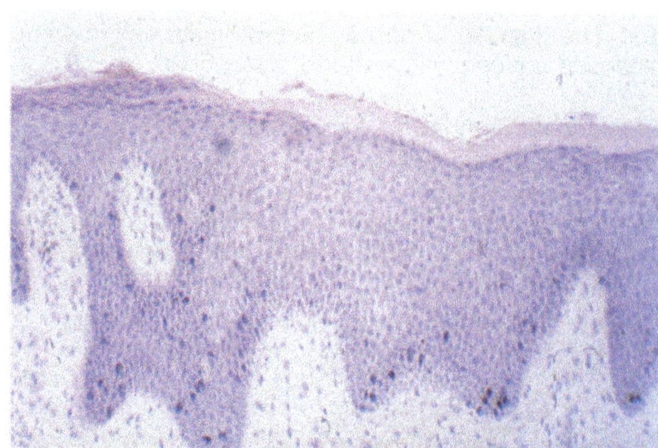

Figure 6.6 Autoradiograph of lichenification. Tritiated thymidine injected 2 days previously. Note rapid transit of labelled cells through the epidermis

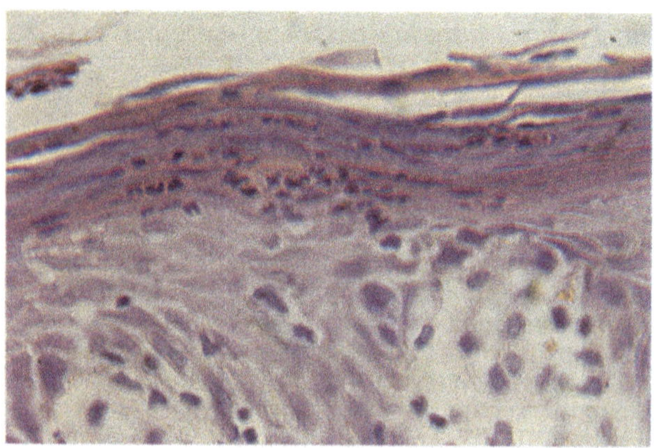

Figure 6.7 Psoriasis. Micro-abscesses in parakeratotic scale. Oedema of epidermis. H & E (C)

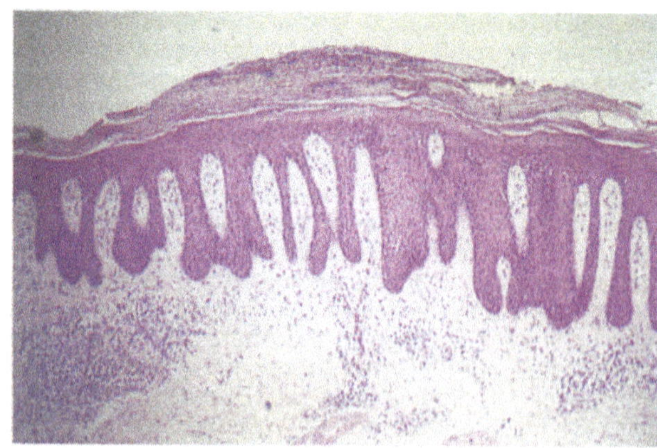

Figure 6.8 Psoriasis. Plaque type. Elongated bulbous epidermal rete pegs. Thinning of epidermis over dermal papillae. Parakeratosis and Munro abscesses in stratum corneum. H & E (B)

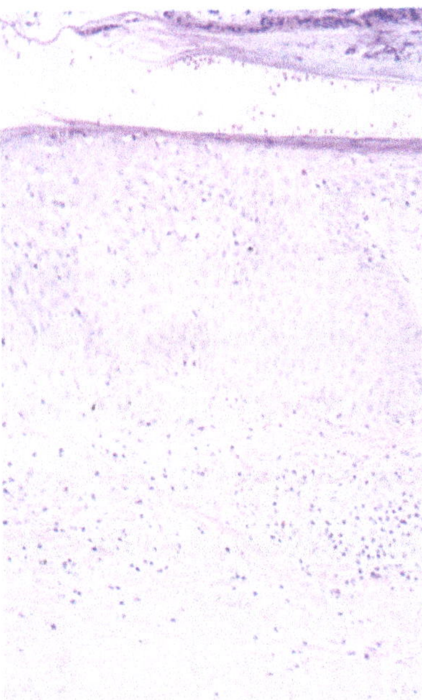

Figure 6.9
Erythrodermic psoriasis. The epidermis is flattened and oedematous. There is parakeratosis and a few neutrophils migrating through the epidermis to collect in the stratum corneum. H & E. (C)

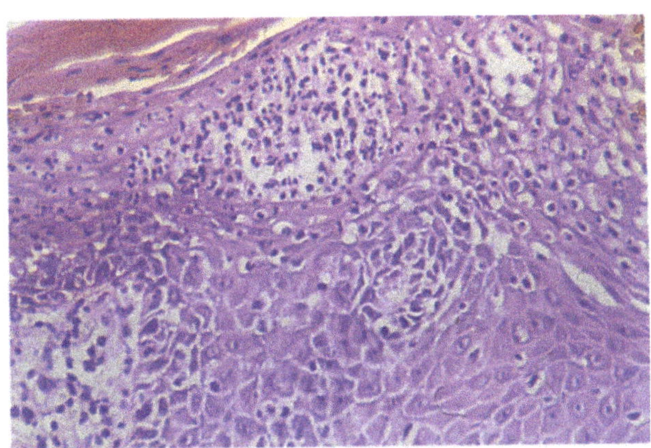

Figure 6.10 Acute pustular psoriasis. The whole of the upper epidermis is invaded by neutrophils. Oedema of the epidermis. H & E (C)

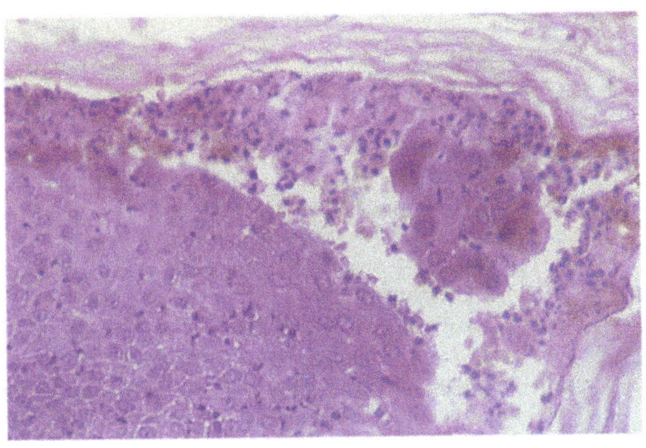

Figure 6.11 Subcorneal pustular dermatosis. A subcorneal collection of neutrophils with some acantholytic epidermal cells. H & E (C)

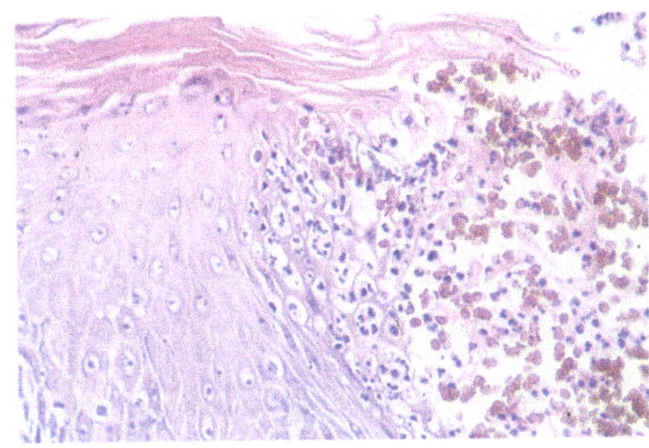

Figure 6.12 Palmar plantar pustular psoriasis. Spongiform pustule within the epidermis. H & E (C)

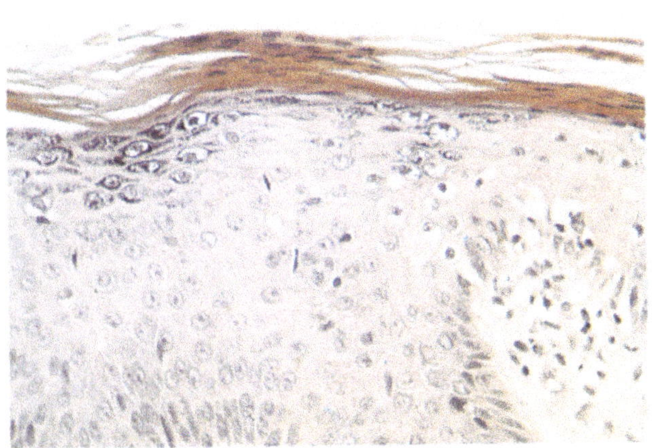

Figure 6.13 Pityriasis rubra pilaris. Focal parakeratosis with spindle-shaped nuclei. Granular cell layer present with some perinuclear vacuolation in the upper epidermis. H & E (C)

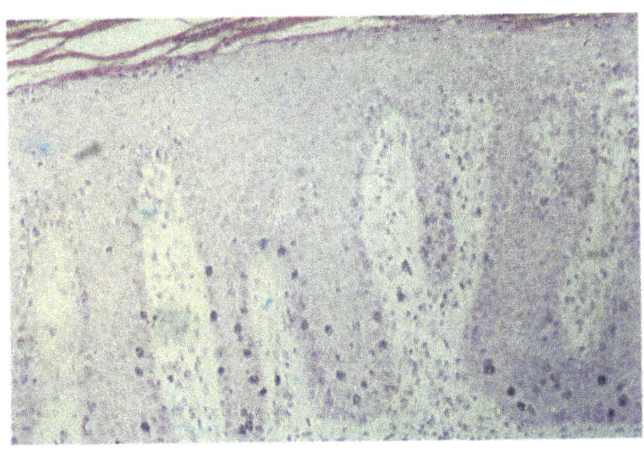

Figure 6.14 Autoradiograph of psoriasis showing mitoses labelled with tritiated thymidine. H & E (B)

Immunofluroescence of lichen planus reveals globular IgG and IgM bodies at the dermo-epidermal junction and in clusters within the upper dermis[10]. A broad ragged band of fibrin traces the basement membrane zone (Figure 6.17).

Differential Diagnosis

This includes lupus erythematosus and lichenoid solar keratosis. In the former there is a deeper perivascular periadnexal infiltrate of lymphocytes and a thickened basement membrane. A lichenoid solar keratosis may closely resemble lichen planus but dyskeratosis will be present within the epidermis and there will be some loss of polarity of the cells. There may also be parakeratosis which does not occur in lichen planus. Drug reactions sometimes result in lichen planus-like rashes and histologically they may closely resemble true lichen planus. However, there will usually be parakeratosis and the lymphocytic infiltrate although tending to hug the epidermis, will also be around the mid dermal vessels. Lichenification is a feature of eczema, the epidermis is thickened but not eroded and the infiltrate is not tight against the basal layer. There is a form of syphilis which is lichenoid but the predominant cells in the infiltrate will be plasma cells and the infiltrate usually invades the epidermis in syphilis. In pityriasis lichenoides typically the lymphocytes migrate into the epidermis causing little disruption and no erosion of the basal layer. The lesions are focal and capped by a parakeratotic scale unlike lichen planus.

Lichen Planopilaris

The changes are limited to the lower parts of the hair follicle (Figure 6.18) and there is erosion of the hair papilla. Damage to the follicle results. Dilatation and horny plugging of the follicle are early features but later they disappear leaving fibrosis in the dermis.

Differential diagnosis. Keratosis pilaris simply shows a horny plug in the follicle and no infiltrate or erosion at the base. A follicle in lupus erythematosus will show changes similar to lichen plano-pilaris but there will be evidence of basal epidermal liquefaction degeneration.

Lichen Nitidus

Clinically this is a micro-papular form of lichen planus in children. Histologically unlike typical lichen planus, solitary dermal papillae are affected. The overlying epidermis is eroded but laterally it elongates to clutch the infiltrate like a claw (Figure 6.19). In some cases epithelioid cells and multi-nucleate giant cells are seen at the dermo-epidermal junction (Figure 6.20).

References

1. Mihm, M. C. Jr, Soter, N. A., Dvorak, H. F. and Austen, K. F. (1976). The structure of normal skin and the morphology of atopic eczema. *J. Invest. Dermatol.*, **67**, 305

2. Marks, R. and Wells, G. C. (1973). Lichen simplex. Morphodynamic correlates. *Br. J. Dermatol.*, **88**, 249

3. Rowland Payne, C. M. E., Wilkinson, J. D., McKee, P. H., Jurecka, W. and Black, M. M. (1985). Nodular prurigo – a clinicopathological study of 46 patients. *Br. J. Dermatol.*, **113**, 431

4. Pinkus, H. and Mehregan, A. H. (1966). The primary histological lesion of seborrhoeic dermatitis and psoriasis. *J. Invest. Dermatol.*, **46**, 109

5. Gordon, M. and Johnson, W. C. (1967). Histopathology and histochemistry of psoriasis. *Arch. Dermatol.*, **95**, 402

6. Cox, A. J. and Watson, W. (1972). Histological variations in lesions of psoriasis. *Arch. Dermatol.*, **106**, 503

7. Baker, H. and Ryan, T. J. (1968). Generalised pustular psoriasis. *Br. J. Dermatol.*, **80**, 771

8. Uehara, M. and Ofuji, S. (1974). The morphogenesis of pustulosis palmaris et plantaris. *Arch. Dermatol.*, **109**, 518

9. Ellis, F. A. (1967). Histopathology of lichen planus based on an analysis of one hundred biopsies. *J. Invest. Dermatol.*, **48**, 143

10. Abell, E., Presbury, D. G. and Marks, R. (1974). The diagnostic significance of immunoglobulin and fibrin deposition in lichen planus. *Br. J. Dermatol.*, **93**, 17

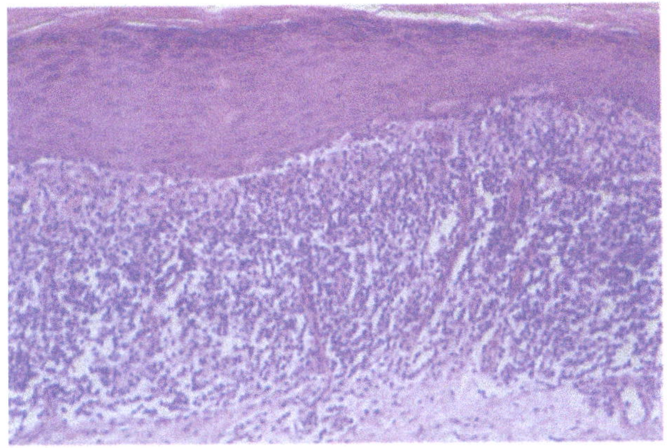

Figure 6.15 Lichen planus. Hyperkeratosis, hypergranulosis. Infiltrate in upper dermis closely applied to the epidermis. H & E (B)

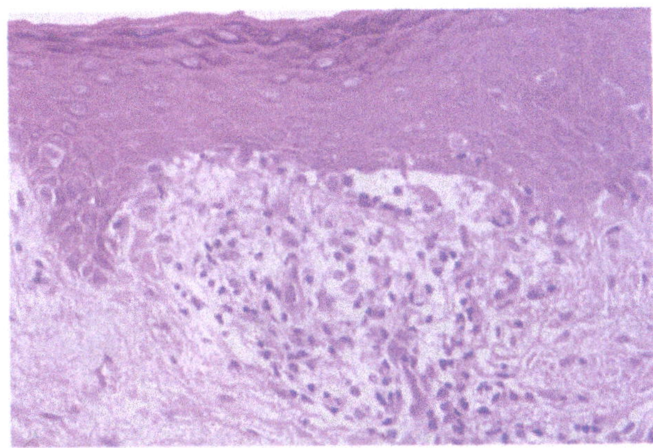

Figure 6.16 Lichen planus. Hypergranulosis. Focal cleft between epidermis and upper dermal lymphocytic infiltrate. Erosion of lower epidermis and resultant 'saw tooth' appearance with colloid bodies. H & E (C)

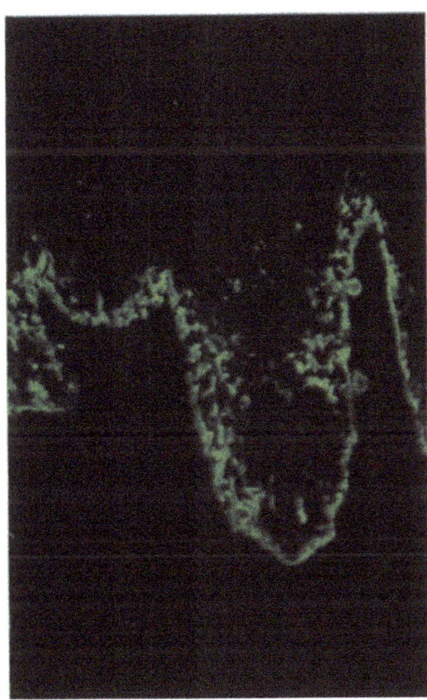

Figure 6.17 Immunofluorescence of lichen planus. Anti-fibrin. Thick ragged fluorescent band traces the lower border of the epidermis. Some round colloid bodies are visible along the band. (B)

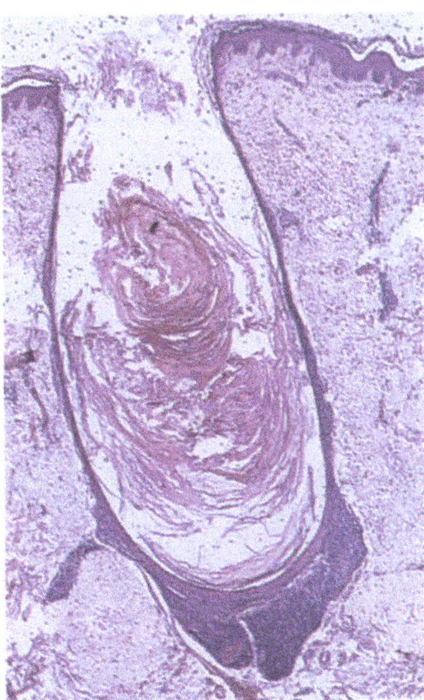

Figure 6.18 Lichen planopilaris. A dilated plugged follicle with an infiltrate tightly applied to the eroded lower border. H & E (B)

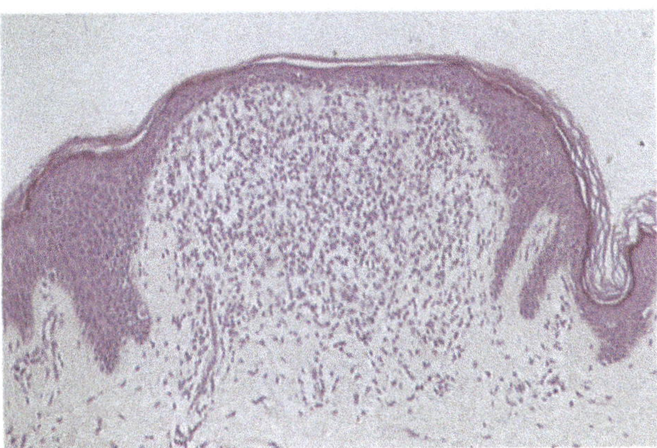

Figure 6.19 Lichen nitidus. Erosion of epidermis by upper dermal infiltrate which fills and expands the dermal papilla. The epidermis clutches the infiltrate like a claw. H & E (B)

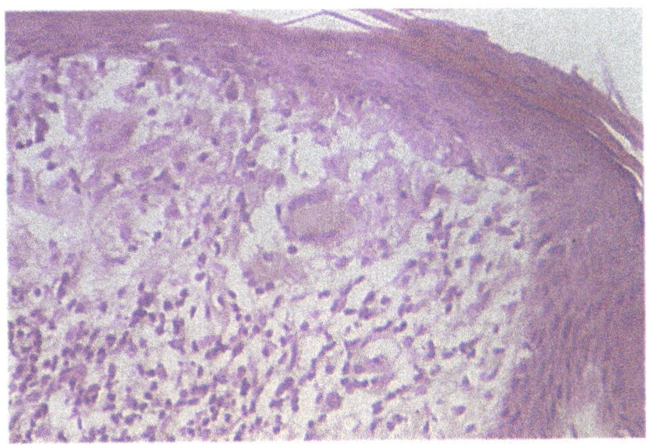

Figure 6.20 Lichen nitidus showing the multinucleate giant cells in the upper part of the infiltrate. H & E (C)

Other Inflammatory Diseases **7**

Acute Febrile Neutrophilic Dermatosis

This recently described condition[1], also known as Sweet's disease after its discoverer, consists of tender papules and plaques up to 2 cm in diameter. The papules are erythematous and are associated with the development of leukocytosis and fever. The face, neck and upper limbs are involved most. There may be an accompanying arthralgia or arthritis. The disorder rapidly responds to systemic corticosteroids but may relapse. Nothing is known of the aetiology or pathogenesis of Sweet's disease although it may be related to erythema multiforme.

Histologically, Sweet's disease consists of a dense, homogeneous neutrophil polymorphonuclear leukocyte infiltration of the dermis (Figure 7.1). Appearances differ from those of an abscess in that necrosis is not seen, there are also many fragments of neutrophil nuclei (leukocytoclasis) and no organisms can be demonstrated by special stains. The overlying epidermis is usually only involved by the acute inflammatory infiltrate to a mild degree, but there is always severe oedema of the papillary dermis.

The histological picture in Sweet's disease bears some similarity to erythema elevatum diutinum. Vascular ectasia and leukocytoclasia are common in both these conditions, but there is no evidence of vasculitis in Sweet's disease. Furthermore, perivascular fibrin is commonplace in erythema elevatum diutinum but not in Sweet's disease.

Sarcoidosis

Sarcoidosis is a systemic disease characterized by the widespread distribution of non-caseating granulomas[2]. Although the aetiology of sarcoidosis in unknown, there is a suspicion that altered immunity plays some part in the disease. Although humoral hypersensitivity is unaffected in sarcoidosis, there does appear to be inhibition of cellular immunity. For instance, lymphocyte transformation by phytohaemagglutinin is impaired in sarcoidosis[3] and there is demonstrable anergy to substances which cause contact hypersensitivity in unaffected persons. It has been suggested that suppressor T lymphocytes may produce the anergy described in sarcoidosis.

This altered state of immunity can be demonstrated by the Kveim test[4]. Intradermal injection of heat-treated sarcoidal tissue evokes a typical sarcoid reaction in patients with sarcoidosis. The granulomas take some 6 to 8 weeks to develop, and must be demonstrated by biopsy. Early biopsy (before 6 weeks have elapsed) may yield a false positive result due to a non-specific macrophage response to the injected Kveim material.

About one-third of cases of systemic sarcoidosis show cutaneous manifestations. The lesions are usually intradermal; a subcutaneous nodule is unusual. The clinical appearance of the lesions is varied. Macular, plaque-like, deep-tumorous, papular and micropapular lesions may all occur. They are typically brown or purple or some shade between these two. The papule of sarcoidosis may become circinate or erythrodermic, and ulcerating or ichthyosiform forms have been described.

The most important point to bear in mind in considering the histological appearances of sarcoidosis is that there are no pathognomonic features. Reliable diagnosis can only be arrived at after considering all the pathological and clinical signs. Sarcoid granulomas are typically well delineated and are composed of plump rounded rather eosinophilic histiocytes (Figures 7.2–7.4). Giant cells are few and there is little or no necrosis. Only a moderate number of lymphocytes are seen and these are to be found at the periphery of the granulomas. However, both central necrosis and marked lymphocytic infiltrate may occur in some cases. The disorder is usually 'focal' in that the inflammation occurs in a series of rounded collections of cells.

The giant cells of sarcoidosis occur most commonly in well-established lesions and may contain one or other of two distinctive inclusions in their cytoplasm. Schaumann bodies are laminated, calcific bodies which appear dark blue in ordinary haematoxylin and eosin stained sections. Asteroid bodies are irregular in outline and appear star-shaped with a central dense core and radiating thin homogeneous spikes. Neither of these two bodies are specific for sarcoidosis and are also found in tuberculosis, leprosy and foreign body granulomas including berylliosis.

Cutaneous sarcoidosis has many differential diagnoses. Apart from the comparative lack of necrosis, sarcoid granulomas are characterized by the plump histiocytes and the relatively mild lymphocytic infiltrate. The granulomas are distributed throughout the dermis. On the other hand, the granulomas in lupus vulgaris are surrounded by a well-marked inflammatory response and they are usually more superficial in distribution than in sarcoidosis. The granulomas of tuberculoid leprosy form around nerves, giving them an elongated oval appearance to contrast with the circular, spherical granulomas of sarcoidosis. Acid-fast bacilli are demonstrable in over 90 per cent of cases of tuberculoid leprosy, but they are infrequent and a prolonged and careful search of specially stained sections is usually required. Other differential diagnoses include deep fungus infection, leishmaniasis, and horn/hair granulomas. Silica granulomas can usually be distinguished by demonstrating birefringent particles within the histiocytes. Zirconium and beryllium granulomas are indistinguishable from those of sarcoidosis and diagnosis may only be possible after analysis of skin biopsies by atomic absorption spectrometry. Apart from infective (Chapter 3) and foreign-body causes of granulomas, the principal differential

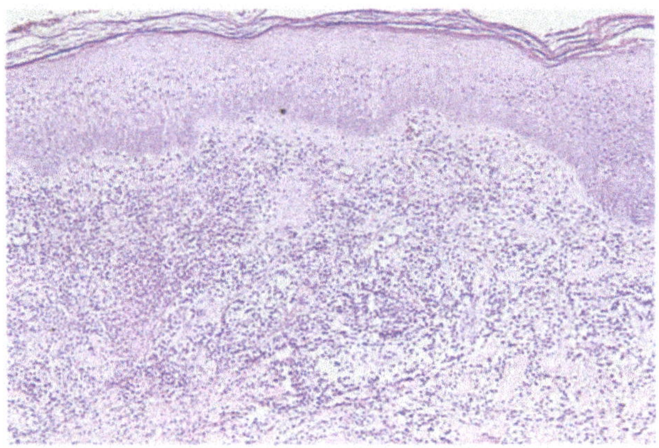

Figure 7.1 Acute febrile neutrophilic dermatosis (Sweet). A diffuse infiltrate of neutrophil polymorphonuclear leukocytes throughout the dermis is typical of Sweet's disease.   H & E (B)

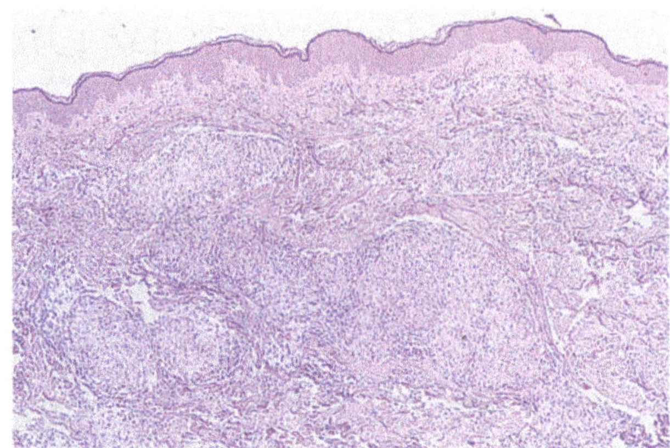

Figure 7.2 Sarcoidosis. Clusters of pale, eosinophilic granulomas are scattered throughout the dermis.   H & E (A)

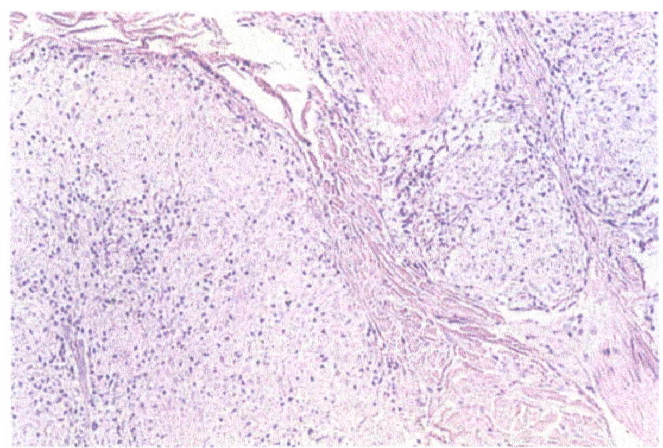

Figure 7.3 Sarcoidosis.   H & E (B)

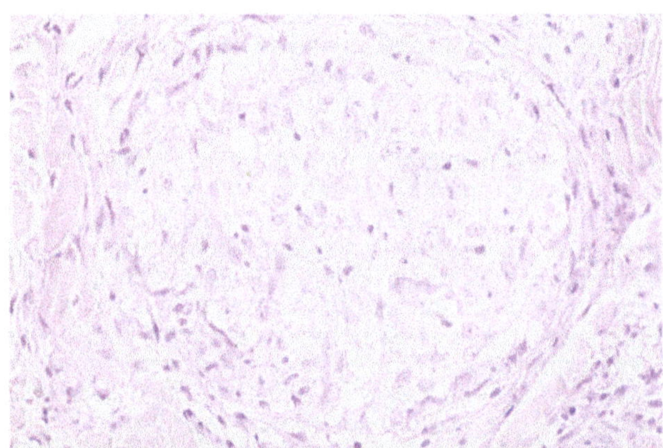

Figure 7.4 Sarcoidosis. The granuloma in sarcoidosis typically shows only a scanty lymphocytic infiltrate. There is no evidence of necrosis at the centre of the clusters of histiocytes.   H & E (C)

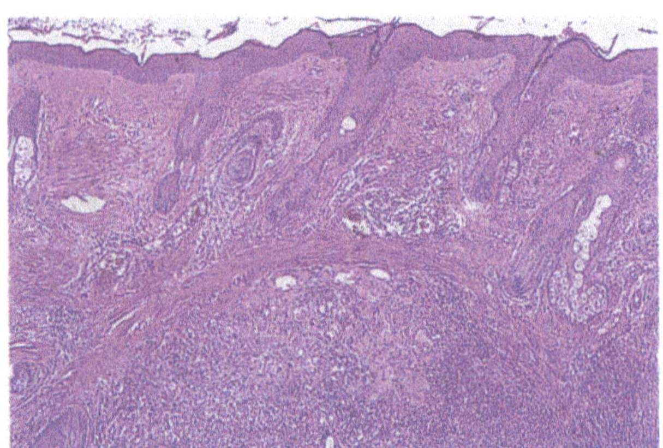

Figure 7.5 Foreign body granuloma. A nodular inflammatory infiltrate in the dermis is a reaction to a ruptured hair follicle.   H & E (A)

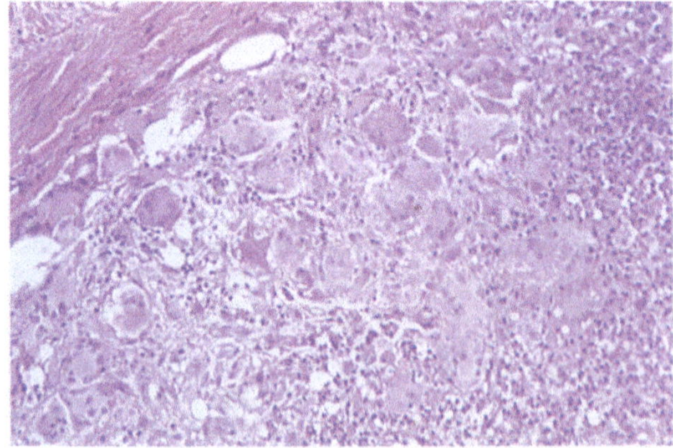

Figure 7.6 Foreign body granuloma. The granuloma is typically poorly formed and contains considerable numbers of lymphocytes.   H & E (B)

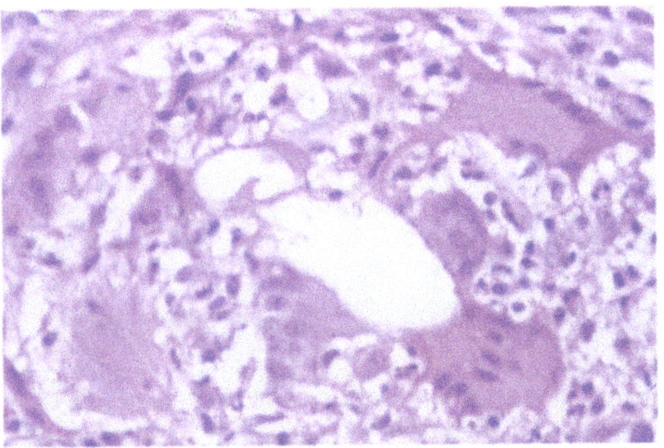

Figure 7.7 Foreign body granuloma. Foreign body giant cells. H & E (C)

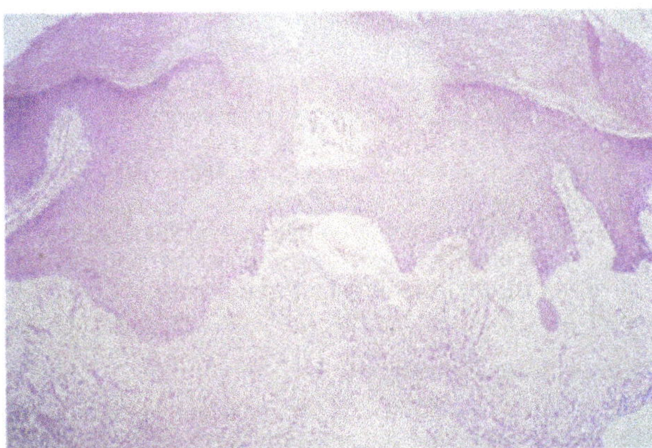

Figure 7.8 Chondrodermatitis nodularis chronica helicis. Marked epidermal hyperplasia and hyperkeratosis overlying an area of inflammation and telangiectasia. H & E (B)

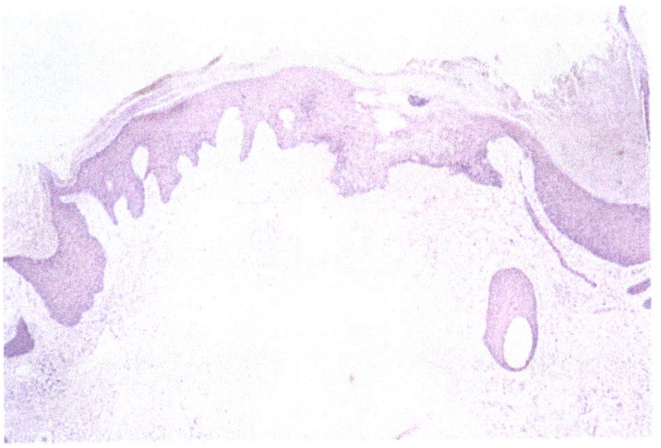

Figure 7.9 Chondrodermatitis nodularis chronic helicis. There is irregular hyperplasia and hyperkeratosis overlying eosinophilic material subepidermally, inflammation and telangiectasia. The cartilage of the ear is also involved by the inflammatory process. H & E (B)

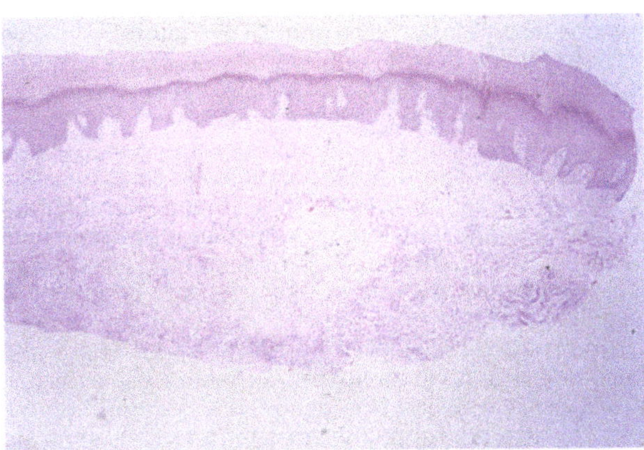

Figure 7.10 Granuloma annulare. An area of altered connective dermal tissue can be seen in the mid and lower dermis. H & E (A)

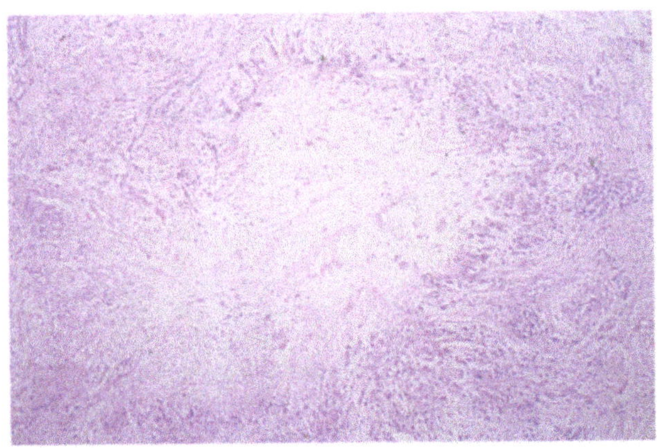

Figure 7.11 Granuloma annulare. There is a palisade of histiocytes around the necrobiotic area. H & E (B)

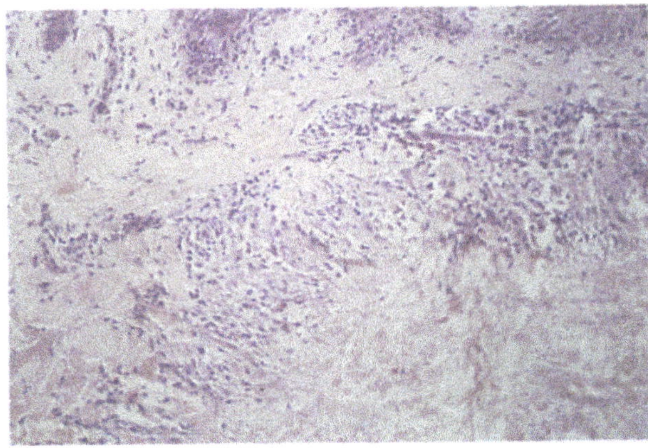

Figure 7.12 Granuloma annulare. Histiocytes and giant cells around necrobiotic focus. H & E (C)

diagnoses of sarcoidosis are necrobiosis lipoidica diabeticorum and granuloma annulare[5].

In summary, although sarcoid granulomas may have a typical appearance, the diagnosis should never be made until sections have been examined for birefringent particles by polarized light and stained for acid/alcohol-fast or, if appropriate, acid-fast organisms.

Foreign-body Granuloma

Foreign body reactions are common in the skin. They may be due to endogenous material such as the products of rupture of an epidermoid cyst or gouty crystals in a tophus or alternatively exogenous, due to vegetable material (such as wooden splinters, thorns and so on), animal material such as bee stings or minerals such as beryllium[6], paraffin[7] and zirconium[8].

The histological appearances of the foreign body reaction depend on the nature of the foreign material. A typical foreign body reaction includes only poorly formed granulomas with an associated well-marked lymphocytic response (Figures 7.5 and 7.6). Histiocytic giant cells are characteristically commonplace (Figure 7.7). This sort of reaction is that seen typically around a ruptured epidermoid cyst, a hair in a pilonidal sinus or a splinter of wood. Many foreign bodies are birefringent and crossed polaroid lenses are very useful in identifying the foreign material. Insect bites usually only show a scanty histiocytic response and a well-marked lymphocytic infiltrate which can produce a pseudolymphomatous appearance. Beryllium, zirconium and other minerals produce sarcoid-like granulomas with often only a scanty lymphocytic response.

A distinctive histological appearance may follow the injection of paraffin mineral oils, vegetable oils or silicon into the skin. The site of injection may become 'tumourous' or ulcerated many years later and may simulate the development of neoplasia. Histologically, an oil granuloma consists of rounded spaces, somewhat larger than adipocytes, which are surrounded by collagen interspersed with lymphocytes, histiocytes and foreign-body giant cells. In frozen sections the rounded spaces stain with oil red O, but usually less strongly than normal adipose tissue.

Chondrodermatitis Nodularis Chronica Helicis

The cause of this odd inflammatory disorder of the external ear is believed to be ischaemia from the minor trauma of pressure during sleep[9]. It mostly occurs in elderly men but has also been described in nuns, due to the pressure from their whimples. The lesion is generally a solitary painful and tender nodule affecting the upper part of the margin of the pinna. The nodule may have a central discharging crypt.

Pathology

There is a striking and characteristic series of changes in the skin. The epidermis may be eroded over the centre of the lesion but is markedly thickened elsewhere. There is oedema and pronounced telangiectasia throughout the dermis which also contains a variably dense mixed inflammatory cell infiltrate (Figure 7.8). A pink band or zone of fibrin is found beneath the epidermis and maybe elsewhere in the dermis (Figure 7.9). The adjoining cartilage may show eosinophilia and infiltration by inflammatory cells. Occasionally debris from the inflammation is expelled to the surface by the process of transepidermal elimination.

The Necrobiotic Disorders

In this group of disorders are included granuloma annulare, necrobiosis lipoidica and rheumatoid nodule. The term indicates a particular change within connective tissue in which the dermis appears damaged and contains less cells than usual.

Granuloma Annulare

This is a common disorder often found in childhood and adolescence but at other ages too. In the common types small pink or skin-coloured plaques (which may appear annular) occur on the backs of the hands and fingers. A superficial type which has a wider distribution also occurs and this may be associated with diabetes. The cause is unknown but may have an immunopathogenesis and be due to a type of hypersensitivity vasculitis[10].

Histopathology. The presence of foci of altered connective tissue characterizes this disorder (Figure 7.10). Around these there are annular areas of inflammatory cell infiltrate with a prominent histiocytic component. Histiocytes often form a peripheral palisade to the inflamed areas (Figure 7.11). Giant cells are often, but not invariably, present (Figure 7.12). In the centre of the rings there is featureless connective tissue that is paler but more eosinophilic and less cellular than usual (necrobiotic). Special stains reveal the presence of mucin in the damaged areas. The condition has to be distinguished from necrobiosis lipoidica and rheumatoid nodules (see later).

Necrobiosis Lipoidica

This disorder is found predominantly in patients with diabetes or a predisposition to diabetes. Some 80 to 90 per cent of patients with necrobiosis lipoidica fall into this category[11]. It occurs on the legs in the majority of patients but lesions occasionally occur at other sites. The lesions are yellowish, irregular plaques that may reach several centimetres in diameter. Ulceration and scarring sometimes occur. The condition persists and may extend before finally becoming inactive and atrophic. The pathogenesis is unclear but it has been reported that immunoglobulins are deposited in the lesions[12].

Histopathology. The histopathology has an overall similarity to that of granuloma annulare. The inflammatory foci tend to be larger and more oval than annular (Figure 7.13). The inflammation also tends to be less intense and there is less tendency to giant cell formation and to palisading by histiocytes. It has been suggested that diabetic patients tend to have a palisaded granuloma while the changes in non-diabetics are more like those of sarcoidosis or tuberculosis[11]. Fat stains reveal the presence of lipid in the histiocytes and in the necrobiotic area.

Rheumatoid Nodules

These nodules appear over the extensor aspects of the small and medium-sized joints in chronic rheumatoid arthritis. Histopathologically they consist of a central acellular 'necrobiotic area' with palisaded histiocytes and giant cells surrounding these sites.

Pityriasis Lichenoides

This is a disorder of unknown cause that may present acutely (pityriasis lichenoides varioliformis et acuta) or develop insidiously and persist for long periods (pityriasis

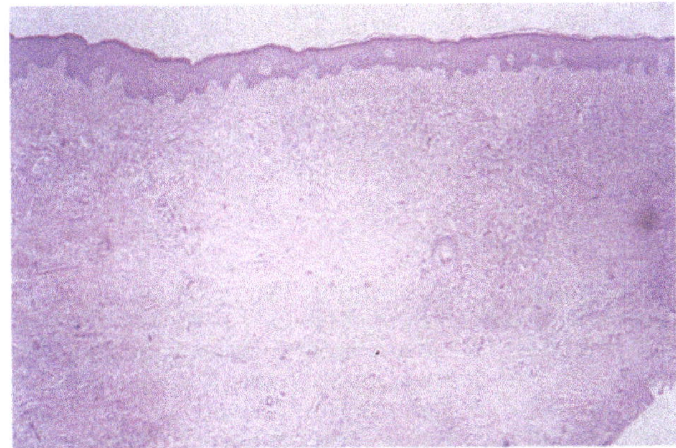

Figure 7.13 Necrobiosis lipoidica. There is a large area of altered connective tissue in the dermis around which is an inflammatory band.   H & E (A)

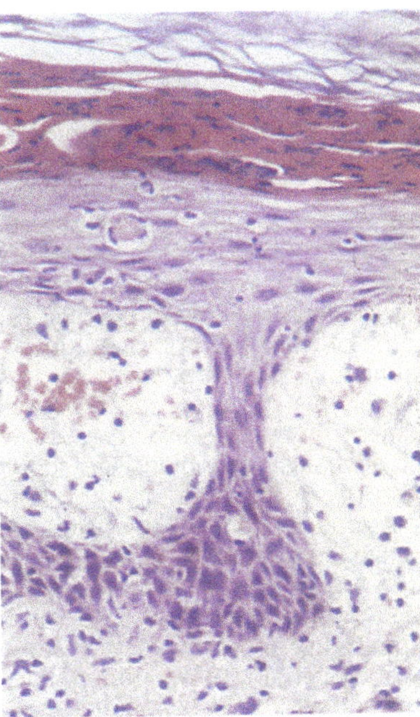

Figure 7.14 Pityriasis lichenoides acuta. The epidermis is surmounted by a crust containing parakeratotis stratum corneum and inflammatory cells. The epidermis contains necrotic keratinocytes and inflammatory cells. H & E (C)

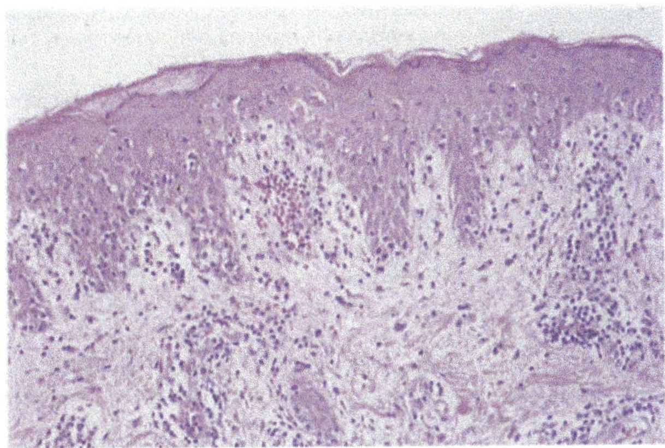

Figure 7.15 Pityriasis lichenoides chronica. Thickened epidermis overlies an area of inflammation within the dermis. There are several necrotic epidermal cells scattered throughout the epidermis.   H & E (B)

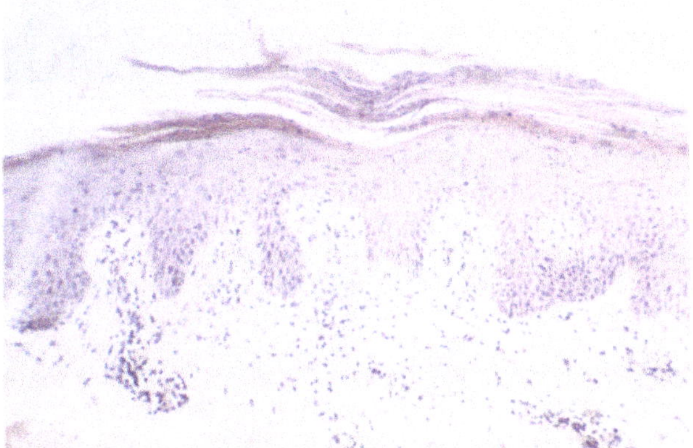

Figure 7.16 Pityriasis lichenoides chronica showing typical parakeratotic scale.   H & E (B)

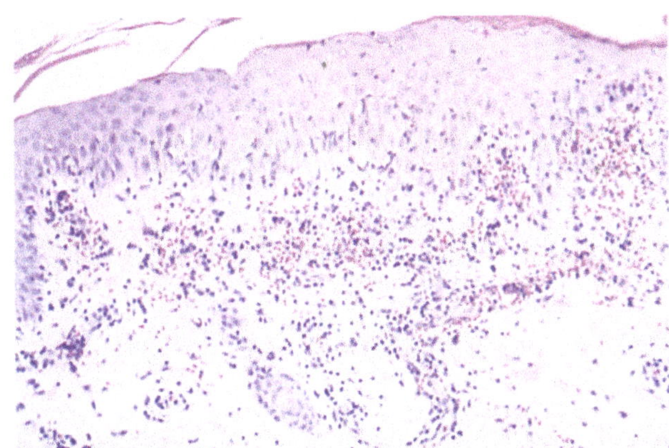

Figure 7.17 Pityriasis lichenoides chronica. Marked inflammatory cell infiltrate around the blood vessels and some haemorrhage into the dermis. H & E (B)

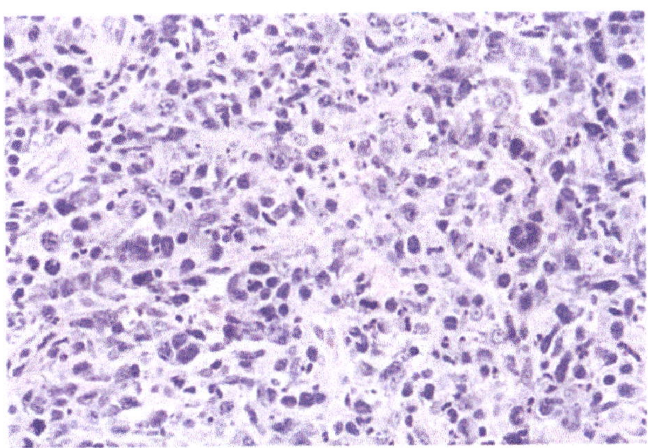

Figure 7.18 Lymphomatoid papulosis. Extensive inflammation – some of the cells are markedly abnormal.   H & E (C)

lichenoides chronica). It was grouped at one time, together with sundry other uncommon scaling disorders, into the parapsoriasis group of skin diseases because of their occasional resemblance to psoriasis[13]. The other conditions in this group included parapsoriasis en plaque, poikiloderma vasculare atrophicans and parakeratosis variegata. These disorders were supposed to possess one particular feature in common – the propensity to develop into a lymphoma of the skin. Improved understanding of the natural history of each of the disorders has obviated the need for this grouping and the term parapsoriasis is not used in this text. Sometimes acute and chronic lesions of pityriasis lichenoides are found simultaneously in patients. Both types present with numerous generalized lesions. Lesions in the acute form are papular and often have central necrosis, sometimes with crusting. Lesions in the chronic form often have a characteristic scale that is detached peripherally (a 'mica-like' scale). In both the acute and chronic forms the lesions appear in crops over many years though ultimately the disease does appear to remit spontaneously.

Histopathology

There is a focal inflammatory disturbance of both the skin and the upper dermis in both acute and chronic lesions. The epidermis may be eroded and crusted in the acute lesions (Figure 7.14) but in the chronic lesions characteristic changes are found in the epidermis, which is slightly thickened and shows marked spongiosis and individual cell necrosis (Figure 7.15). There is marked parakeratosis and in addition exocytosis of monocytic cells (Figure 7.16). A detailed study of the epidermal changes demonstrated increased hydrolase activity within the epidermis and an increased rate of epidermal cell production[14]. The dermis is oedematous and there is often pronounced extravasation of red cells into the dermis although the blood vessels are not obviously damaged (Figure 7.17). There is a marked inflammatory cell infiltrate which is subepidermal and loosely perivascular. It consists of lymphocytes and histiocytes predominantly although they may be a few neutrophils in the acute form of the disease. Also in the acute type there is admixed with the lymphocytes and histiocytes the occasional larger cell with a large dark indented nucleus, reminiscent of the abnormal cells found in larger numbers in lymphomatoid papulosis (see below).

Lymphomatoid Papulosis

The relationship of this quite uncommon disorder to pityriasis lichenoides is uncertain[15]. The two diseases share certain clinical features, notably the appearance of inflamed papules with central necrosis. The papules are less uniform in size than in pityriasis lichenoides and quite large lesions may be seen. As in pityriasis lichenoides crops of lesions appear. The abnormal cells of the cellular infiltrate (see below) is suggestive of lymphoma and the relationship of the disorder to lymphoma is uncertain. It seems that some patients do in fact progress to frank lymphoma and it would seem unwise to accept the condition as a type of 'pseudolymphoma'.

Histopathology

The dominating feature of the histological picture is the presence of many bizarre large cells in the inflammatory cell infiltrate that cluster around blood vessels in the upper and mid dermis (Figure 7.18). The cells possess large reniform or crenated nuclei and are not unlike mycosis fungoides cells (see page 140). Studies with cell markers identify these cells as T lymphocytes[16].

References

1. Sweet, R. D. (1979). Acute febrile neutrophilic dermatosis. *Br. J. Dermatol.*, **100**, 93

2. Mitchell, D. N., Scadding, J. G., Heard, B. E. and Hinson, K. F. W. (1977). Sarcoidosis: histopathological definition and clinical diagnosis. *J. Clin. Pathol.*, **30**, 395

3. Langner, A., Moskalewska, K. and Proniewska, M. (1979). Studies on the mechanism of lymphocyte transformation inhibition in sarcoidosis. *Br. J. Dermatol.*, **81**, 829

4. Steigleder, G. K., Silva, A. Jr and Nelson, C. T. (1961). Histopathology of the Kveim test. *Arch. Dermatol.*, **84**, 828

5. Hirsh, B. C. and Johnson, W. C. (1984). Pathology of granulomatous diseases. Epithelioid granulomas. Part II. *Int. J. Dermatol.*, **23**, 306

6. Dutra, F. R. (1949). Beryllium granulomas of the skin. *Arch. Dermatol. Syphilol.*, **60**, 1140

7. Dertel, V. C. and Johnson, F. B. (1977). Sclerosing lipogranuloma of the male genitalia. *Arch. Pathol.*, **101**, 321

8. Epstein, W. L, Skahen, J. R. and Krasnobrod, H. (1963). The organised epithelioid cell granuloma: differentiation of allergic (zirconium) from colloidal (silica) types. *Am. J. Pathol.*, **43**, 391

9. Newcomber, V. D., Steffen, C. G., Sternberg, T. H. and Lichtenstein, L. (1953). Chondrodermatitis nodularis chronica helicis. *Arch. Dermatol. Syphilol.*, **68**, 241

10. Dahl, M. V., Ullman, S. and Goltz, R. W. (1977). Vasculitis in granuloma annulare. *Arch. Dermatol.*, **113**, 463

11. Muller, S. A. and Winkelmann, R. K. (1966). Necrobiosis Lipoidica Diabeticorum. *Arch. Dermatol.*, **93**, 272

12. Ullman, S. and Dahl, M. (1977). Necrobiosis lipoidica: An immunofluorescence study. *Arch. Dermatol.*, **113**, 1671

13. Lambert, W. C. and Everett, M. A. (1981). The nosology of parapsoriasis. *J. Am. Acad. Dermatol.*, **5**, 373

14. Marks, R. and Black, M. M. (1972). The epidermal component of pityriasis lichenoides. *Br. J. Dermatol.*, **87**, 106

15. Willemze, R. and Scheffer, E. (1985). Clinical and histologic differentiation between lymphomatoid papulosis and pityriasis lichenoides. *J. Am. Acad. Dermatol.*, **13**, 418

16. Bing, G., Hoffman-Fezer, G., Nikolouski, J., Schmoeckel, C., Braun-Falco, O. and Stunkel, K. (1981). Lymphomatoid papulosis. A cutaneous T cell pseudo lymphoma. *Acta Dermatovener (Stockholm)*, **61**, 491

Lupus Erythematosus

The syndrome of lupus erythematosus (LE) has a spectrum of disease activity from the purely cutaneous discoid type to the rapidly progressive systemic form with internal organ involvement. Antinuclear antibodies circulate in the systemic form but the demonstration of cutaneous immunological abnormalities by immunofluorescence is important to all types.

It is not possible on a histological basis to differentiate between the cutaneous manifestations of systemic and discoid LE with certainty.

Discoid LE

Localized red scaly plaques appear on sun-exposed areas particularly the face. They are chronic and heal very slowly resulting in scarring and loss of hair follicles.

Histologically the important features of cutaneous LE are (1) hyperkeratosis with follicular plugging, (2) atrophy of the epidermis, (3) liquefaction degeneration of the basal cells, (4) a deep lymphocytic infiltrate around the dermal blood vessels and adnexal structures (Figure 8.1) (5) oedema of the upper dermis, vasodilatation and some extravasation of red cells[1].

The most significant feature of LE is a focal liquefaction degeneration of the basal layer of the epidermis and hair follicles. Without this a specific diagnosis is difficult. Colloid bodies are seen in the region of the basal layer (Figure 8.2). These are pink round homogenous bodies which are degenerated epidermal cells. Rarely the epidermis becomes hyperplastic and verrucous and may result in carcinoma. The basement membrane is thickened and is best identified by a PAS stain (Figure 8.3) though H and E staining may be sufficient (Figure 8.4). Hyperkeratosis occurs without parakeratosis and horny plugs are found in the follicular openings and in the orifices of sweat glands. Involvement of hair follicles is a common feature and may result in total destruction and resultant replacement by scar tissue (Figure 8.5). The erector pili muscles remain and an elastic stain is helpful in localizing the scarred follicles (see page 80).

Acute LE

Pathological features resemble discoid LE but without hyperkeratosis or follicular plugs. The epidermis is atrophic, the papillae are oedematous and the dermal infiltrate is sparse[2]. The diagnostic features are found predominantly in the epidermis. They are basal liquefaction degeneration and colloid body formation.

Panniculitis of LE

In some cases of LE there is a panniculitis in addition to the more usual features. A lymphocytic infiltrate extends between fat-cells. Occasionally histiocytes and giant cells may give a granulomatous character to the infiltrate. Fatty necrosis can occur. True LE profundus is a pure panniculitis of LE but without the normal epidermal or follicular changes[3].

Immunofluorescence tests for LE

Direct immunofluorescence of affected skin shows deposits of IgM, IgG or complement at the dermo-epidermal junction[4] in a homogeneous or granular band (Figure 8.6). Normal skin in acute LE may show the same features.

Differential diagnosis of LE

The main conditions to be differentiated histologically are lichen planus, lichen planopilaris, dermatomyositis, Jessner's lymphocytic infiltrate of the skin and a drug reaction. In lichen planus epidermal features may be similar but there is usually hypergranulosis and in addition there is saw toothing and cleft formation at the dermo-epidermal junction. The lymphocytic infiltrate is packed up against the epidermis and does not surround dermal blood vessels and adnexal structures. Lichen planopilaris may resemble discoid LE as both show erosion of the follicles but no changes are seen in the interfollicular epidermis. Dermatomyositis may closely resemble acute LE with papillary oedema, some basal cell liquefaction degeneration and a mild upper dermal perivascular infiltrate. However there may be dermal deposits of mucopolysaccharide in dermatomyositis. Indeed immunofluorescence may be necessary to differentiate these conditions as the immunofluorescent changes of LE are not seen in dermatomyositis. A perivascular and periadnexal lymphocytic infiltrate occurs in both LE and Jessner's disease (Figure 8.7) but in the latter no epidermal or follicular changes occur[5]. A lichenoid drug reaction may be similar to LE but the basal cell damage is more spotty and eosinophils may be seen in the dermal infiltrate.

Morphoea and Scleroderma

Definition and Description

In both conditions there is a woody thickening of the skin. Morphoea is a localized and non-progressive type and scleroderma is generalized with systemic manifestations including renal, cardiac and swallowing difficulties leading eventually to severe morbidity or death. Raynaud's disease often precedes scleroderma[6].

Histologically the two conditions are similar. There is an early inflammatory and a late sclerotic change. A deep biopsy is important as many features are in the subcutis. Elastic fibres are preserved.

In the early inflammatory stage, the collagen bundles

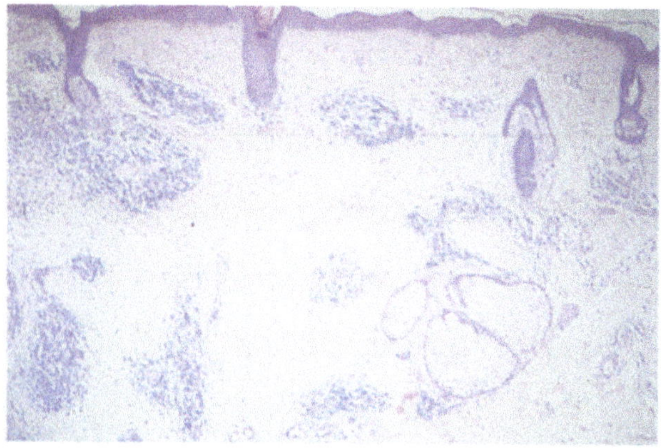

Figure 8.1   Lupus erythematosus. Low power showing deep dense perivascular and periadnexal infiltrate.   H & E (A)

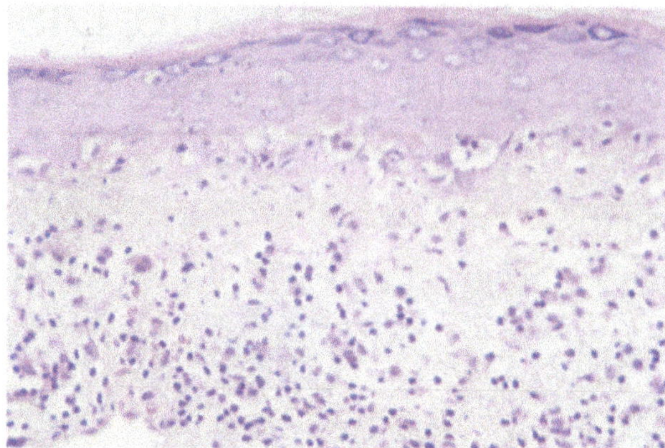

Figure 8.2   Lupus erythematosus. Basal liquefaction and colloid body formation at the dermo-epidermal junction.   H & E (C)

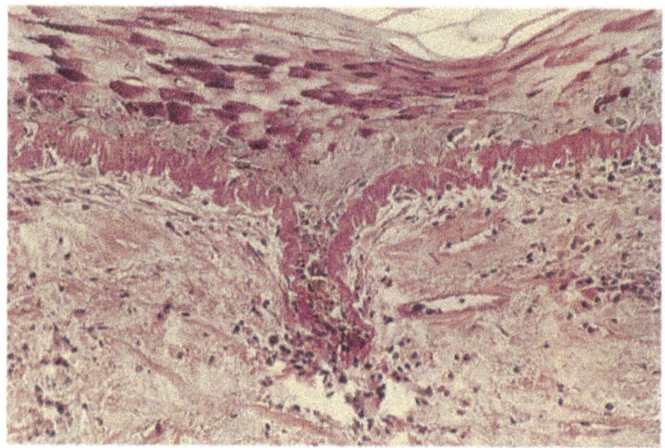

Figure 8.3   Lupus erythematosus. Thickened basement membrane seen as red band along lower border of epidermis.   PAS (C)

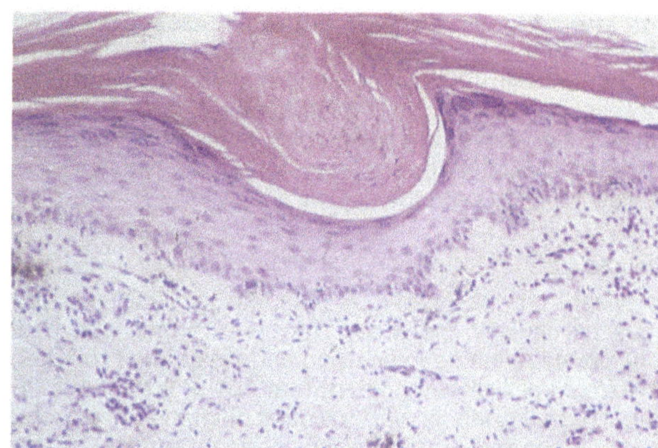

Figure 8.4   Lupus erythematosus. Follicular plugging and thickened basement membrane seen as a clear band along the lower border of epidermis.   H & E (C)

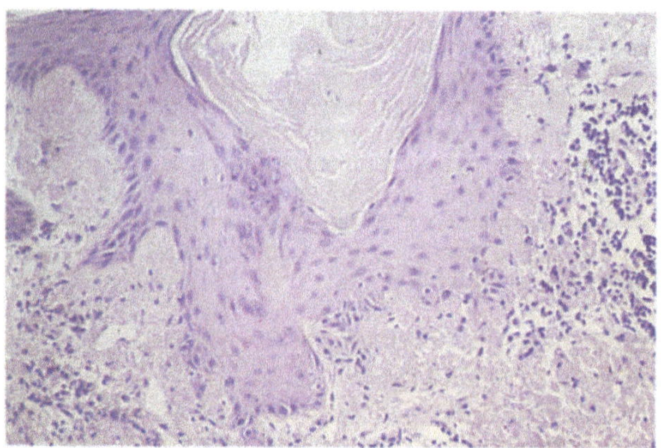

Figure 8.5   Lupus erythematosus. Follicular involvement. Erosion of basal cells and large numbers of colloid bodies below the epidermis.   H & E (C)

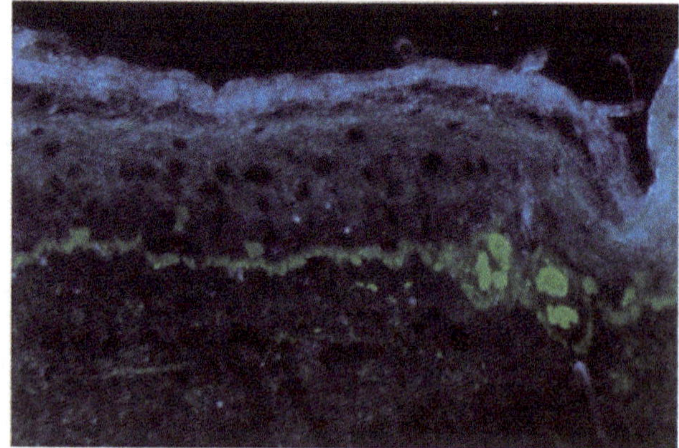

Figure 8.6   Lupus erythematosus. Direct immunofluorescence to show linear basement membrane fluorescence and a group of colloid bodies at one edge. Anti IgM reagent.   (C)

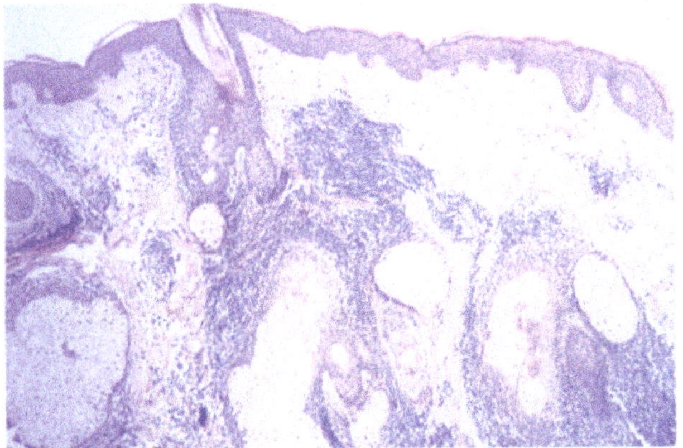

Figure 8.7 Jessner's lymphocytic infiltrate of the skin. Dense perivascular periadnexal lymphocytic infiltrate with no epidermal changes. H & E (B)

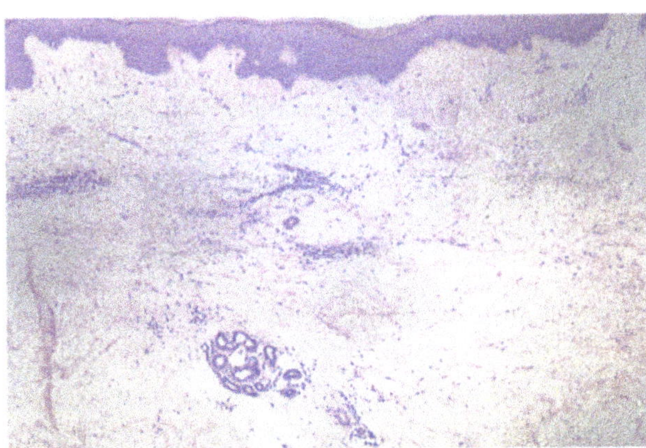

Figure 8.8 Scleroderma. Early infiltrate phase. Mild lymphocytic perivascular infiltrate. Normal epidermal pattern. H & E (B)

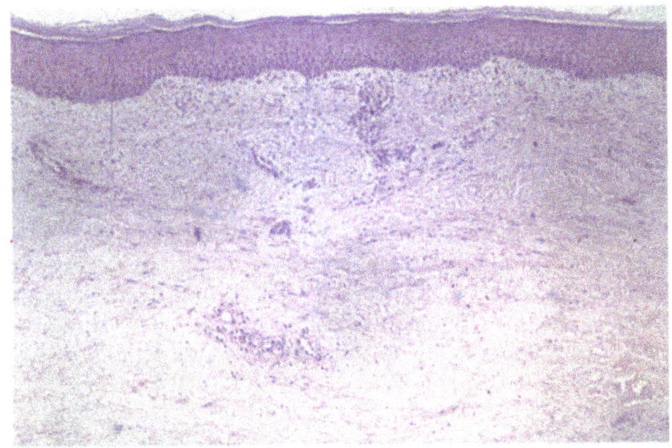

Figure 8.9 Scleroderma. Late sclerotic phase. Loss of epidermal rete pattern. Acellular dermis with loss of adnexal structures. H & E (B)

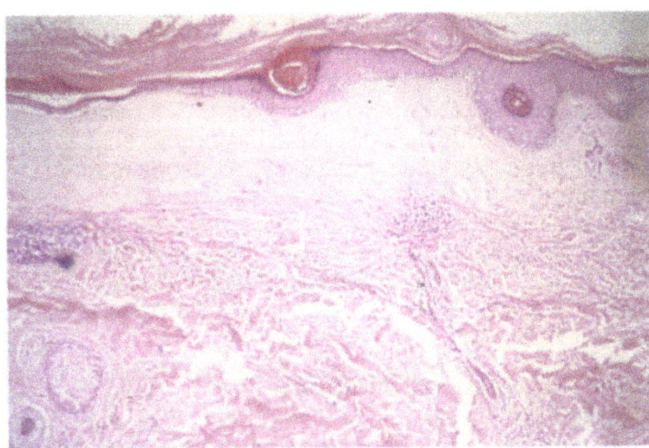

Figure 8.10 Lichen sclerosus et atrophicus. Normal skin to right of photomicrograph. On left hyperkeratosis, thin atrophic epidermis, follicular plugging and a band of pale acellular dermis below the epidermis. H & E (B)

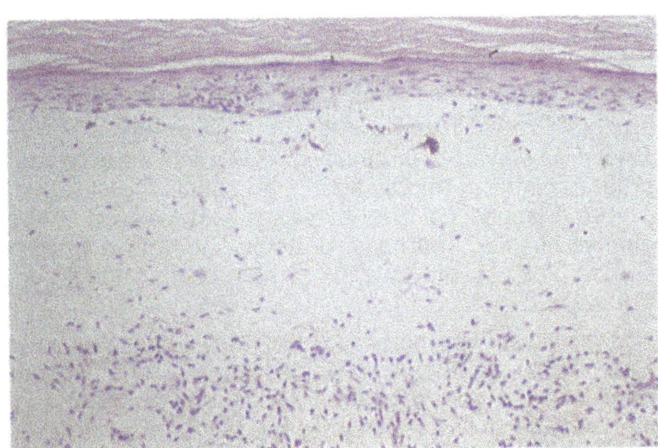

Figure 8.11 Lichen sclerosus et atrophicus. Hyperkeratosis, thin atrophic epidermis and some dermo-epidermal separation. Pigmentary incontinence, pale acellular upper dermis. A band of lymphocytes in mid dermis. H & E (B)

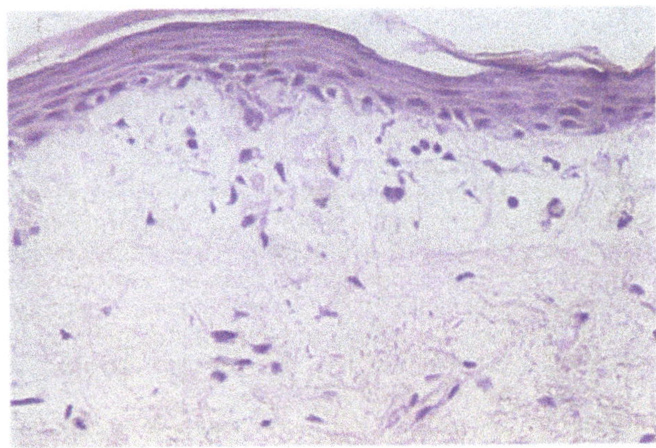

Figure 8.12 Dermatomyositis. Gross upper dermal oedema with groups of colloid bodies 'hanging' below the epidermis. H & E (B)

are thickened and there is a lymphocytic infiltrate between them and around the blood vessels. (Figure 8.8). Similarly the infiltrate extends around eccrine sweat glands in the subcutis. The fat trabeculations are infiltrated and thickened by deposition of new collagen[7].

In the late sclerotic stage the infiltrate disappears from the dermis but a trace may remain in the subcutis. The epidermis may be normal or flattened (Figure 8.9). In the papillary dermis the collagen will be homogenous instead of the usual loosely arranged fibres. Collagen bundles in the mid dermis are thickened, tightly packed and also homogeneous. The eccrine sweat glands atrophy and the surrounding fat disappears. Those that remain appear to be higher in the dermis than normal because the subcutaneous fat is replaced by new collagen.

A late feature in scleroderma is vascular change in the subcutis. Fewer, thicker blood vessels are seen and they have narrow lumina. The epidermis in systemic sclerosis is thin and flattened but is usually normal in morphoea. Calcium deposits in the subcutis are a later feature.

Differential Diagnosis. In scars and keloids elastic fibres are generally absent but are usually present in morphoea and scleroderma. The collagen in a keloid is arranged in whorled bundles. Scleredema is exceedingly rare and difficult to detect histologically. The woody feel to the skin is due to increased hyaluronic acid in the ground substance and mucopolysaccharide stains are necessary.

Scleromyxoedema histologically may resemble a fibroma because of the increased number of fibroblasts with little increase in ground substance. A mucin stain will be positive in scleredema and scleromyxoedema but not morphoea and scleroderma.

Lichen Sclerosus et Atrophicus

An uncommon chronic skin disease occurring in middle-aged women particularly around the neck and on the vulva. The skin becomes slightly thickened, ivory white with follicular hyperkeratosis and a tendency to haemorrhagic blisters. Rarely it is found in children. The male counterpart is balanitis xerotica obliterans – affecting the skin of the inside of the foreskin and glans penis.

Histologically, the diagnosis is readily made under low power examination (Figure 8.10). The findings are (a) hyperkeratosis with follicular plugging, (b) epidermal thinning and basal cell liquefaction, (c) subepidermal separation, (d) upper dermal homogenization and oedema of connective tissue, (e) an infiltrate of lymphocytes in the mid dermis. The stratum corneum is constantly thickened in contrast to a thin atrophic epidermis. Clumps of colloid bodies are seen near the dermo-epidermal junction. The basement membrane is initially thicker and then disintegrates.

A band of oedema develops below the epidermis and on histological sections separation of epidermis from dermis may be seen as artefacts from fixation shrinkage (Figure 8.11). The upper dermis become homogenous and relatively acellular giving a very typical clear pale zone below which is a band of lymphocytes with some perivascular disposition. The hair follicles, sweat and sebaceous glands are normal.

Differential Diagnosis. Although clinically morphoea and lichen sclerosus may be indistinguishable there should be no difficulty histologically[8,9]. It is unlikely that other conditions can be mistaken for lichen sclerosus.

Dermatomyositis

Definition and Description

Dermatomyositis is a rare clinical condition of proximal muscle weakness and tenderness with a purple red rash on the face, particularly the eyelids, V of the neck and backs of hands. Oedema of the skin is characteristic. Underlying neoplasia may be found in adults.

Histologically, the typical features are best seen in clinically affected skin rather than skin from a muscle biopsy site. They are (a) lymphoid infiltrate, (b) upper dermal oedema, (c) basal cell liquefaction degeneration and colloid bodies in the papillary dermis[10]. The lymphocytic infiltrate is sparse in the papillary dermis and cuffs the larger dermal blood vessels. Oedema is always present (Figure 8.12) and may be seen in clinically normal skin. It is prominent in the papillary dermis and is associated with increase of acid mucopolysaccharides demonstrated by the alcian blue stain. Basal cell liquefaction is often seen and groups of colloid bodies are found in the papillary dermis just below the dermo-epidermal junction. The basement membrane as demonstrated by the PAS stain is of normal thickness.

Differential Diagnosis. Lupus erythematosus has to be differentiated and both conditions demonstrate basal cell liquefaction and colloid bodies. Oedema however is not usually a prominent feature and the basement membrane is frequently thickened in LE except in the acute type. Immunofluorescence examination of the skin in dermatomyositis is not diagnostic but immunofluorescence is important in the diagnosis of LE.

Vasculitis

The term implies organic damage to the vascular wall in the form of necrosis, hyalinization, fibrinoid change or granulomatous involvement. All inflammatory processes involve blood vessels and simple cuffing by lymphocytes or neutrophils does not necessarily mean vasculitis.

Leukocytoclastic Vasculitis

This is a pathological term for a reaction which occurs in a number of clinical conditions. These include Henoch–Schönlein purpura, erythema elevatum diutinum, allergic vasculitis, some urticarias and some drug reactions.

Histologically they all show fragmented neutrophil nuclei and nuclear dust in and around the small blood vessel walls. In addition there is hyalinization of small vessel walls (Figure 8.13), perivascular oedema, some eosinophils, neutrophils and lymphocytes[11].

Henoch-Schönlein purpura. This is a palpable purpura mainly affecting the extensor surfaces. It may follow a streptococcal sore throat and may be associated with intestinal haemorrhagic oedema, arthritis and nephritis.

Erythema elevatum diutinum. This is a rare disease seen predominantly in middle-aged men consisting of brownish-red plaques on the extensor surfaces of knees, elbows, hands, feet and buttocks. It runs a chronic course. The vessels have toxic hyaline within and around the walls (Figure 8.14).

Allergic vasculitis. This is a clinical term which may cover a number of conditions including Henoch–Schönlein purpura. The cutaneous lesions may or may not be associated with vasculitis in other organs. In the more common type the legs are mostly involved with haemorrhagic papules, necrosis, purpura and some ulceration papules.

Granuloma Faciale

This is a rare disease consisting of solitary reddish-brown plaques on the face of middle-aged persons. *Histologically* there is a low-grade form of leukocytoclastic vasculitis but also there are histiocytes, lymphocytes, plasma cells and eosinophils in large numbers. These fill the upper and mid dermis except for a clear zone (Grenz zone) (Figures 8.15 and 8.16) between the infiltrate and the epidermis and between the hair follicles and the infiltrate[12]. The blood vessels are clad in a fibrinoid material. There may be foamy or giant cells within the dense infiltrate, thus combining a leukocytoclastic vasculitis and granulomatous reaction.

Periarteritis Nodosa (Polyarteritis nodosa)

This affects the larger and deeper blood vessels resulting in a necrotizing inflammatory periarteritis. *Clinically* nodules occur along the course of superficial arteries. They are due to segmental necrosis of the arterial wall and at bifurcations and healing may result in aneurysmal swellings. Embolization of thrombi leads to peripheral gangrene. There is widespread internal organ involvement.

Histopathologically there is a widespread leukocytoclastic vasculitis but there is actual necrosis of vessel walls (Figure 8.17) and occlusion by thrombi which are not seen in Henoch–Schönlein purpura[13]. The skin may not show the typical lesions of systemic periarteritis nodosa and a renal biopsy would then be most useful.

Granulomatous Vasculitis

This is seen in Wegener's granulomatosis and temporal arteritis.

Wegener's granulomatosis. This is a rare disease with granulomatous destruction of the respiratory tract and generalized necrotizing arteritis with glomerulitis. Pathologically there are two types of lesions, necrotizing granulomas and necrotizing vasculitis.

Temporal arteritis. This is a disease of the elderly. The patient has tenderness and pain over the temple. The temporal artery pulsation may be reduced and there are tender nodules along its surface. The ESR is always markedly elevated. Pathologically the arterial intima is thickened with some obliteration of the lumen. The internal elastic lamina is disrupted with fibrinoid necrosis and an infiltrate of neutrophils and giant cells (Figure 8.18). Around the vessel is an extensive histiocytic and giant cell infiltrate which clears as fibrosis of the vessel wall extends[14].

Erythema Nodosum

This is a relatively common disease predominantly seen in young women. Patients have raised red tender nodules on the shins. Some systemic symptoms occur and the disease lasts 4–6 weeks, with the nodules fading through the colour changes of a bruise. The aetiology includes streptococcal infection, sarcoidosis, tuberculosis, inflammatory bowel disease and drugs.

Histopathology

The condition is an inflammation in the subcutaneous tissues. The primary involvement is in the small blood vessels and interlobular fat septa[15]. Multinucleate giant cells are a constant feature and the infiltrate is mainly lymphocytes with some neutrophils but no plasma cells or eosinophils. The infiltrate extends into the fat lobules from the periphery and gives a lace-like appearance. Necrosis does not occur and there are no epithelioid tubercles.

Erythemas

The simple toxic erythema seen clinically is a generalized reddening of the skin which may be due to drugs, viral infection or pregnancy.

Histologically no epidermal changes will be seen and the main features are mild dermal oedema and a loosely arranged perivascular lymphocytic infiltrate. Erythema annulare centrifugum is slightly different because the infiltrate is deeper and denser resembling that seen in Jessner's lymphocytic infiltrate of the skin. Generally however the erythemas do not have a characteristic histology and must be differentiated from secondary syphilis, pigmented purpuric eruptions and mild eczema or a dermatophyte infection.

Urticaria

The wheals of urticaria have no characteristic histology. There is dermal oedema which is difficult to identify on paraffin sections and a mild perivascular infiltrate perhaps with some eosinophils. Occasionally a clinical case of urticaria has the histology of leukocytoclastic vasculitis (so called urticarial vasculitis).

References

1. Clark, W. H. Jr, Reed, R. J. and Mihm, M. C. (1973). Lupus erythematosus. Histopathology of cutaneous lesions. *Hum. Pathol.*, **4**, 157

2. Pruniéras, M. and Montgomery, H. (1956). Histopathology of cutaneous lesions in systemic lupus erythematosus. *Arch. Dermatol.*, **74**, 177

3. Sánchez, N. P., Peters, M. S. and Winkelmann, R. K. (1981). The histopathology of lupus erythematosus panniculitis. *J. Am. Acad. Dermatol.*, **5**, 673

4. Dantzig, P. I., Mauro, J., Rayhanzadeh, S. *et al.* (1975). The significance of a positive cutaneous immunofluorescence test in systemic lupus erythematosus. *Br. J. Dermatol.*, **93**, 531

5. Jessner, M. and Kanof, N. B. (1953). Lymphocytic infiltration of the skin. *Arch. Dermatol. Syph.*, **68**, 447

6. Sharp, G. C. and Anderson, P. C. (1980). Current concepts in the classification of connective tissue diseases. Overlap syndromes and mixed connective tissue disease (MCTD). *J. Am. Acad. Dermatol.*, **2**, 269

7. D'Angelo, W. A., Fries, J. F., Masi A. T. *et al.* (1969). Pathological observations in systemic sclerosis (scleroderma). *Am. J. Med.*, **46**, 428

8. Jablonska, S. (1980). Relationship between morphoea and lichen sclerosus et atrophicus. *Am. J. Dermatopathol.*, **2**, 285

9. O'Leary, P. A., Montgomery, H. and Ragsdale, W. E. (1957). Dermatohistopathology of various types of scleroderma (Review). *Arch. Dermatol.*, **75**, 78

10. Janis, J. F. and Winkelmann, R. K. (1968). Histopathology of the skin in dermatomyositis. *Arch. Dermatol.*, **97**, 640

11. Mackel, S. E. and Jordon, R. E. (1982). Leukocytoclastic vasculitis. *Arch. Dermatol.*, **118**, 296

12. Johnson, W. C., Higdon, R. S. and Helwig, E. B. (1959). Granuloma faciale. *Arch. Dermatol.*, **79**, 42

13. Diaz-Perez, J. L., Schroeter, A. L. and Winkelmann, R. K. (1980). Cutaneous periarteritis nodosa. *Arch. Dermatol.*, **116**, 56

14. Goodman, B. W. Jr (1979). Temporal arteritis. (Review). *Am. J. Med.*, **67**, 839

15. Winkelmann, R. K. and Förström, L. (1975). New observations in the histopathology of erythema nodosum. *J. Invest. Dermatol.*, **65**, 441

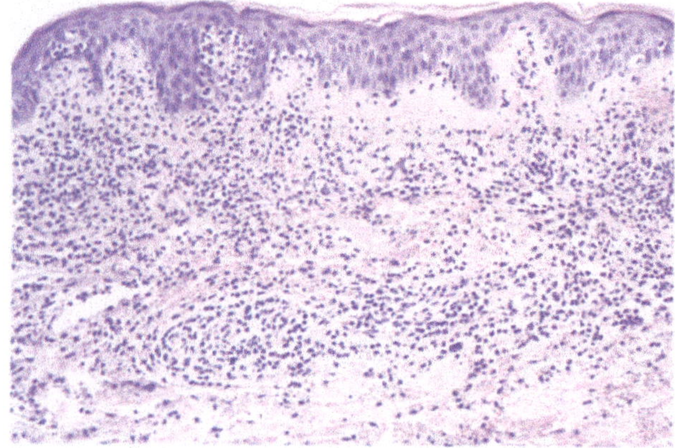

Figure 8.13 Leukocytoclastic vasculitis. Swelling and fibrinoid change of vessel wall, large numbers of neutrophils and nuclear dust within and around the vessel walls.   H & E (B)

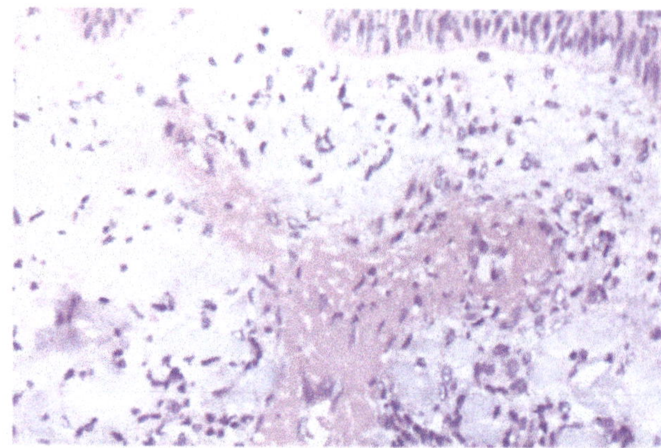

Figure 8.14 Erythema elevatum diutinum. Cellular infiltrate of neutrophils and eosinophils. There is 'toxic hyaline' around the blood vessel – this is similar to fibrinoid in staining reactions.   H & E (B)

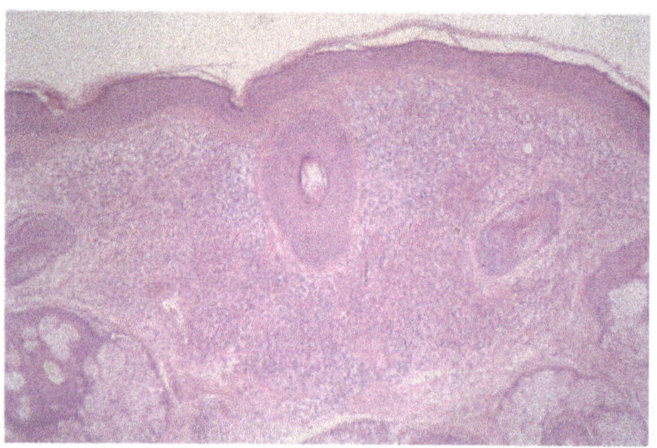

Figure 8.15 Granuloma faciale. Note the dense infiltrate in the mid dermis but with a clear zone between it and the epidermis and adnexal structures.   H & E (A)

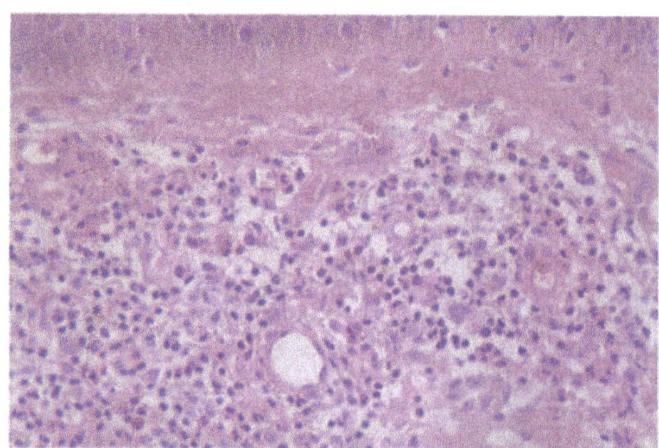

Figure 8.16 Granuloma faciale. There is a Grenz zone between the epidermis and dermal infiltrate. The infiltrate is mixed with neutrophilis, nuclear dust and eosinophils.   H & E (C)

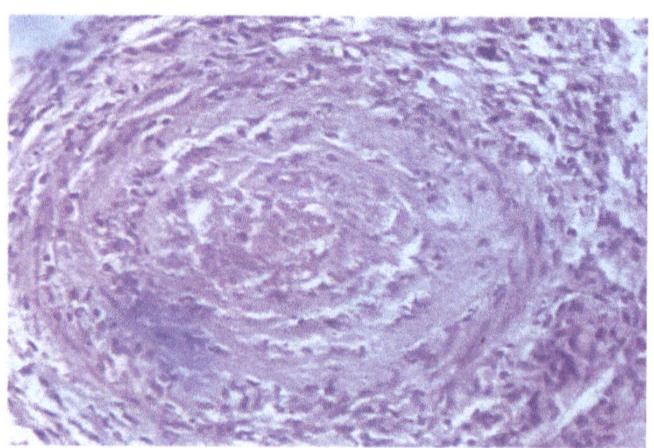

Figure 8.17 Periarteritis nodosa. A medium-sized artery is necrotic and swollen. It is blocked with fibrim and there are neutrophils within and around the vessel.   H & E (D)

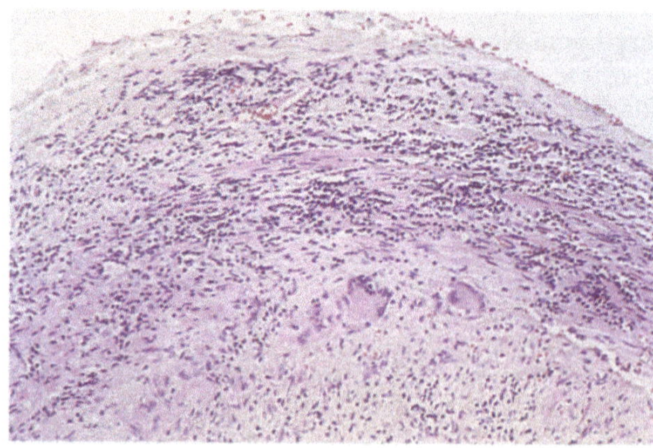

Figure 8.18 Temporal arteritis. Extensive histiocytic and giant cell infiltrate within the vessel wall. There are also a large number of neutrophils within and around the vessel.   H & E (C)

Acne, Rosacea, Perioral Dermatitis and Related Disorders

9

Acne

Acne is an inflammatory disorder of hair bearing skin, characterized initially by hyperkeratosis of follicular canals and an increased rate of sebum secretion and subsequently by the development of inflamed papules and abscesses ('cysts'). It affects the majority of individuals mildly during adolescence, but can give rise to serious disease in a relatively small proportion of individuals. The lesions observed clinically are comedones (blackheads) which are really casts of the follicular canal and arise on the face, chest and upper back, papules and pustules, which are inflammatory lesions arising from obstructed follicles, and cysts, which are in reality cold abscesses, the result of colliquative necrosis around several follicles. The more inflamed and destructive lesions cause unsightly scarring.

Aetiology and Pathogenesis

The ultimate cause of acne is unknown, but two elements are important in its pathogenesis – an increased rate of sebum production (seborrhoea) and follicular hyperkeratosis (and maybe abnormal keratinization)[1], resulting in obstruction to the follicular canal. Whether increased production of androgens, changes in androgen receptor binding, or alterations in the metabolism of androgens (or any combination of these) is responsible for the seborrhoea is unclear.

Histopathology

The pathological picture is dependent on the type of lesion biopsied and its duration. When areas of skin containing comedones are biopsied, the follicular canals contain abundant lamellated horn, which may be impacted in the follicular canals (Figure 9.1). The follicular epithelium may show a curious type of irregular hypertrophy, particularly involving the external root sheath. If inflamed papules are sampled, there is a quite dramatic picture of follicular breakdown and ultimate destruction, with an intense and mixed inflammatory cell infiltrate focussed on the follicle (Figure 9.2). In earlier lesions there are sheets of polymorphonuclear neutrophils and cell debris. In lesions that are more mature, histiocytes, epithelioid cells and foreign body giant cells make their appearance (Figure 9.3). In some cases it is evident that the liberation of follicular contents (and in particular, horn) into the dermis following follicular rupture has played a substantial role in producing the inflammation. Later in the process scarring occurs. The new fibrous tissue tends to invest follicular structures in particular. In many examples follicular debris and collections of closely applied inflammatory cells are surrounded by irregular hypertrophied outgrowths of the follicular wall in the process of transepidermal elimination (Figure 9.4).

In the condition of sycosis nuchae, which appears to be a variant of scarring acne affecting the back of the neck, there are broad strands of new connective tissue with an admixture of clusters of various inflammatory

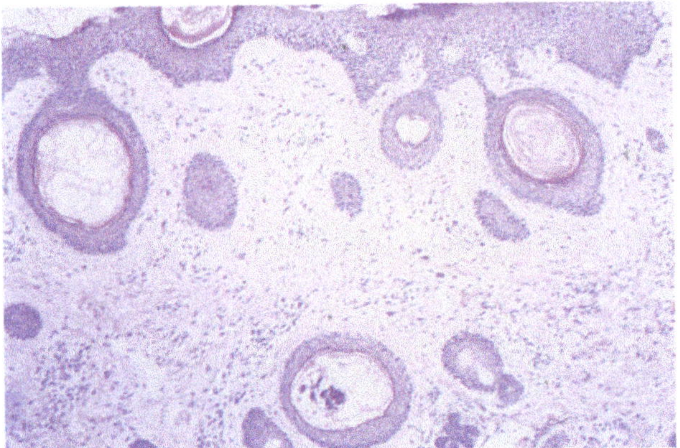

Figure 9.1 Oblique section to show follicular blocking in several follicles in acne. H & E (B)

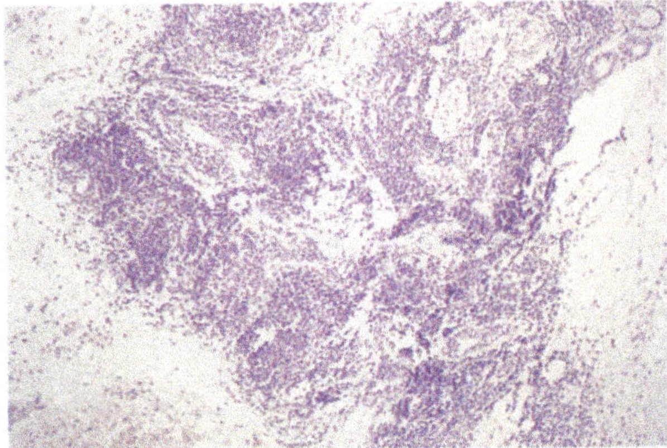

Figure 9.2 Mixed inflammatory cell infiltrate deep in the dermis in acne. H & E (B)

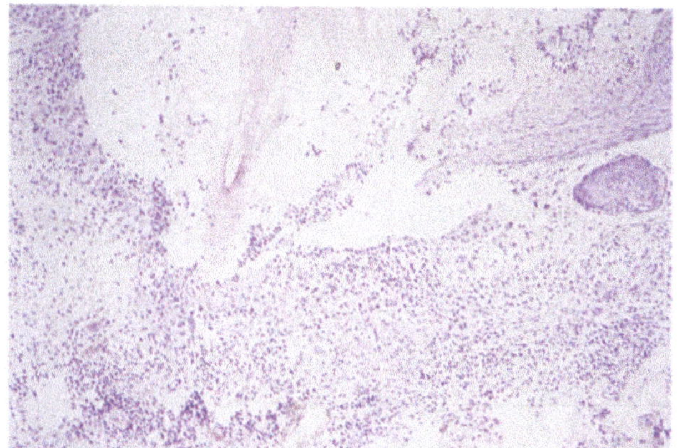

Figure 9.3 Granulomatous response by a destroyed hair follicle in acne. H & E (B)

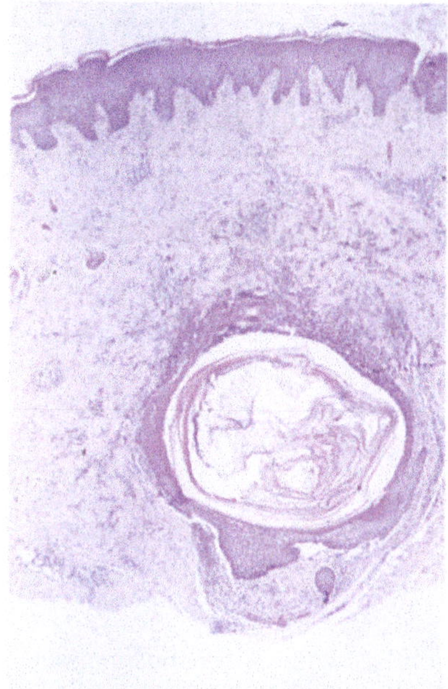

Figure 9.4 Acne. To show abnormal follicular hypertrophy and severe inflammation resulting in transepidermal elimination. H & E (B)

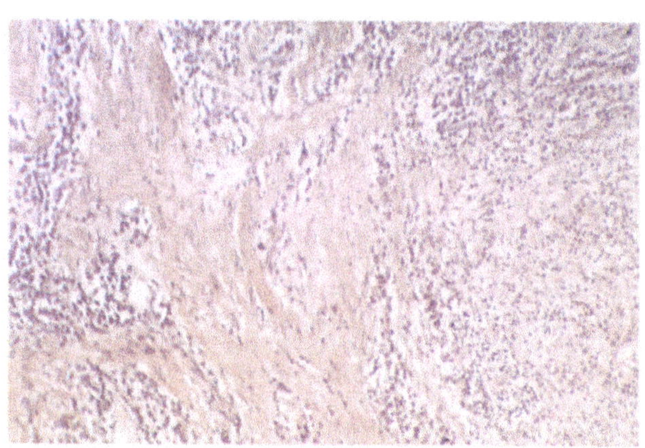

Figure 9.5 Sycosis nuchae. Scarring and mixture of inflammatory cells including many plasma cells. H & E (C)

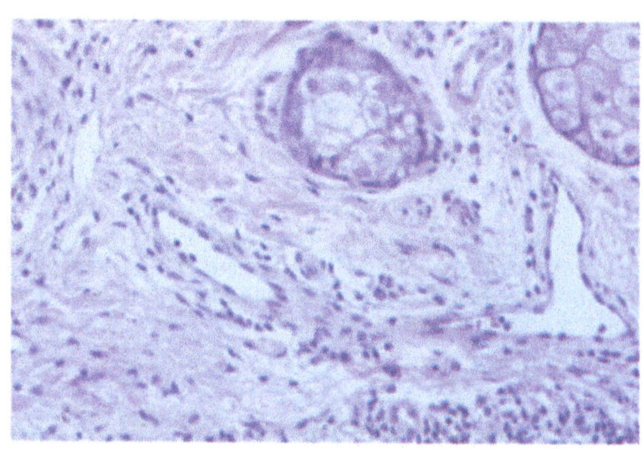

Figure 9.6 Rosacea. There is marked solar elastotic degenerative change in the upper dermis and several dilated blood vessels. H & E (C)

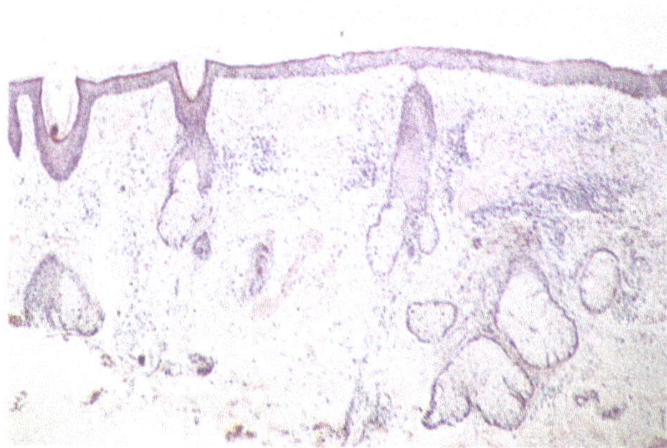

Figure 9.7 Rosacea. Plan view to show oedema and telangiectasia and scattered inflammatory cell infiltrate. H & E (B)

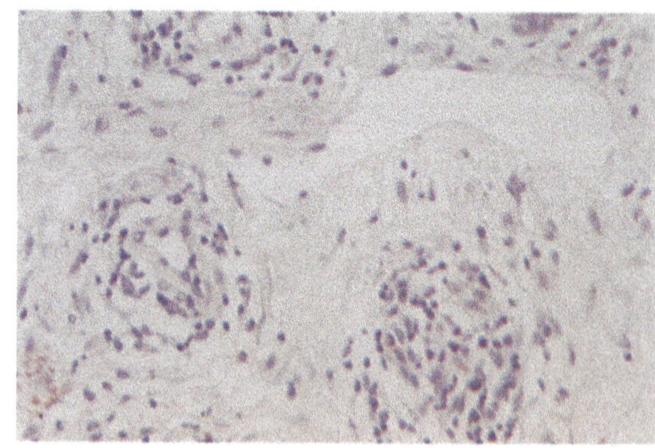

Figure 9.8 Rosacea. Perivascular inflammatory cells. H & E (B)

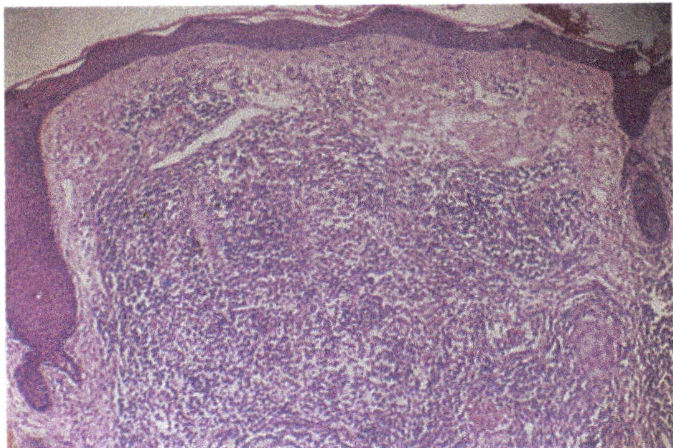

Figure 9.9 Rosacea. Dense mixed inflammatory cell infiltrate. H & E (B)

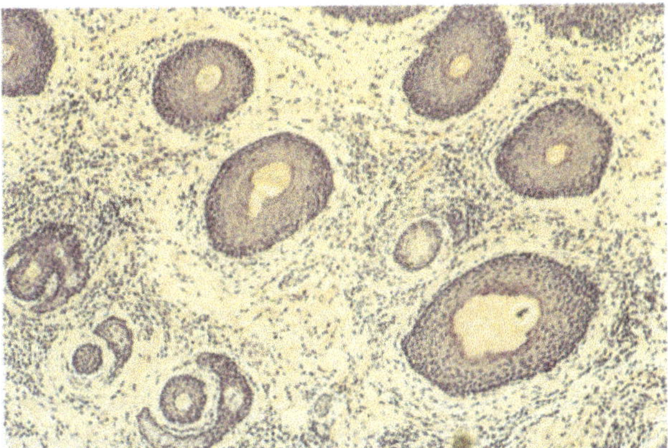

Figure 9.10 Rosacea. Apparent perifollicular distribution of inflammatory cells due to inflammatory cells investing the perifollicular capillaries. H & E (B)

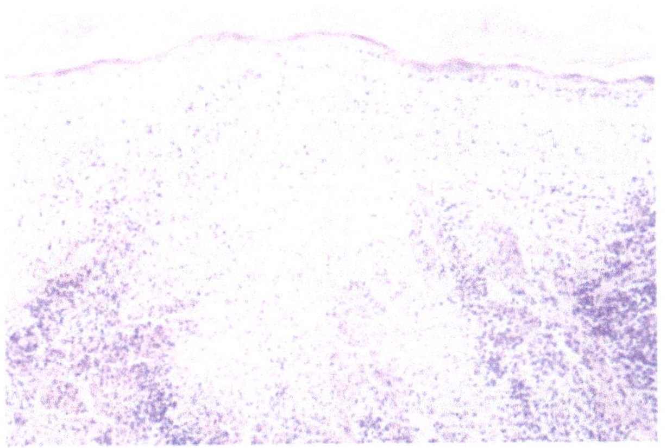

Figure 9.11 Rosacea. Marked granulomatous cell infiltrate. H & E (B)

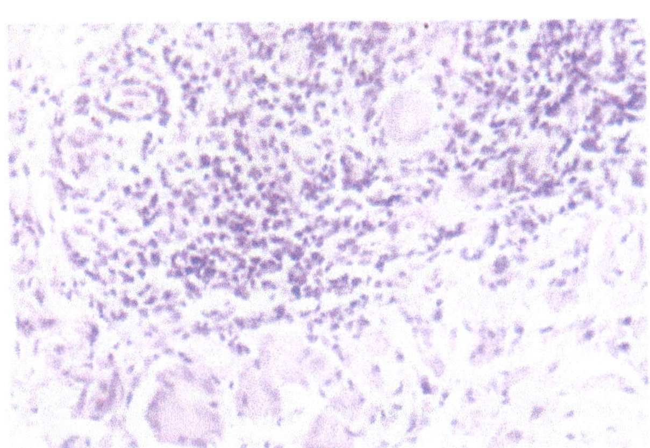

Figure 9.12 Rosacea. Several giant cells in granulomatous focus. H & E (C)

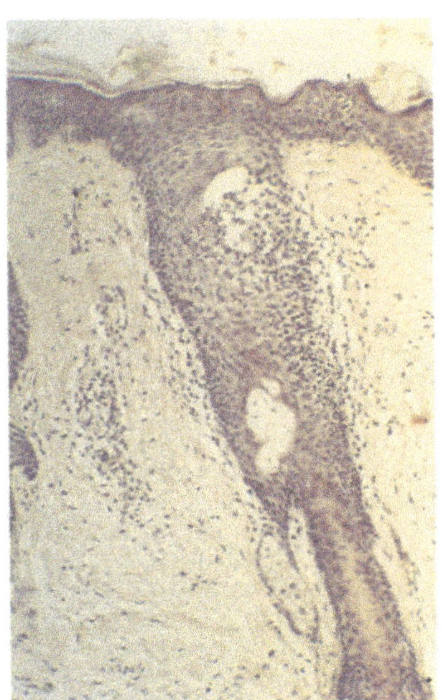

Figure 9.13 Perioral dermatitis. There is spongiosis of the follicular wall and invasion by inflammatory cells. H & E (B)

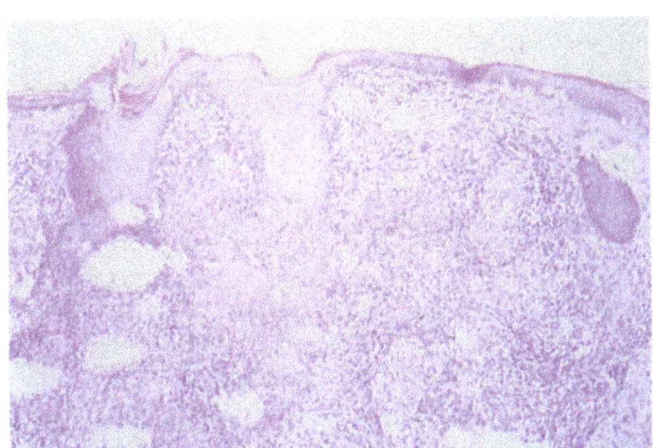

Figure 9.14 Acne agminata showing granulomatous inflammation and necrosis. H & E (B)

cells. Large numbers of plasma cells are sometimes also present in this odd disorder (Figure 9.5).

Acne cysts are inappropriately named as they have no epithelial lining but are actually cold abscesses. Areas of colliquative dermal necrosis contain numerous polymorphonuclear leukocytes and leukocyte debris, and are surrounded by fibrotic dermal collagen.

Rosacea

Rosacea is a common chronic disorder of the light exposed area of facial skin of unknown cause, characterized by persistent erythema of the facial convexities and episodes of inflammation with papules and swelling.

Aetiology and Pathogenesis

Despite our lack of understanding with regard to the entire sequence of events in the development of rosacea, recent observations are starting to clarify the nature of the disease. Firstly, it is now clear that rosacea has only the most tenuous of connections with acne. Secondly, its predominance in fair complexioned Caucasians, its distribution over the face and the degree of dermal damage suggest that climatic factors (particularly the sun) play an important role[3]. Finally, there appears to be an immunological component in which there is depressed delayed hypersensitivity and the deposition of immunoglobulins at the dermo-epidermal junction[4,5].

Clinical Picture

The disorder is most frequently seen in fair complexioned women in the third, fourth and fifth decade, but is by no means confined to this group. Typically the cheeks, chin, nose and forehead are affected by erythema and telangiectasia. Swelling, papules and maybe pustules develop at times. Comedones, cysts and scars are not seen. It also differs from acne in that rosacea does not affect the chest, shoulders or back, although lesions are occasionally observed on the neck. Increased blushing is a frequent symptom. A complication in middle-aged and elderly men affected by the disorder is rhinophyma. In this odd complaint the soft tissues of the nose enlarge irregularly, so that the nose becomes thickened, craggy and dull red or mauve in colour.

Histopathology[8]

When the only clinical changes are erythema and telangiectasia, the microscopic abnormalities are mainly in the upper dermis. The dermal connective tissue appears more disorganized than usual, with individual fibres separated by oedema. There is also more solar elastotic degenerative change than is to be expected for the age and history of sun exposure (Figure 9.6). Set amongst the dystrophic dermal connective tissue are dilated vascular channels (Figure 9.7). Most appear to be thin-walled blood capillaries, but some are trefoil in shape with button-shaped nuclei projecting into the lumen so that they resemble lymphatics.

Around the vessels there is a variable amount of inflammatory cell infiltrate consisting of lymphocytes and histiocytes (Figure 9.8). Inflamed lesions are marked histologically by larger collections of inflammatory cell infiltrate (Figure 9.9). These often appear to be perifollicular, but detailed examination has shown that this appearance is due to the profusion of perifollicular capillaries rather than any primary disorder of the follicles (Figure 9.10). This is a major distinction between rosacea

and acne, and explains our preference for the term rosacea, rather than the older term 'acne rosacea'. The inflammatory cell infiltrate tends to be more granulomatous the larger the collections of cells. In about 10 per cent of such infiltrates, giant cell systems are found (Figure 9.11). Such granulomata contain no foreign particles and special stains do not reveal the presence of micro-organisms.

In rare instances the granulomata are frankly tuberculoid in appearance, and the term *granulomatous rosacea* is used to describe this situation (Figure 9.12). When the lesions clinically are indolent and dull red or mauvish in colour, and histologically the picture is predominantly that of tuberculoid granulomata, the condition has been called rosaceous tuberculid, but it is doubtful whether it represents anything other than one end of the rosacea spectrum. Despite its name it has no association with tuberculosis.

Immunofluorescent examination of affected skin often reveals the immunoglobulins IgG and IgM in a band at the dermo-epidermal junction. However, the findings are not sufficiently consistent to be of diagnostic assistance.

Perioral Dermatitis

Perioral dermatitis is an inflammatory dermatosis of unknown aetiology that typically occurs around the mouth and in the nasolabial clefts in young women. Although the lesions are predominantly small papules and pustules it is not believed to be related to either acne or rosacea. It appears to be aggravated (and some believe precipitated) by the use of topical corticosteroids[7]. The disorder was quite common in the 1960s and early 1970s but is much less frequently seen at the time of writing.

Histopathology

The only consistent feature is the presence of spongiotic change in the upper part of the external root sheath of the hair follicles[8] (Figure 9.13). Moderate numbers of lymphocytes and histiocytes are found perivascularly in the upper dermis. The dermal dystrophy and oedema characteristic of rosacea are not found.

Acne Agminata (Acnitis; lupus miliaris disseminata facei)

Acne agminata is an uncommon persistent granulomatous disorder of unknown aetiology that affects the face alone. It is characterized by the appearance of brownish-red papules over the cheeks, nose and forehead. Typically it affects young or middle-aged individuals and lasts some months, eventually leaving small pock-like scars.

Histopathology

The characteristic feature of this disorder is the presence of foci of tuberculoid granulomata. The papillary dermis and epidermis remain unaffected (Figure 9.14). Numerous epithelioid cells and giant cell systems are often present and there may be caseation necrosis at the centre of the foci. Special stains do not reveal the presence of micro-organisms and the cause of this dermatosis remains a mystery.

Lupus vulgaris (see page 33), leprosy and leishmaniasis should be excluded by examining appropriately stained sections for micro-organisms. The condition may be difficult to distinguish from granulomatous rosacea although the absence of the dermal connective changes in acne agminata should be helpful.

References

1. Lavker, R. M., Leyden, J. J. and McGinley, K. J. (1981). The relationship between bacteria and the abnormal follicular keratinization in acne vulgaris. *J. Invest. Dermatol.*, **77**, 325

2. Dalziel, K., Kingston, T. and Marks, R. (1985). The effects of isotretinion on the pathology of early acne papules. *Clin. Exp. Dermatol.*, **10**, 365

3. Marks, R. (1976). Rosacea. In *Common Facial Dermatoses.* pp. 8–24. (Bristol: John Wright)

4. Manna, V., Marks, R. and Holt, P. (1982). Involvement of immune mechanisms in the pathogenesis of rosacea. *Br. J. Dermatol.*, 203-8

5. Nunzi, E., Rebora, A., Harmerlinck, F. and Cormane, R. H. (1980). Immunopathological studies on rosacea. *Br. J. Dermatol.*, **103**, 543

6. Marks, R. and Harcourt Webster, N. (1969). Histopathology of rosacea. *Arch. Dermatol.*, **100**. 683

7. Wilkinson, D. S. (1981). What is perioral dermatitis? *Int. J. Dermatol.*, **20**, 485

8. Marks, R. and Black, M. M. (1971). Perioral dermatitis. A histopathological study of 26 cases. *Br. J. Dermatol.*, **84**, 242

Miscellaneous Disorders of Connective Tissue

10

Congenital Disorders

Pseudoxanthoma Elasticum[1]

Pseudoxanthoma elasticum is a disorder of elastic fibres and is inherited as both an autosomal recessive and occasionally an autosomal dominant trait. A variety of clinical syndromes with different inheritances exist. The tissue distribution of the abnormality is patchy. Abnormal elastic fibres may be found generally in the walls of arteries or in the skin, where the abnormality is most frequently located in the middle and lower thirds of the dermis. Appearing as groups of soft, yellow papules or macules, the skin lesions are normally first observed in the second or third decade of life. The macules slowly progress in extent and are usually found at the sides of the neck and in the groin. The involvement of elastic tissue in the arteries is most easily seen in the angioid streaks of the retina, and this alteration may progress to cause impairment of vision.

In ordinary haematoxylin and eosin sections of a lesion of pseudoxanthoma elasticum, the accumulation of thickened elastic fibres in the dermis is seen particularly in the lower two thirds of the dermis (Figures 10.1 and 10.2). These abnormal elastic fibres are basophilic, resembling the staining pattern observed in solar elastosis of the dermis, but in the case of pseudoxanthoma elasticum this colour change is due to calcification of the elastic fibres, which can be demonstrated by using von Kossa's stain. The best demonstration of the abnor-

mal elastic tissue is achieved by using Verhoeff's stain (Figure 10.3) which reveals that the abnormal fibres are thickened, curled and appear to have a frayed, irregular edge. In thin histological sections, the abnormal curling of the fibres results in frequent transections, giving an appearance which has been likened to chopped spaghetti. If calcification is marked, there has been reported to be a giant-cell histiocytic response with occasional transepidermal elimination of the abnormal elastic.

Ehlers–Danlos Syndrome

Hyperextensibility of the skin is the chief characteristic of Ehlers–Danlos syndrome. The skin is also susceptible to trauma and heals by abnormal atrophic scars with frequent haematomas. The fundamental disorder is of collagen, and there is hyperextensibility of the joints leading to an abnormally high incidence of dislocations[2]. Ehlers–Danlos syndrome is classified according to the mode of inheritance, the clinical manifestations and the biochemical defects, if known (Table 10.1).

Skin biopsies in Ehlers–Danlos syndrome may show little abnormality in the absence of trauma. If the skin is stretched before fixation to the length it occupied in life, there may be evidence of thinning of the dermal collagen with an increase in the proportion of elastic fibres. However, in most biopsies these abnormalities are undetectable. Traumatized skin from patients with Ehlers–Danlos

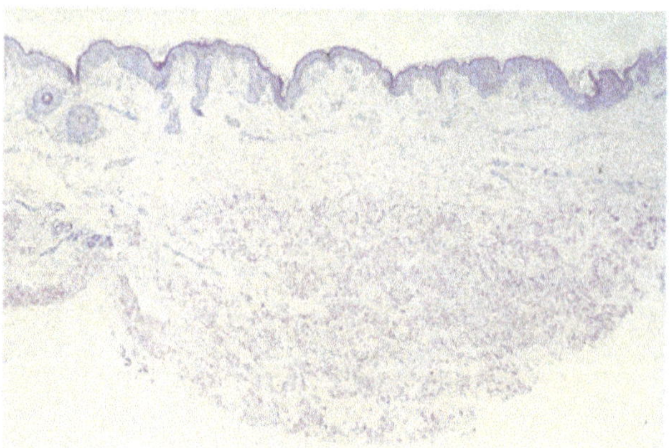

Figure 10.1   Pseudoxanthoma elasticum.   H & E (A)

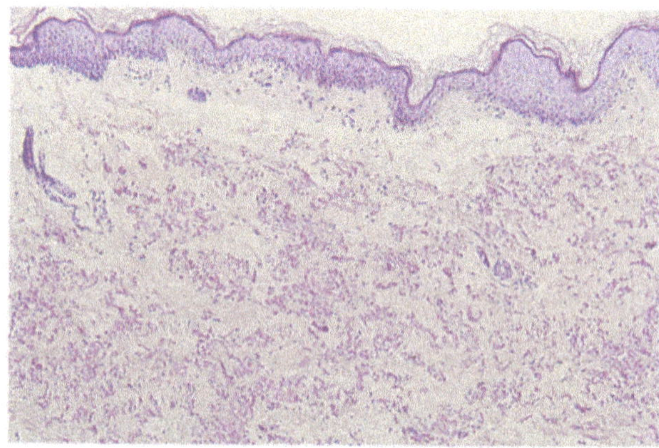

Figure 10.2   Pseudoxanthoma elasticum. The abnormal elastic tissue is to be found in the deeper layers of the dermis.   H & E (B)

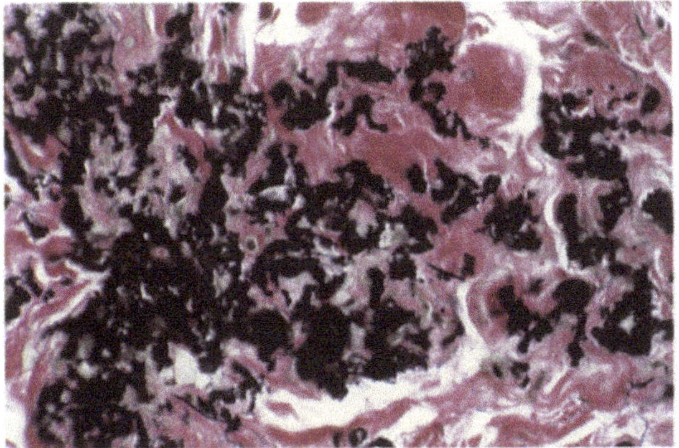

Figure 10.3 Pseudoxanthoma elasticum. In specially stained sections, the fragmented elastic fibres can be more easily identified. Elastic Van Gieson stain. (B)

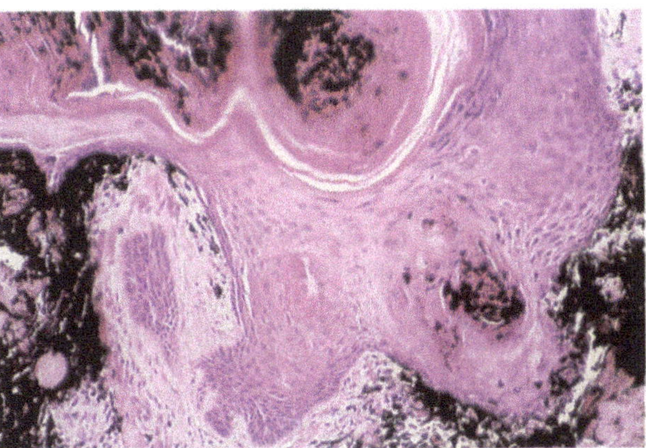

Figure 10.4 Transepidermal elimination of injected foreign material. Black particles of marking ink are seen in the superficial dermis, within a hair follicle and in the horny layer of the epidermis. H & E (B)

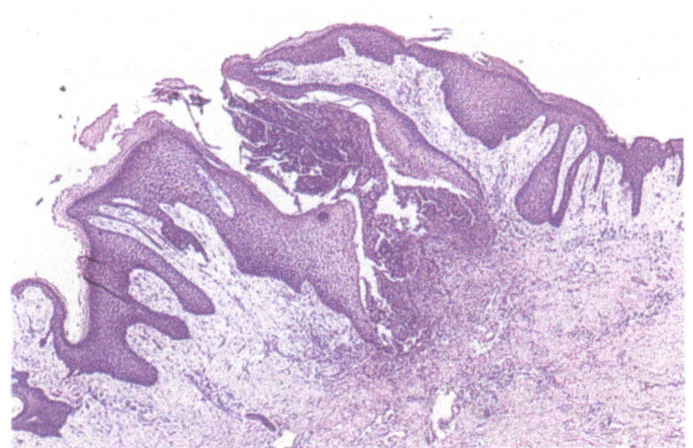

Figure 10.5 Elastosis perforans serpiginosa. A cup-shaped area of transepidermal elimination. H & E (A)

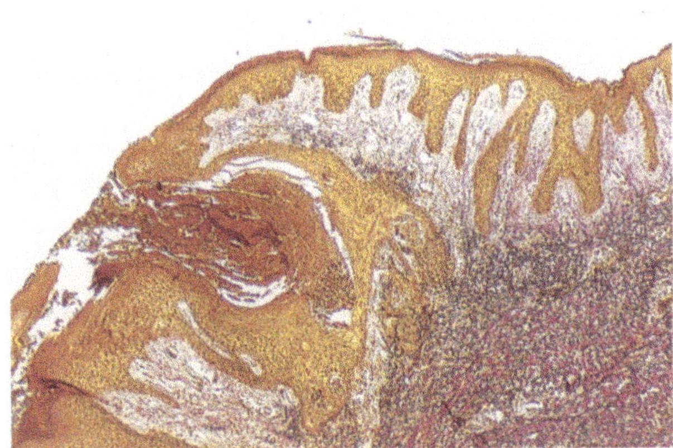

Figure 10.6 Elastosis perforans serpiginosa. Special stains show that elastic fibres extend into the area of transepidermal elimination. EVG (A)

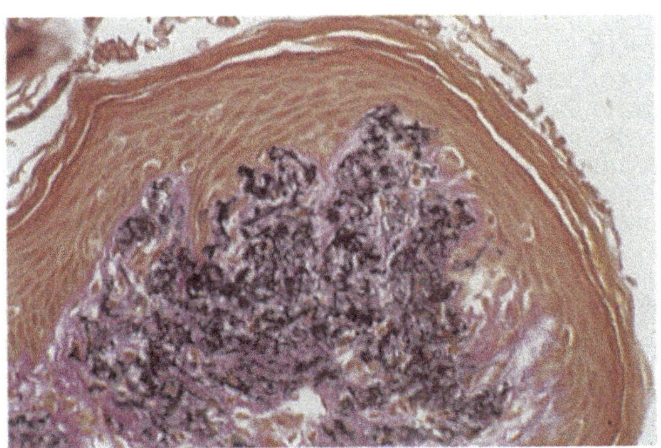

Figure 10.7 Elastosis perforans serpiginosa, showing hyperplasia of elastic fibres in dermal papillae. EVG (B)

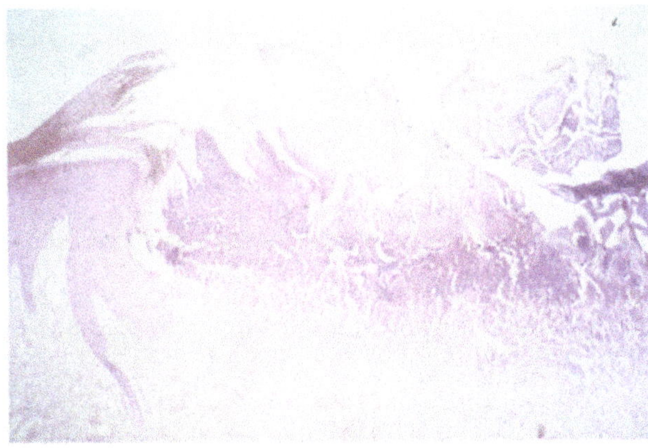

Figure 10.8 Perforating folliculitis. H & E (A)

syndrome may show abnormally prominent haematomas with extensive fat necrosis and areas of dystrophic calcification.

Cutis Laxa (Dermatochalasis, Generalized Elastolysis)

Both congenital and acquired types of cutis laxa have been described. The congenital type is inherited autosomally and is usually a recessive trait, although a milder dominant form has been described. There are systemic manifestations of cutis laxa in both the inherited and non-inherited forms. Frequent complications include pulmonary emphysema, gastrointestinal and urogenital diverticula and hernias; both umbilical, inguinal and hiatus in type[3]. The histological changes of cutis laxa are of breakdown of elastic fibres and deposition of mucopolysaccharides. The changes vary greatly from one area to another and some areas may appear essentially normal. If skin is biopsied from the early stages of cutis laxa the principal change may be of diminished elastic fibres rather than the granular fragmentation typical of the fully developed lesions.

Table 10.1 Classification of Ehlers–Danlos syndrome

Type	Clinical manifestation	Inheritance	Deficiency
I	Gravis; marked skin fragility	Autosomal dominant	Unknown
II	Mitis; frequent skin haematomas	Autosomal dominant	Unknown
III	Benign hypermobile	Autosomal dominant	Unknown
IV	Arterial ecchymoses	Autosomal recessive	Type III collagenase
V	X-linked; similar to Type I	X-linked recessive	Lysyl oxidase
VI	Ocular; intra-ocular haemorrhage	Autosomal recessive	Lysyl hydroxylase
VII	Arthrochalasis; multiple dislocations	Autosomal recessive	Alpha-collagen
VIII	Periodontal	Autosomal dominant	Unknown
IX	Striae, platelet aggregation defect	Autosomal recessive	Plasma fibronectin

Tuberous Sclerosis

Tuberous sclerosis is an autosomal dominant inherited disorder in which there is the variable coincidence of mental deficiency, epilepsy and small, reddish papules at the centre of the face, around the nasolabial folds, cheeks and chin[4]. Subungual fibromata and hypopigmented macular areas are also seen. Although the skin papules have been termed 'adenoma sebaceum of Pringle' they are angiofibromas[5], which consist of areas of fibrosis of the dermis associated with dilated capillary blood vessels[6]. The collagen in these lesions may contain proliferating stellate fibroblasts which tend to compress adnexal structures to produce atrophy of hair follicles and sebaceous glands. There may also be so-called shagreen patches occurring as thickened areas of skin, in the lumbosacral region. These lesions are connective tissue naevi and may be the earliest manifestation of tuberous sclerosis. Although variable in appearance, the most typical histological appearance of a shagreen patch is of concentric hyperplasia of collagen bundles around the adnexal structures in the lower third of the dermis. In other cases, the principal histological finding is of abnormally orientated fibres of collagen in the dermis, so that the normal parallel orientation of collagen is lost and the fibres become interwoven.

Connective Tissue Naevus

Connective tissue naevi occur as one or more pale or yellow plaques of widespread distribution. When genetically determined, they are inherited in an autosomal dominant manner[7]. Some such naevi are essentially abnormalities of elastic fibres, and there may be great variation within individual lesions[8]. The fibres may be absent or sparse, or greatly increased in number. Occasionally, the increased elastic fibres may coalesce into clusters, giving some similarity to pseudoxanthoma elasticum. However, unlike pseudoxanthoma elasticum there are neither degenerative changes nor evidence of calcification in connective tissue naevi.

Werner's Syndrome

Although inherited, this autosomal recessive condition is only manifested between the ages of 10 and 30 years. The skin of the arms and legs is tense. There are signs of progeria such as cataracts and greying hair and premature death from atheroma of the arteries is a common complication.

Histologically, there is atrophy of sweat glands, fibrosis of the dermis and hyalinization of the collagen. The epidermis is atrophic and the dermal papillae are flattened. These appearances are very similar to those of scleroderma, except in that there is no inflammatory infiltration, even in the early stages of the disease.

Perforating Diseases with Transepithelial Elimination

Transepidermal elimination is a phenomenon in which material is expelled from the dermis through the epidermis to the surface. This process is seen as a response to the injection of foreign bodies (Figure 10.4) or spontaneously in certain skin disorders[9] (Table 10.2), in which degraded connective tissue acts as the foreign material. The effete connective tissue may be eliminated either through the epidermis or through a follicle. Of these conditions, pseudoxanthoma elasticum is considered at the beginning of this chapter, and granuloma annulare and necrobiosis lipoidica are considered in Chapter 7. The remaining conditions are described below.

Elastosis Perforans Serpiginosa

This unusual disorder occurs in two closely related forms[10,11]. Clinically, both forms have a similar appearance, consisting of annular clusters of scaling papules up to 0.5 cm in diameter. The idiopathic form is often associated with inherited disorders such as Down's or Marfan's syndromes or pseudoxanthoma elasticum. The other form of elastosis perforans serpiginosa is that associated with prolonged penicillamine treatment.

The histological features of elastosis perforans serpiginosa of either of the above types are hyperplasia of dermal elastic tissue, with transepidermal elimination (Figure 10.5). Although these changes are appreciable in ordinary histological sections they are best seen in sections stained for elastic tissue with Verhoeff's reagents (Figure 10.6). Most characteristic of elastosis perforans serpiginosa is the presence of hyperplastic elastic fibres in the dermal papillae (Figure 10.7). Transepidermal elimination of elastic fibres is through deep, narrow and hyperplastic follicular channels. Characteristically, the elastic within the channels is degenerate and loses its affinity for Verhoeff's stain, but small numbers of elastic fibres are usually seen at the base of the channel. Similar changes may be seen in Kyrle's disease

Table 10.2 Diseases with spontaneous transepidermal elimination of dermal content

Elastosis perforans serpiginosa
Kyrle's disease
Perforating folliculitis
Perforating collagenosis
Granuloma annulare
Necrobiosis lipoidica
Pseudoxanthoma elasticum
Sarcoidosis
Foreign bodies
Amyloid

and perforating folliculitis, but in neither of these is there the characteristic hyperplasia of elastic fibres in dermal papillae.

Pencillamine-induced elastosis perforans serpiginosa tends to show rather less hyperplasia of elastic tissue in the papillary dermis than the idiopathic form. The hyperplastic fibres show lateral protuberances at right angles to the main axis of the fibre. Such changes are thought to be specific for the pencillamine-induced form of elastosis perforans serpiginosa.

Kyrle's Disease (Hyperkeratosis Follicularis et Parafollicularis in Cutem Penetrans)

This rare disorder consists of the formation of hyperkeratotic papules up to 0.7 cm in diameter, which may fuse into a plaque[12]. Each papule contains a conical plug which in histological sections can be seen to consist of degenerate parakeratotic material. The epidermis at the depths of the plug lacks a granular layer and consists of vacuolated parakeratotic cells. In some cases, this part of the parakeratotic column may penetrate into the dermis and evoke a foreign-body giant cell histiocytic response. Beneath the lesion of Kyrle's disease there may be condensation of elastic fibres due to compression, but there is no hypertrophy of elastic of the type seen in elastosis perforans serpiginosa.

Perforating Folliculitis

Although there are some features of similarity between Kyrle's disease and perforating folliculitis, there are sufficient differences to establish them as separate entities[13]. Clinically, although the lesions of perforating folliculitis are similar to those of Kyrle's disease, they usually arise after injury and are always on the elbows, knees or buttocks, always involve a hair follicle and do not coalesce to form plaques.

Histologically, the perforating folliculitis plug consists of basophilic debris which often contains convoluted hair shafts (Figure 10.8). Unlike Kyrle's disease there is degeneration of the surrounding dermis. The elastic fibres no longer stain with Verhoeff's reagents or orcein but are eosinophilic and homogeneous. No hyperplasia of elastic can be demonstrated.

Perforating Collagenosis

This rare disorder may be sporadic and non-familial or may show autosomal recessive inheritance. Trauma may play a part in the aetiology of some cases.

The area of transepithelial elimination in this disorder is characteristically cup-shaped. The degenerate collagen is basophilic, shows no increase in the amount of elastic fibres and chiefly occupies the papillary dermis. Numerous points of perforation through the overlying epidermis are seen.

References

1. Lund, H. Z. and Gilbert, C. F. (1976). Perforating pseudoxanthoma elasticum. Its distinction from elastosis perforans serpiginosa. *Arch. Pathol. Lab. Med.*, **100**, 544
2. Sulica, V. I., Cooper, P. H., Pope, F. M., Hambrick, G. W. Jr, Gerson, B. M. and McKusick, V. A. (1979). Cutaneous histologic features in Ehlers–Danlos syndrome. *Arch. Dermatol.*, **115**, 40
3. Goltz, R. W., Hutt, A.–M., Goldfarb, M. and Gorlin, R. J. (1965). Cutis laxa. *Arch. Dermatol.*, **92**, 373
4. Bender, B. L. and Yunis, E. J. (1982). The pathology of tuberous sclerosis. *Pathol. Annu.*, **17**, 339
5. Bhawan, J. and Edelstein, L. (1977). Angiofibromas in tuberous sclerosis: a light and electron microscopic study. *J. Cutan. Pathol.*, **4**, 300
6. Sanchez, N. P., Wick, M. R. and Perry, H. O. (1981). Adenoma sebaceum of Pringle: a clinicopathologic review, with a discussion of related pathologic entities. *J. Cutan Pathol.*, **8**, 395
7. Raque, C. J. and Wood, M. G. (1970). Connective tissue nevus. Dermatofibrosis lenticularis disseminata with osteopoikilosis. *Arch. Dermatol.*, **102**, 390
8. Uitto, J., Santa Cruz, D. J. and Eisen, A. Z. (1980). Connective tissue nevi of the skin. Clinical, genetic and histopathologic classification of hamartomas of the collagen, elastin, and proteoglycan type. *J. Am. Acad. Dermatol.*, **3**, 441
9. Batres, E., Klima, M. and Tschen, J. (1982). Transepithelial elimination in cutaneous sarcoidosis. *J. Cutan. Pathol.*, **9**, 50
10. Pedro, S. D. and Garcia, R. L. (1974). Disseminate elastosis perforans serpiginosa. *Arch. Dermatol.*, **109**, 84
11. Brachfeld, J. H. and Wolf, J. E. Jr (1980). Elastosis perforans serpiginosa. *Cutis*, **26**, 503
12. Constantine, V. S., Carter, V. H. (1968). Kyrle's disease. II. Histopathologic findings in five cases and review of the literature. *Arch. Dermatol.*, **97**, 633
13. Mehregan, A. H. (1977). Perforating dermatoses: A clinicopathologic review. *Int. J. Dermatol.*, **16**, 19

Scarring Alopecia of the Scalp

This condition may be the end result of discoid lupus erythematosus, lichen planus, a deep fungus or bacterial infection and pseudopelade of Brocq, although there is some doubt as to whether the last is a separate entity. There is localized scarring atrophy of the scalp with permanent loss of hair follicles.

Histopathology

In pseudopelade of Brocq there is a mononuclear cell infiltrate around the upper part of the hair follicles. The lower part is clear. There will also be an upper dermal perivascular lymphocytic infiltrate. The cells invade the follicle and sebaceous glands leading to their destruction. In the late stages the follicles are replaced by fibrous cords, and there is extensive fibrosis in the dermis[1]. An elastic stain will demonstrate the site of scarred follicles.

Discoid lupus erythematosus differs because the inflammatory infiltrate is also scattered throughout the dermis and not just around the follicles. In addition there will be basal cell liquefaction and cytoid body formation at the dermo-epidermal junction. However in the late stages where no inflammatory changes are present the fibrotic result will be very similar to pseudopelade of Brocq.

Elastic stains are useful in demonstrating scarred areas in the scalp. Elastic fibres are lost in scarred dermis and localized clumping of elastic tissue occurs around the sites of previous follicles[2] (Figure 11.1).

Alopecia Mucinosa (Follicular Mucinosis)

A rare condition having two clinical forms. A benign type occurs on the face or scalp as boggy follicular plaques devoid of hair. Lesions resolve spontaneously. The malignant form is associated with mycosis fungoides and may be very widespread.

Histopathology

Mucinous change occurs in the outer root sheath and sebaceous glands. Accumulation of mucin appears in and between the cells which degenerate resulting in cystic spaces[3] (Figure 11.2). An inflammatory infiltrate of lymphocytes, histiocytes and eosinophils is present within and around the affected follicles (Figure 11.3). The mucin can be demonstrated with the PAS stain, Hale procedure or by Alcian blue[4] (see page 13). A search should be made for evidence of mycosis fungoides cells in the dermis and migrating into the epidermis.

Trichotillomania

Compulsive hair pulling can lead to patches of alopecia. However, in trichotillomania there is a stubble of regrowth and in alopecia areata the bald patches are uniformly smooth.

Histopathology

Empty hair follicles are found among normally growing hairs in a dermis having no inflammatory infiltrate. Traumatic damage results in retention of partially extracted hairs, clefting in the hair matrix and pigment debris in affected follicles[5,6] (Figure 11.4). Perifollicular haemorrhage is sometimes seen. Sometimes there is an eosinophilic membrane around the follicles. All the follicles are of normal size unlike alopecia areata in which miniature hair structures are the main feature. There is no lymphocytic infiltrate around the hair bulb in trichotillomania.

Alopecia Areata

A common disorder particularly in children and young adults. Localized bald areas are found in the scalp. The typical exclamation mark hairs are short dark hairs which taper towards the follicle. Regrowth occurs in 4–6 months. The condition is sometimes associated with vitiligo and thyroid disease.

Histopathology

Miniature hair structures are characteristic of alopecia areata. They may be dystrophic early anagen or telogen hairs. The early anagen hairs are more common in fresh lesions. The bulb is higher than mature anagen hair structure and keratinization of the hair is incomplete. Dystrophic telogen hair structures are smaller, have a thin cord of epithelium at their base and are surrounded by a thick convoluted fibrous root sheath. Around many of the miniature hair structures is a prominent dermal infiltrate of lymphocytes during the active stage of the disorder[7,8]. They may invade the bulb and outer root sheath of the early anagen hairs. This 'swarm of bees' appearance of lymphocytes around the hair follicles is quite characteristic of the disorder (Figure 11.5).

Tinea (Pityriasis) Amiantacea

A localized scaly disease of the scalp associated with temporary alopecia. It generally occurs in young people and is probably of an eczematous aetiology.

Histopathology

Spongiosis, parakeratosis, acanthosis and lymphocytic migration into the epidermis are prominent features. These occur on the epidermal surface and in the follicular canal[9]. No features of psoriasis are seen – in particular no Munro abscesses are present in the stratum corneum. Parakeratotic corneum is layered around the hair like an onion skin. The sebaceous glands may be shrunken. Eczematous changes are therefore characteristic.

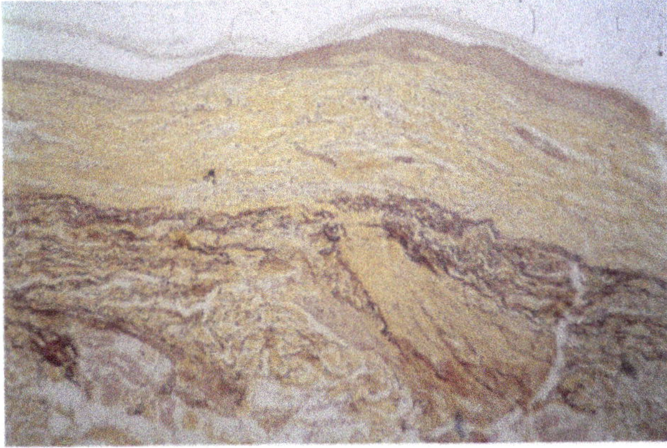

Figure 11.1 Scarring alopecia. Section of scalp, elastic fibres stain black. Note absence of elastic fibres at site of scarred hair follicle in mid dermis. Also loss of elastic fibres in upper dermis. Weigert's stain counterstained with Van Gieson. (C)

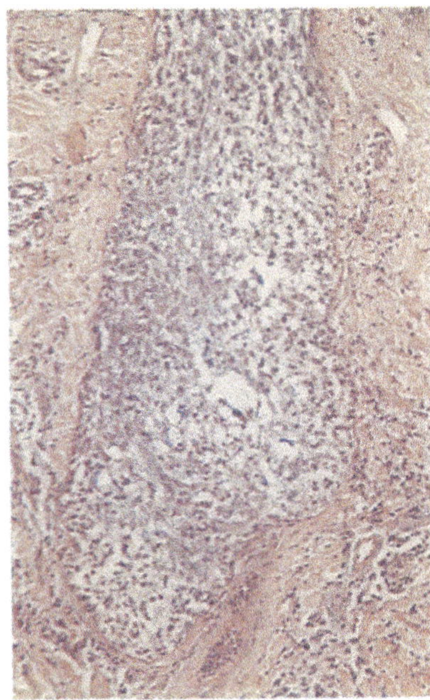

Figure 11.2 Follicular mucinosis. Mucinous degeneration of hair follicle and inflammatory infiltrate within the follicle. Mucin stains blue. Alcian blue. (C)

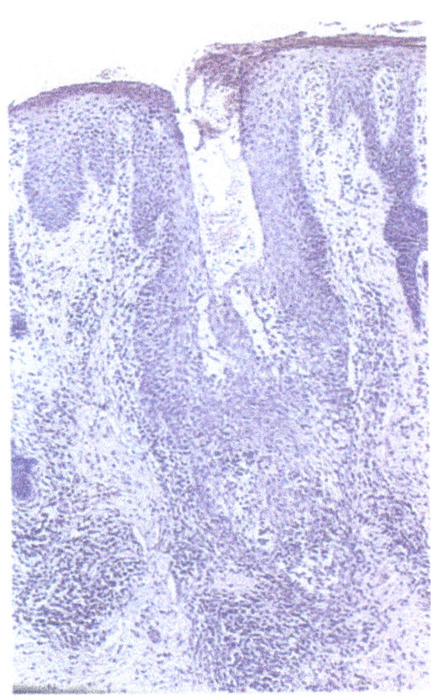

Figure 11.3 Follicular mucinosis. Mucinous degeneration of follicle with intense inflammatory infiltrate within and around the follicle. H & E (B)

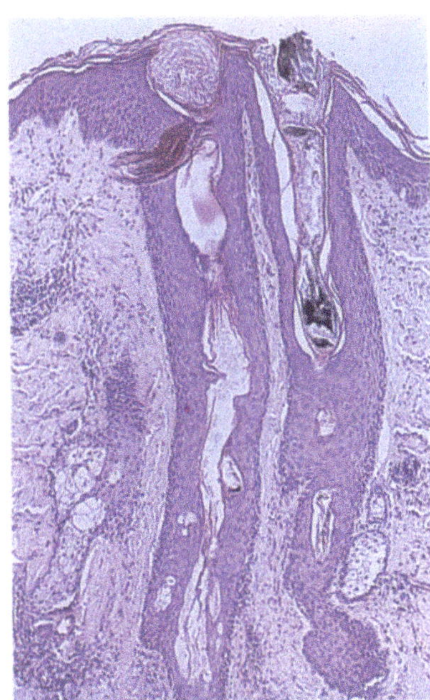

Figure 11.4 Trichotillomania. Note normal size of hair follicles. Some pigment debris within follicles. H & E (B)

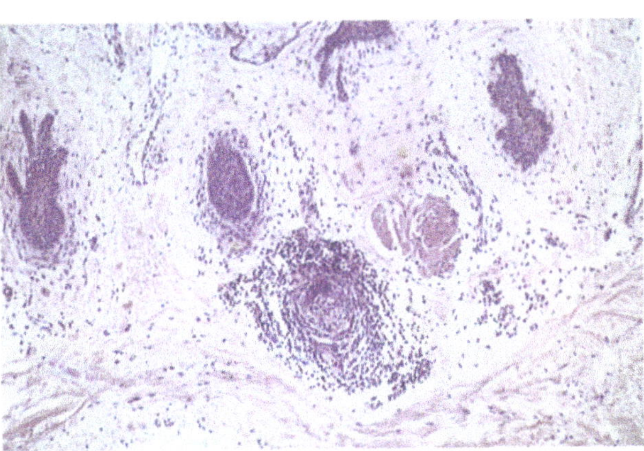

Figure 11.5 Alopecia areata. 'Swarm of bees' appearance around miniature hair bulb. The infiltrate is mostly lymphocytes. H & E (B)

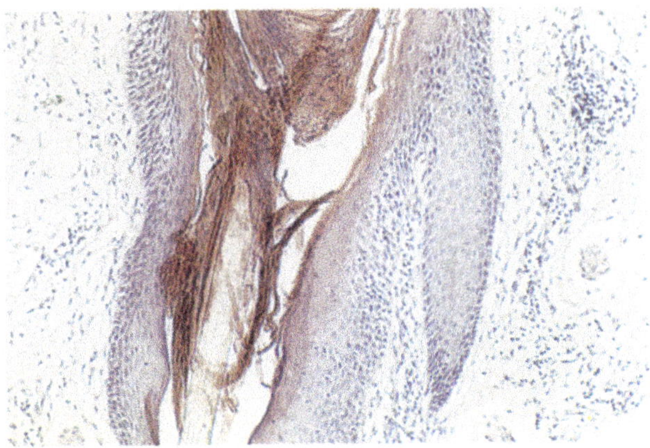

Figure 11.6 Pityriasis amiantacea. Parakeratotic corneum is layered around the hair. Some spongiosis in the follicular wall. H & E (B)

References

1. Pinkus, H. (1980). Alopecia: clinicopathologic correlations. *Int. J. Dermatol.*, **19**, 245

2. Pinkus, H. (1978). Differential patterns of elastic fibres in scarring and non-scarring alopecias. *J. Cutan. Pathol.*, **5**, 93

3. Emmerson, R. W. (1969). Follicular mucinosis. *Br. J. Dermatol.*, **81**, 395

4. Pinkus, H. (1957). Alopecia mucinosa. *Arch. Dermatol.*, **76**, 419

5. Lachapelle, J. M. and Pierard, G. E. (1977). Traumatic alopecia in trichotillomania. *J. Cutan. Pathol.*, **4**, 51

6. Muller, S. A. and Winkelmann, R. K. (1972). Trichotillomania. *Arch. Dermatol.*, **105**, 535

7. Goos, M. (1971). Zur histopathologie der Alopecia areata. *Arch. Dermatol. Forsch.*, **240**, 160

8. Pierard, G. E. and de la Brussinne, M. (1975). Cellular activity in the dermis surrounding the hair bulb in alopecia areata. *J. Cutan. Pathol.*, **2**, 240

9. Knight, A. G. (1977). Pityriasis amiantacea: A clinical and histopathological investigation. *Clin. Exp. Derm.*, **2**, 137

Porphyrias

The dermatological manifestations of porphyria are the result of damage caused by photosensitivity to long-wave ultraviolet light absorbed by porphyrins in the skin[1]. The histological changes in the skin are similar in the various forms of porphyria, but they tend to vary in degrees of severity.

Porphyria Cutanea Tarda

Porphyria cutanea tarda is characterized by the appearance of blisters on light-exposed sites. Pigmentation, hirsutes and scleroderma-like changes may also be seen at these sites. The bullae have a rather characteristic histological appearance[2] with the level of clefting being located in the subepidermal zone (Figure 12.1). The floor of the bulla is irregular due to the persistence of the ridges of the dermal papillae. Capillary blood vessels in the papillae are surrounded by amorphous material which stains with PAS reagents even after pretreatment with diastase (Figure 12.2). Besides the preservation of dermal papillae in the base of the blister, the lesions of porphyria cutanea tarda are typically devoid of a significant inflammatory-cell infiltrate, despite the presence of IgG and complement around the blood vessels of the affected skin of most cases. The immunoglobulin is thought to be merely entrapped in the hyaline deposit, and not to represent an immune response.

Erythropoietic Protoporphyria

This form of porphyria is characterized by the deposition of hyaline material within the affected skin[3]. The hyaline is principally seen in the vicinity of the endothelial cells of superficial capillary blood vessels, but in more severely affected cases the deposit may be seen around adnexal structures and may become so extensive as to obliterate the papillary dermis.

This hyaline substance is considered to be basement membrane material synthesized by capillary endothelial cells. Although the ultrastructural appearances of a multilayered basement membrane arranged around the capillaries is quite distinctive, the changes are not pathognomonic in that similar appearances are seen in electron micrographs of skin biopsies from cases of lipoid proteinosis[4]. Collagen is seen within the hyaline deposits in the skin of patients with erythropoietic porphyria, and the end result of the dermatological manifestation of this disorder is superficial dermal scarring.

Although the hyaline deposits in porphyria can be recognized in ordinary haematoxylin and eosin sections, they are best demonstrated by staining with PAS reagents (Figure 12.3). The deposits also contain mucopolysaccharides and lipids, and can also be demonstrated by alcian blue, colloidal iron and Sudan stains. Similar staining reactions are seen in the cases of hyalin deposition in the skin in lipoid proteinosis.

Amyloidosis

Amyloid can be seen in the skin as part of a systemic disease or as an isolated phenomenon. Although the electron-microscopic appearance of amyloid is the same in the various forms of the disease, there are different biochemical forms of amyloid[5]. In primary and myeloma-associated amyloidosis the amyloid is formed from light-chain immunoglobulin and is called AL amyloid. In secondary amyloidosis the amyloid is derived from alpha-globulin in the serum (AA amyloid). Dermal deposits have been reported in about a third of cases of primary systemic amyloidosis: secondary amyloidosis does not usually affect the skin. Purely cutaneous forms of amyloidosis include lichenoid and macular variants[6].

Systemic Amyloidosis

In secondary amyloidosis, only very small amounts of amyloid material have been demonstrated in the walls of the capillaries of subcutaneous fat, but this may be a useful site for diagnostic biopsy if the usual rectal biopsy is unavailable. Primary amyloidosis, on the other hand, may be associated with the development of cutaneous petechiae due to the development of capillary fragility and the development of discrete amyloid papules, which may also undergo petechial haemorrhage.

In histological sections of skin involved by primary systemic amyloidosis the characteristic amyloid deposits are seen both in the dermis and in the subcutaneous tissue. The dermal deposits usually include some foci immediately beneath the epidermis and within the papillary ridges. Although the earliest deposits occur around the capillary blood vessels, the lesions eventually coalesce and involve dermal collagen and eccrine glands.

Amyloid substance is easily overlooked in routine sections stained with haematoxylin and eosin. Metachromatic stains, such as crystal violet, may be used to demonstrate amyloid, but the most useful special stain is probably Congo red[7]. Although many structures within the skin may stain with Congo red, the apple green dichroism seen when Congo red-stained amyloid material is viewed with polarized light is almost specific. Apart from amyloid, only the hyaline material seen in porphyria, lipoid proteinosis and colloid milium is likely to show orange–green dichroism. These diseases are usually clinically distinctive and are unlikely to be confused with amyloidosis. Electron-microscopic examination may reveal unbranched filaments about 6 nm in diameter, and ultrastructural examination of biopsies may be useful in detecting very small quantities of amyloid substance.

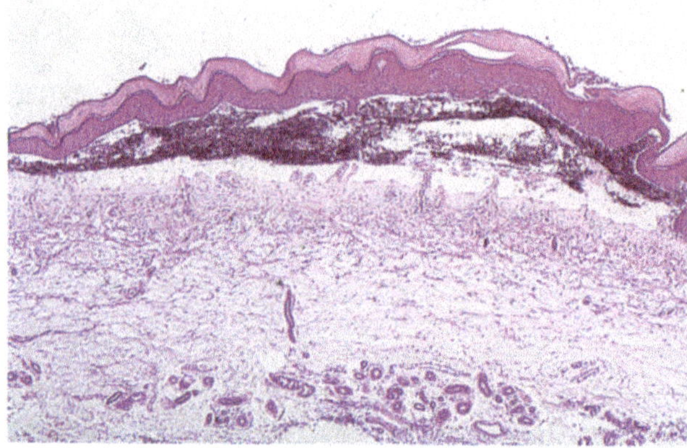

Figure 12.1 Porphyria cutanea tarda. Subepidermal bulla formation without inflammatory reaction. H & E (A)

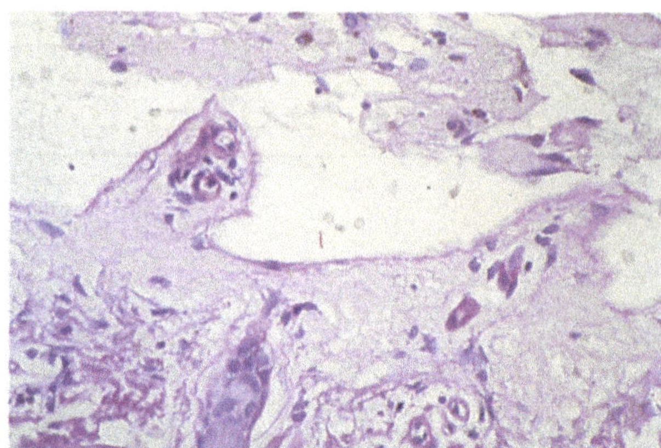

Figure 12.2 Porphyria cutanea tarda. Hyaline in the walls of the capillaries in the base of the bulla stains positively with PAS reagents. PAS (C)

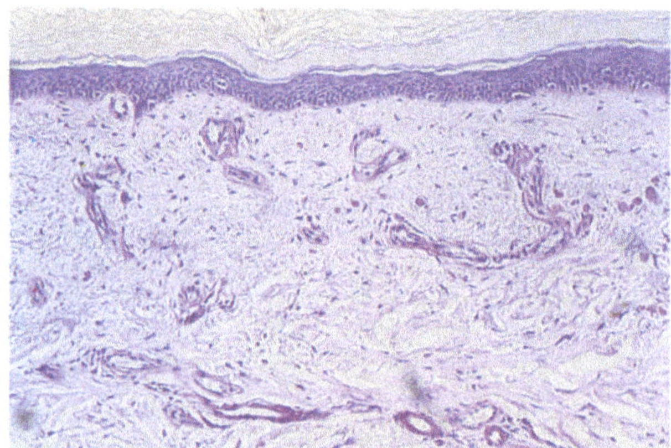

Figure 12.3 Porphyria variegata. No blistering occurs in this form of porphyria, but hyaline material can be demonstrated in the walls of capillary blood vessels in the superficial dermis. PAS (B)

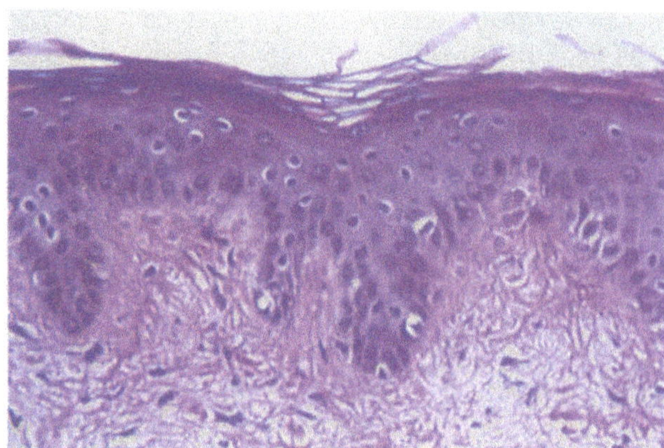

Figure 12.4 Macular amyloidosis. In ordinarily stained sections it is easy to overlook the small amyloid bodies, confined to the tips of the dermal papillae. H & E (B)

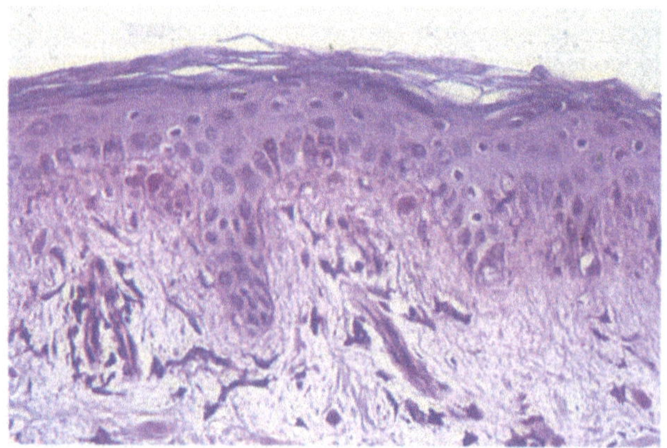

Figure 12.5 Macular amyloidosis. Amyloid bodies are more easily identified in this specially stained section. PAS (B)

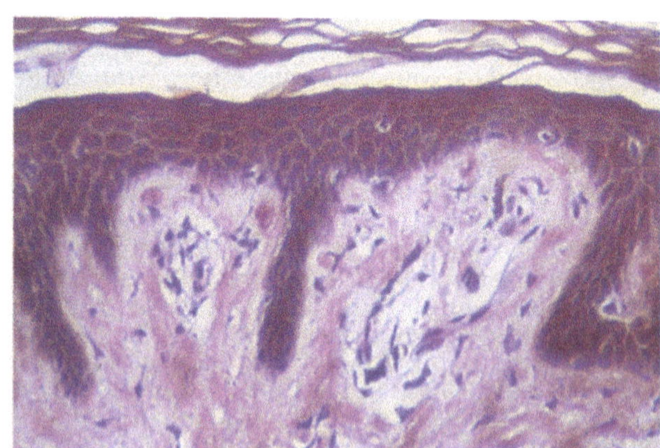

Figure 12.6 Macular amyloidosis. Amyloid bodies in the papillary dermis are identified by being stained with Congo red. (B)

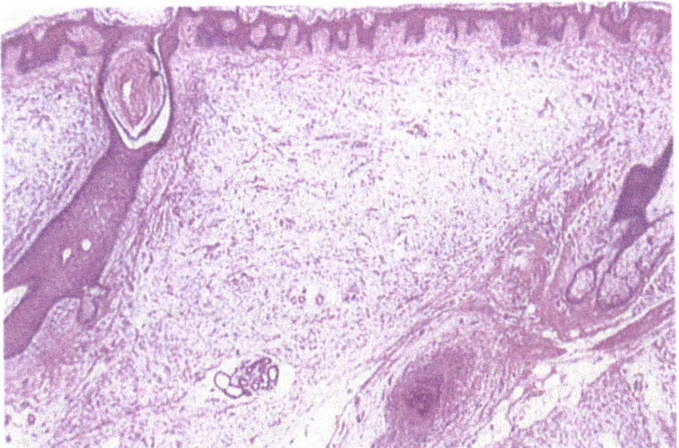

Figure 12.7 Pretibial myxoedema. The collagen bundles of the dermis are separated by pale-staining myxoid ground substance, which can be demonstrated by Hale's colloidal iron or alcian blue staining. H & E (A)

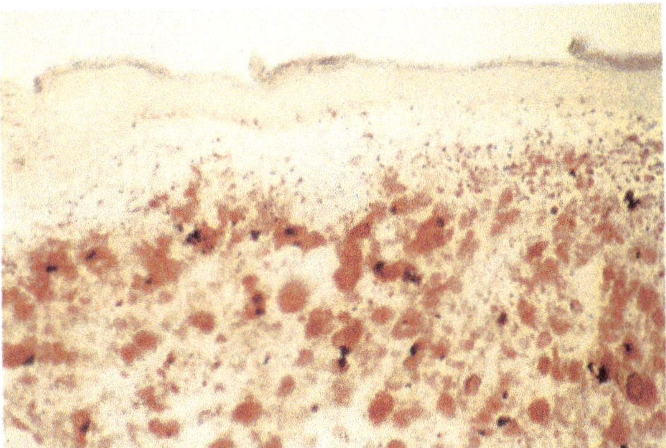

Figure 12.8 Xanthoma. The lipid content is demonstrated by special staining. Oil red O (B)

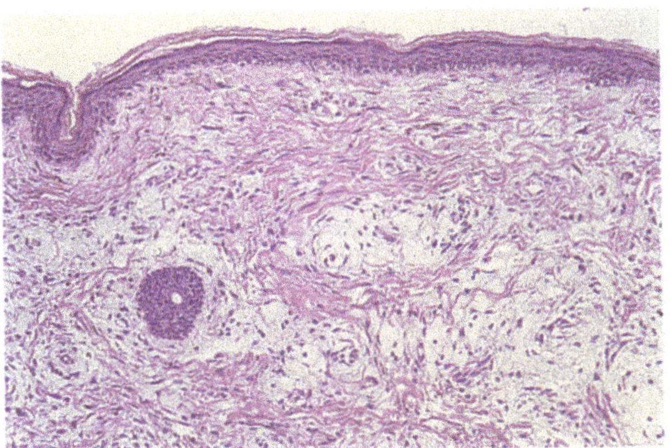

Figure 12.9 Xanthelasma. H & E (B)

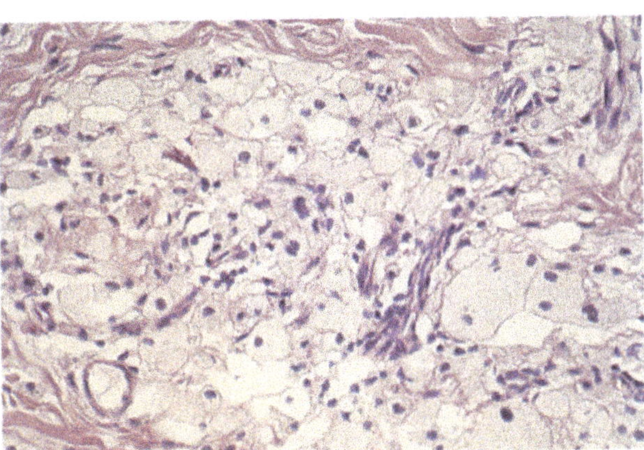

Figure 12.10 Xanthelasma. Foamy macrophages are scattered thoughout the superficial dermis. H & E (C)

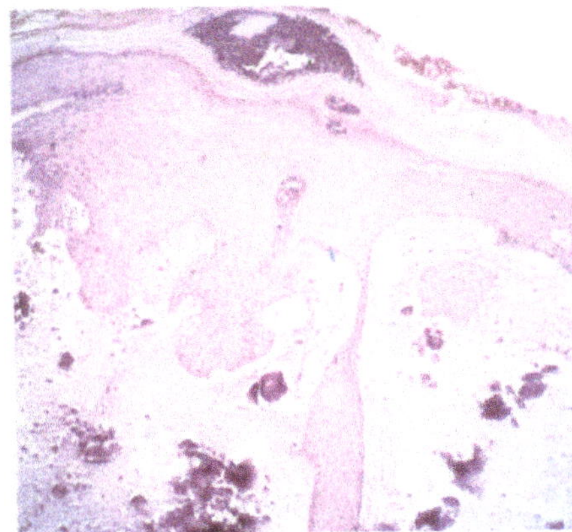

Figure 12.11 Calcinosis cutis. Small foci of haematoxyphil calcium salts can be seen in the reticular dermis. H & E (A)

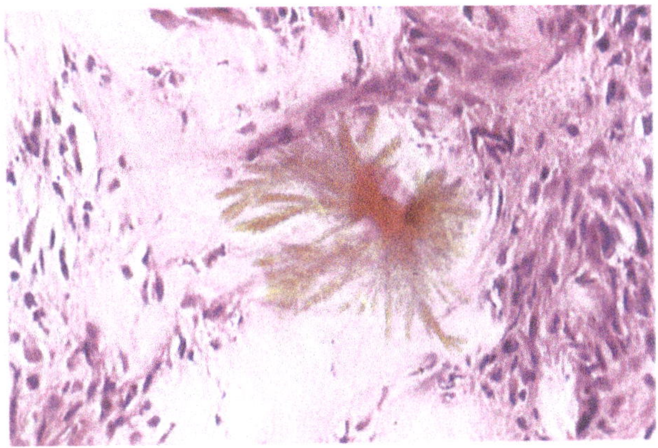

Figure 12.12 Gouty tophus. In ordinary histological sections, most of the urate crystals are dissolved during processing and may be difficult to identify. Nonetheless, the admixture of clumps of amorphous deposit surrounded by a histiocytic and giant-cell inflammatory response is quite characteristic. H & E (B)

Localized Amyloidosis

Although two forms of localized amyloidosis (macular and lichenoid) have been described, they are really varieties of the same process. In macular amyloidosis the lesions are characteristically pigmented and pruritic. The lichenoid lesions also itch, but are papular and hyperkeratotic, red–brown plaques.

Unlike the skin lesions of systemic amyloidosis, the amyloid deposits of both macular and lichenoid amyloidosis are confined to the papillary dermis. The amyloid is most prominent in the lichenoid lesion, which is also characterized by acanthosis and hyperkeratosis of the epidermis. In macular amyloidosis, the deposits of amyloid may be very scanty and are easily overlooked (Figures 12.4–12.6).

Mucinosis[8]

Ground substances in the dermis of the skin include mucins with a high proportion of hyaluranic acid. In several conditions the amount of mucin is increased in the dermis to produce a palpable nodule or plaque. Perhaps most common of these conditions in myxoedema in thyroid disease. Generalised myxoedema is due to thyroid insufficiency and is characterised by a dry, pale skin with a rather firm consistency. In histological sections of skin it is usually difficult to demonstrate the excess of mucins. Pretibial myxoedema, however, usually contains demonstrable mucoid ground substance in the dermis (Figure 12.7). This condition is associated with thyrotoxicosis and is mostly seen on the anterior aspect of the leg and the dorsum of the foot. In the absence of thyroid disease, excessive dermal mucins are most commonly associated with papular mucinosis or scleromyxoedema.

Papular Mucinosis

The papules of papular mucinosis are small, measuring only about 2 mm in diameter, although occasionally larger nodules are seen[9]. Nodules and papules are both soft in consistency. Histological examination of the papules shows a localized area of mucin deposition in the superficial dermis. The surrounding collagen shows a reactive hyperplasia.

Scleromyxoedema

Mucin deposition, similar to that seen in papular mucinosis, is the hallmark of scleromyxoedema[10]. However, the mucin deposition is more widespread and is associated with a greater hyperplasia of dermal collagen fibres. The consequent thickening of the skin can cause such coarsening of the skin folds as to simulate scleroderma, although the immobility of the skin seen in scleroderma is not seen in scleromyxoedema. Immunofluorescence studies may reveal the presence of IgG in the mucin. Almost all cases of scleromyxoedema have a monoclonal paraprotein in the serum, usually of the IgG type. Although the relationship of the IgG to the mucin is unclear, the constant presence of IgG in the serum suggests that a plasma cell dyscrasia may be involved in the pathogenesis of scleromyxoedema. Nonetheless, there have only been one or two cases of scleromyxoedema associated with multiple myeloma.

Xanthoma and Xanthelasma

Xanthoma

The characteristic cell of xanthomas is the foamy histiocyte. The lipid content of the histiocytes gives the xanthoma a yellow colour. Clinical forms of xanthoma include eruptive, tuberous, tendon and plane types[11]. All are associated with the various types of hyperlipoproteinaemia. Eruptive xanthomas are small papules on the buttocks, thighs and elsewhere and are seen in all forms of hyperlipoproteinaemia apart from type IIA (hyperbeta-lipoproteinaemia). On the other hand, tuberous xanthomas are found on the elbows, knees and fingers and are associated with hyperbetalipoproteinaemias of types II, III and IV. Plane and tendon xanthomas occur predominantly in the type III (broad-beta) hyperlipoproteinaemia. The tendons most commonly affected are Achilles tendon and the tendons in the fingers.

In histological sections, the characteristic foamy histiocytes appear empty because the lipid in their cytoplasm has been extracted by the organic solvents used during processing of the section. In frozen sections, however, the lipid is readily demonstrated by Sudan and other lipid stains (Figure 12.8). Giant cells are distinctly unusual in xanthomas, but when they are seen they may be of either foreign-body or Touton types. Although the various clinical types of xanthoma have a similar histological appearance, the proportion of cholesterol is higher in tuberous and tendon xanthomas than in eruptive xanthomas. Accordingly, some histological differentiation on frozen sections can be made between these two groups, because the cholesterol in tuberous xanthomas tends to be birefringent.

The appearance of all xanthomas varies with age. Younger lesions have less foamy cells than mature lesions and a higher proportion of chronic inflammatory cells. Aged lesions consist almost entirely of foam cells but eventually there may be an increase in collagen within the lesion as well. Only the plane xanthoma, usually from the skin of the palms of the hands, is free from fibrosis in a fully matured lesion.

There is a strong correlation between the presence of a xanthoma and hyperlipoproteinaemia[12]. Consequently, all patients with xanthoma should have measurements of fasting concentrations of triglycerides and cholesterol in the serum and maybe lipoprotein electrophoresis.

Xanthelasma

Although very similar to xanthomas, these common lesions differ in some respects. Only about one-third of patients with xanthelasmas have hyperlipoproteinaemia, a far lower proportion than is the case with xanthomas. Nonetheless, the frequent incidence of xanthelasmas makes them the commonest skin lesion in type IIA (hyperbeta) hyperlipoproteinaemia, and testing of the serum, as in patients with xanthomas, is advisable.

Xanthelasmas occur on the eyelids as small, soft, flattened yellow papules and plaques. Histologically, they differ from xanthomas in that the characteristic foamy macrophages are located very superficially and like plane xanthomas, but unlike eruptive, tuberous or tendon xanthomas, there is no evidence of fibrosis (Figures 12.9 and 12.10).

Calcinosis Cutis

Calcification may occur in the skin in a variety of conditions, either due to high circulating levels of calcium or phosphate, or due to local tissue necrosis and precipitation of cytoplasmic calcium[13,14]. When due to hypercalcaemia or hyperphosphataemia, the calcinosis is termed metastatic; when due to tissue necrosis, the term dystrophic calcinosis cutis is used.

In both types of calcinosis histological sections contain haematoxyphil amorphous deposits in the dermis and subcutis (Figure 12.11). The presence of calcium salts in the deposits can be confirmed by using von Kossa's stain or, more specific, alizarin red S. Larger calcium deposits evoke a foreign-body giant cell reaction and may undergo metaplasia into bone. Dystrophic calcinosis may occur in scleroderma[14].

Gouty Tophus

Improvements in the diagnosis and treatment of gout have resulted in a reduction in the number of cases in which urate crystals are deposited in the skin (gouty tophus). When tophi occur, they are most common around the joints of the elbows, fingers and toes and in the pinna of the ears[15]. If they grow to several centimetres in size, there is a tendency for tophi to discharge through the epidermis as a chalk-like powder.

In histological sections prepared by routine methods the urate crystals are largely dissolved during clearing and mounting of the section. Formalin fixation may make some of the crystals amorphous and better preservation is seen in alcohol-fixed tissue. Urate crystals are soluble in the organic solvents used for clearing and mounting histological sections. Accordingly, the usual appearances are of spaces and scanty crystals surrounded by a florid foreign-body giant-cell response (Figure 12.12). The extent of crystal deposition and foreign-body response are quite characteristic, but confirmation of the presence of urate is best obtained by examination of a smear of crystals in a wet preparation under polarized light when the typical needle shape can easily be discerned[16].

References

1. Epstein, J. H., Tuffanelli, D. L. and Epstein, W. L. (1973). Cutaneous changes in the porphyrias. *Arch. Dermatol.*, **107**, 689

2. Cormane, R. H., Szabo, E. and Tio, T. Y. (1971). Histopathology of the skin in acquired and hereditary porphyria cutanea tarda. *Br. J. Dermatol.*, **85**, 531

3. Stretcher, G. S. (1977). Erythropoietic porphyria. *Arch. Dermatol.*, **113**, 1553

4. Wolff, K., Honigsmann, H., Rauschmeier, W., Schuler, G. and Pechlaner, R. (1982). Microscopic and fine structural aspects of porphyrias. *Acta Derm. Venereol. (Stockh.) (Suppl.)*, **100**, 17

5. Glenner, G. G. (1980). Amyloid deposits and amyloidosis. The β-fibrilloses. *N. Engl. J. Med.*, **302**, 1333

6. Habermann, M. C. and Montenegro, M. R. (1980). Primary cutaneous amyloidosis. Clinical, laboratory and histopathological study in 25 cases. *Dermatologica*, **160**, 240

7. DeLellis, R. L. and Bowling, M. C. (1970). The use of Sirius red and Congo red staining in routine histopathology. *Hum. Pathol.*, **1**, 655

8. Reed, R. J., Clark, W. H. and Mihm, M. C. (1973). The cutaneous mucinoses. *Hum. Pathol.*, **4**, 201

9. Farmer, E. R., Hambrick, G. W. Jr and Schulman, L. E. (1982). Papular mucinosis. A clinicopathologic study of four patients. *Arch. Dermatol.*, **118**, 9

10. Rudner, E. J., Mehregan, A. and Pinkus, H. (1966). Scleromyxoedema. A variant of lichen myxedematosus. *Arch. Dermatol.*, **93**, 3

11. Fleischmajer, R., Hyman, A. B. and Weidman, A. I. (1964). Normolipemic plane xanthomas. *Arch. Dermatol.*, **89**, 319

12. Fleischmajer, R. (1971). Diagnosis and treatment of familial lipoproteinemias. *Int. J. Dermatol.*, **10**, 251

13. Cornelius, C. E. III, Tenenhouse, A. and Weber, J. C. (1968). Calcinosis cutis. *Arch. Dermatol.*, **98**, 219

14. Kolton, B. and Pedersen, J. (1974). Calcinosis cutis and renal failure. *Arch. Dermatol.*, **110**, 256

15. Lichtenstein, L., Scott, H. W. and Levin, M. H. (1959). Pathologic changes in gout. *Am. J. Pathol.*, **32**, 871

16. Culling, C. F. A., Allison, R. T. and Barr, W. T. (1984). *Cellular Pathology Technique.* pp. 591-2. (London: Butterworths)

Alterations in the melanin pigmentation of the skin produce abnormal duskiness or whiteness and may be due to many factors. Lightening of the skin may be due to a deficiency of melanin, or a reduction in the number of melanocytes. In albinism there are normal numbers of melanocytes, whereas in vitiligo the number of melanocytes is reduced or absent. This change is difficult to judge in ordinarily stained histological sections but can be assessed by quantitative electron-microscopic studies[1], or by performing a DOPA oxidase histochemical test. In a similar fashion, darkening of the skin may be caused by an increase in epidermal or subepidermal melanin or an increase in the number of melanocytes. Thus in Addison's disease there is an increase of activity of the cutaneous melanocytes without an alteration in their number, whereas in naevi and melanoma the abnormal pigmentation is associated with melanocytic hyperplasia.

Lentigo and Ephelis

Ephelides (freckles) are seen in histological sections to consist of foci of increased pigmentation of the basal layer of the epidermis. Lentigines are also areas of hyperpigmentation, but there is also elongation of the rete ridges of the epidermis. Two types of benign lentigo have been described. Lentigo simplex shows only moderate extension of rete ridges and there are sometimes small nests of naevus cells indicating gradation of lesions from lentigo simplex into junction naevus (Figure 13.1). Lentigo senilis appears to be stimulated by sun exposure. Elongation of rete ridges is more marked than in lentigo simplex. In some cases the elongation of rete ridges may be so well marked as to produce an appearance very similar to that of reticulated seborrhoeic keratosis (Figure 13.2).

Melanocytic Naevi[2]

On clinical examination, benign melanocytic naevi ('moles') can be flat, dome-shaped or even pedunculated. Flat lesions tend to be pigmented and are usually junctional naevi, whereas dome-shaped and pedunculated lesions may be non-pigmented and are usually intradermal naevi. Naevi arise in adolescence, new 'moles' appearing in later adult life should be viewed with suspicion.

There appears to be a cycle of growth, maturation and involution in melanocytic naevi. In any individual naevus there may be evidence of any or all of these stages of growth, giving the naevus either a junctional, compound or intradermal appearance.

Junctional Naevus

This type of naevus is most common at a young age and is thought of as the earliest phase in the growth cycle.

The characteristic feature is the presence of nests of epitheloid melanocytes in the basal layers of the epidermis (Figure 13.3). These nests are usually concentrated at the tips of the rete ridges. Coarsely clumped melanin is commonplace within the naevus cells and often spills out into the superficial dermis where it is engulfed by macrophages. These so-called melanophages may become so deeply pigmented that proper recognition of their histiocytic nature may be difficult in histological sections, unless they are bleached before staining. Occasional junctional naevi may show a chronic inflammatory cellular infiltrate and, particularly in young patients, there may be significant hyperplasia of the junctional melanocytes nearby.

Intradermal Naevus

In older patients, naevi are usually of the intradermal type. No junctional component is seen, the melanocytes appear as nests and cords of small cells between the collagen bundles of the dermis (Figure 13.4). These nests (or theques) typically contain close-packed, facetted naevus cells. Deeper in the dermis, the naevus cells become elongated and spindle-shaped and appear as cords rather than nests. There is plentiful collagen between the naevus cells so that appearances may resemble those of a neurofibroma. When this change is particularly marked, the lesion is often referred to as a neuroid naevus.

This apparent maturation of the naevus towards its base deep in the dermis is a useful marker of benign behaviour. There are two other common features of intradermal naevi that must not be misinterpreted as indicating malignancy. First is the tendency for the more epithelioid, superficial nests of cells to shrink during processing and produce an appearance that gives a false impression of lymphatic invasion. Second, there is the tendency for mature intradermal naevi to contain large, bizarre naevus giant cells. These cells contain multiple nuclei arranged around the periphery of the cytoplasm or in a single clump at the centre of the cell. Fortunately, this type of cell is rarely seen in malignant melanoma.

Some intradermal naevi may contain components other than melanocytes. Papillomatous naevi may contain hair follicles which can undergo rupture and cause acute inflammation within the naevus. In such cases, the inflammation may eventually be replaced by dystrophic calcification and even ossification.

Compound Naevus

These naevi are commonest in young adult life. They show a combination of the changes described above in junctional and intradermal naevi (Figure 13.5). Melanin pigmentation is rather variable in compound naevi, but is usually confined to the superficial parts of the naevus,

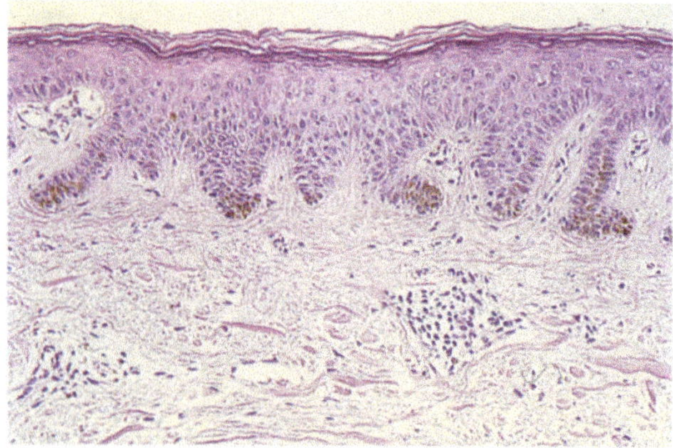

Figure 13.1   Lentigo simplex, showing elongation of rete ridges with an increase in melanin pigmentation at the junction zone.   H & E (B)

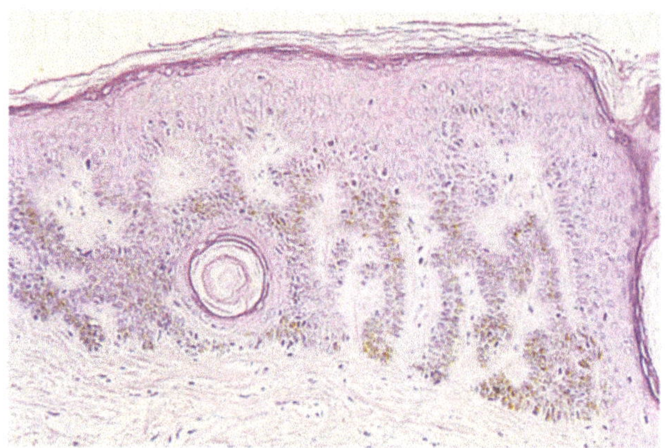

Figure 13.2   Lentigo senilis. The elongation of the rete ridges produces an appearance reminiscent of a reticulated seborrhoeic keratosis.   H & E (B)

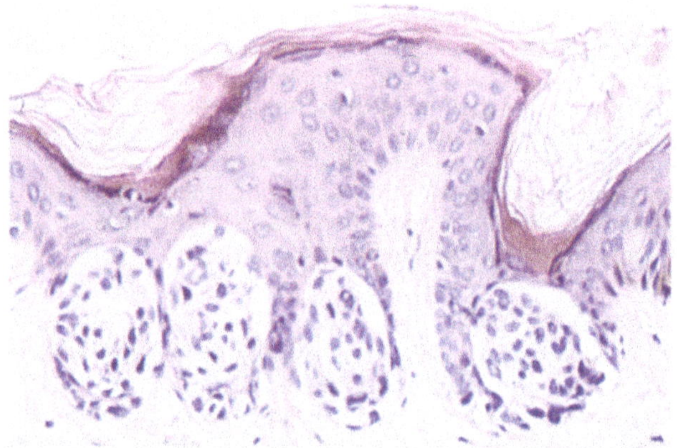

Figure 13.3   Junctional naevus. Nests of naevocytic cells are located at the tips of the rete ridges.   H & E (B)

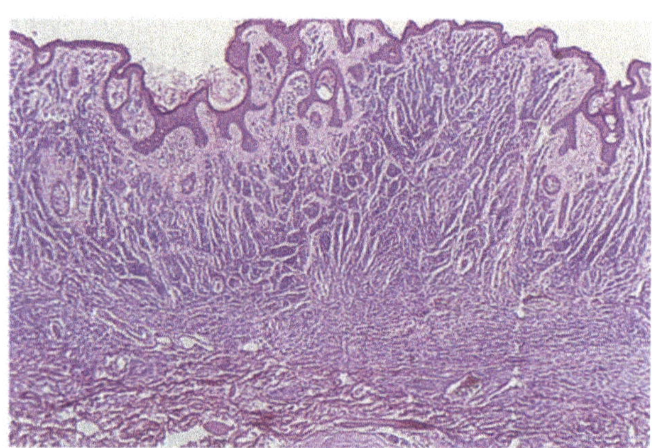

Figure 13.4   Intradermal naevus. Cords of tightly packed naevus cells extend down into the reticular dermis. The symmetry of the lesion is demonstrated at this low magnification.   H & E (A)

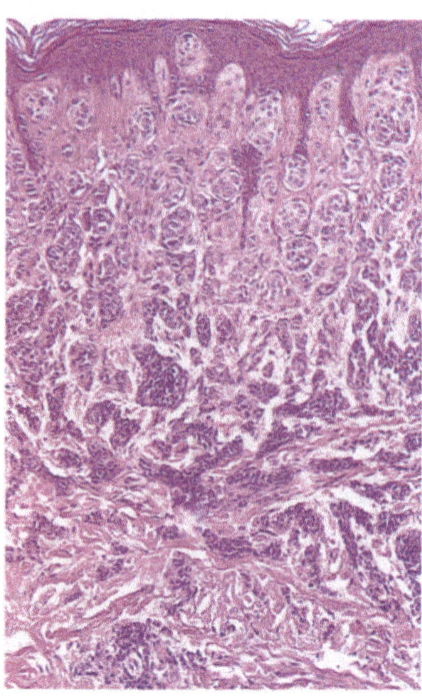

Figure 13.5   Compound naevus. Both junctional and intradermal naevus cells are seen. Compound naevi are typically lightly pigmented. H & E (A)

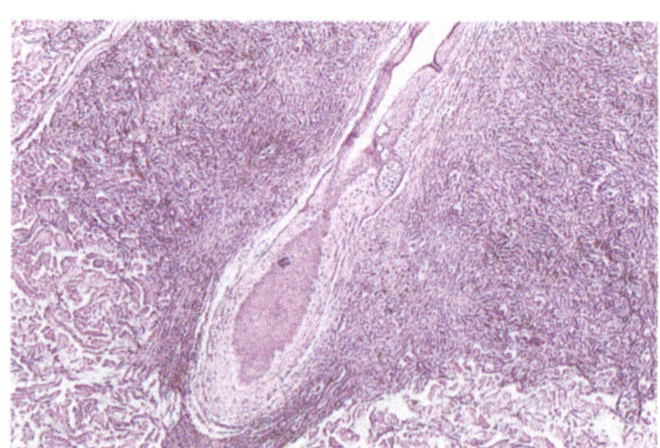

Figure 13.6   Blue naevus. Spindle-shaped, heavily pigmented melanocytes surround a hair follicle.   H & E (A)

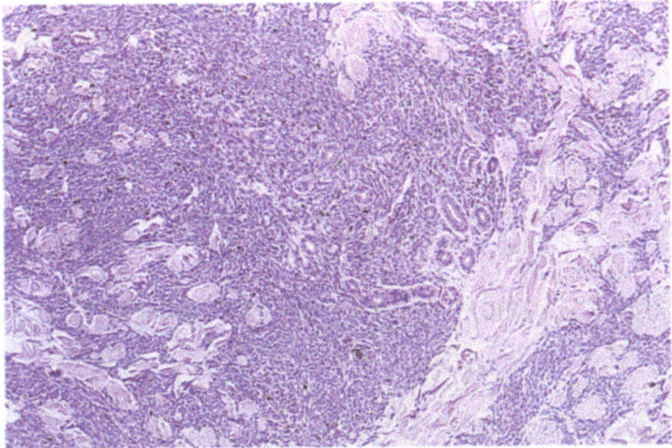

Figure 13.7 Cellular blue naevus. The infiltrative pattern seen at low magnifications does *not* imply malignancy.   H & E (A)

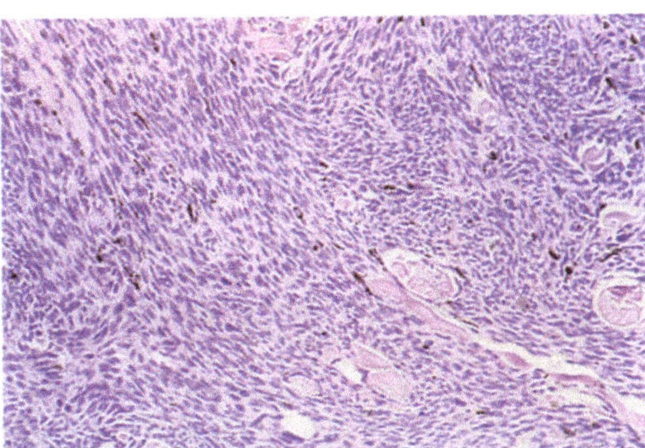

Figure 13.8 Cellular blue naevus. Pigmentation is typically scanty, and mainly within histiocytes.   H & E (A)

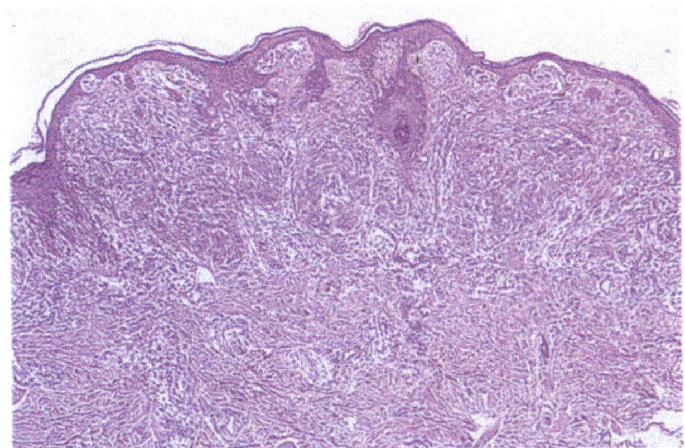

Figure 13.9 Spitz naevus. The lesion is symmetrical, depigmented and has a scanty, perivascular inflammatory-cell infiltrate at the base.   H & E (A)

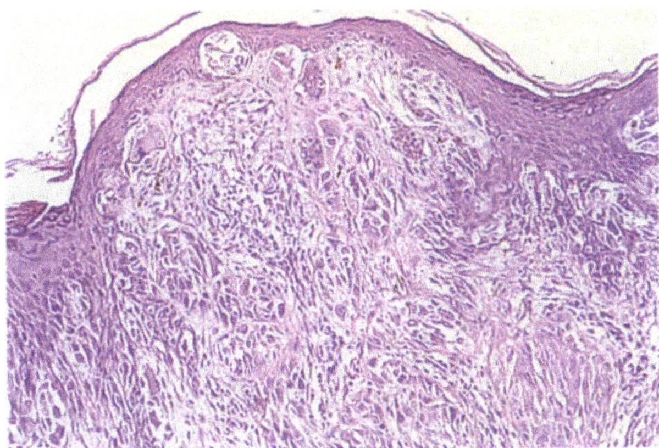

Figure 13.10 Spitz naevus. At higher magnification, the spindle and epithelioid character of the naevus cells can be seen.   H & E (B)

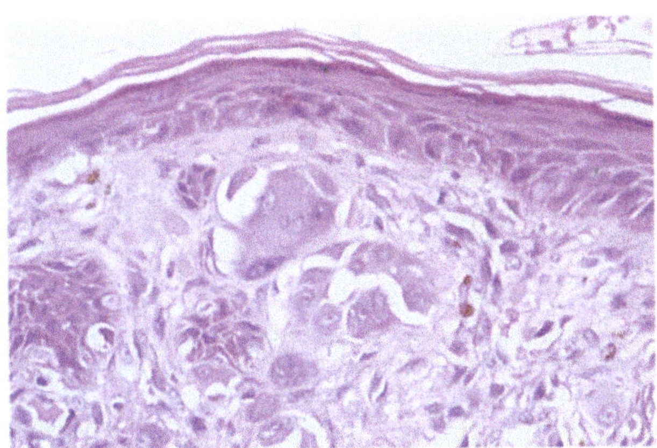

Figure 13.11 Spitz naevus. Junctional giant cells.   H & E (C)

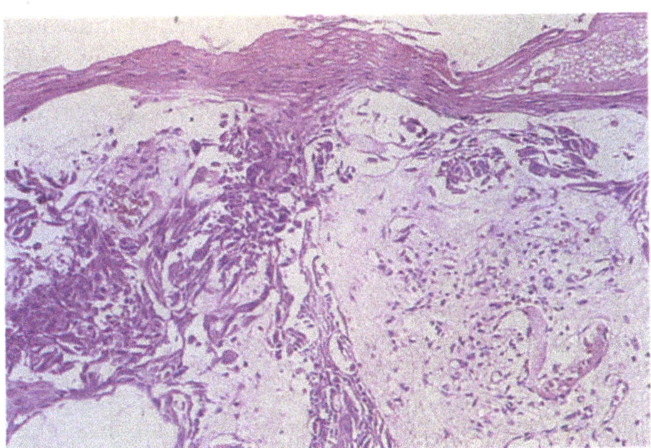

Figure 13.12 Spitz naevus. Considerable oedema of the papillary dermis is seen in some examples of this entity.   H & E (B)

and is rarely in sufficient quantities to spill over into macrophages.

Blue Naevus[3]

Blue naevi are so-called because of their rather dusky grey/blue rather than brown appearance. This characteristic colour is the result of the greater depth of melanin within the dermis than in junctional or compound naevi. Absorption of the red part of the spectrum by the superficial layers of the skin causes the usually brown pigment in the naevus to appear blue–grey in colour. Although the commoner blue naevus is typically highly pigmented, the rarer cellular blue naevus is often paradoxically almost colourless or pink in colour.

Histologically, the common blue naevus is composed of dendritic melanocytes which are diffusely arranged around adnexal structures and between bundles of dermal collagen (Figure 13.6). The melanocytes themselves are elongated and spindle-shaped with moderate amounts of melanin pigment and these cells are interspersed between more rounded and densely pigmented macrophages. It is unusual to be able adequately to examine the cytological characteristics of a common blue naevus without first bleaching the section.

The cellular blue naevus has a rather different appearance[4]. Characteristically, these lesions are almost spherical in outline and are found at the junction between the dermis and the subcutis. They are composed of two different types of cell, giving the lesion a distinctive biphasic appearance. The major component consists of intersecting bundles of large, epithelioid or spindle-shaped cells which contain little or no melanin (Figures 13.7 and 13.8). These cells may show nuclear pleomorphism and frequent mitotic activity; but none of the mitoses are atypical. The minor component has a cytological architecture resembling that seen in a common blue naevus and deeply pigmented cells of this minor component tend to surround the bundles of melanin-free cells. This second component is useful in helping to distinguish cellular blue naevi from dermal deposits of metastatic melanoma.

About 1 per cent of naevi show an association of compound and blue naevi[5]: the so-called combined naevi. Such combined naevi appear to behave no differently from the more common naevi, although clinically they appear more deeply pigmented. Melanoma arising in a cellular blue naevus has been described but is rare. As nuclear pleomorphism and mitotic activity are seen in cellular blue naevi, diagnosis can be very difficult. However, the presence of necrosis or ulceration in a cellular blue naevus appears to be the principal distinguishing feature of malignancy.

Spitz Naevus

Spitz naevi, also known as juvenile melanoma or spindle and epithelioid-cell naevi are most commonly found in young adults and children[6]. They are pink or tan-coloured nodules usually less than 1 cm in diameter and often have an irregular or peau d'orange type of surface. Their importance largely depends on distinguishing them from melanoma, a task which may be very difficult in that Spitz naevi frequently show cellular pleomorphism, an inflammatory infiltrate and may contain mitotic figures. There may be well-marked junctional activity and even single cell infiltration of the epidermis to add even greater difficulty to achieving a correct diagnosis. Typical features of Spitz naevi include (Figures 13.9–13.12):

(1) Well-circumscribed nesting of the naevus cells, both in the junctional and intradermal components.
(2) Large spindle-shaped or epithelioid naevus cells with prominent cytoplasm.
(3) Oedema and telangiectasia in the dermis.
(4) Maturation of the naevus cells at the base of the lesion.
(5) The presence of mitoses, but without atypical mitotic forms.
(6) The presence of spherical nodules of eosinophilic hyaline material[7]. These so-called Kamino bodies are periodic acid–Schiff positive, diastase resistant.
(7) Relatively scant or absent melanin pigmentation.

Although single-cell infiltration of the epidermis is seen in some Spitz naevi, the infiltration is only seen over the intradermal component of the lesion. Pagetoid infiltration of the epidermis lateral to the lesion is rarely seen in Spitz naevi and if it occurs is highly suspicious of melanoma.

Occasionally, intradermal Spitz naevi are associated with a well-marked fibroblastic reaction, which masks the underlying naevocytic nature of the lesion (Figures 13.13–13.15). Such lesions have been termed 'desmoplastic naevi'[8]. The naevus cells of desmoplastic naevi show the features described in ordinary Spitz naevi, and the lesion should be carefully distinguished from desmoplastic melanoma, in which it is usual to find an atypical junctional component at some point in the lesion. Desmoplastic naevi are most common in children and young adults, desmoplastic melanoma is generally a disease of old age.

Pigmented Spindle-cell Naevus[9]

This recently described entity may be confused with superficial spreading melanoma. It may be a variant of Spitz naevus and is characterized by its small diameter (less than 6 mm), sharply delineated edge and intense pigmentation. The commonest age of patients presenting with a pigmented spindle-cell naevus is 20-30 years, but the described age range is large, from 2 years to 56 years in one series. The commonest sites were thigh and arm.

In histological sections, the principal features are a well-delineated nested junctional component of spindle-shaped melanocytes (Figures 13.16 and 13.17). Occasionally, upward migration of nests of melanocytes can be seen but single melanocytes within the epidermis are an unusual finding which should raise the suspicion of melanoma. Pigmented spindle-cell naevi are thin lesions and characteristically the base of the lesion is surrounded by a band of pigment macrophages. Inflammation is scanty, and when seen is perivascular rather than band-like in distribution. Nuclear pleomorphism is not a feature of pigmented spindle-cell naevus and mitoses are rare.

Congenital Melanocytic Naevi

The common melanocytic naevi acquired during childhood and adolescence are generally smaller than congenital melanocytic naevi, some of which may be very large: the so-called giant congenital melanocytic naevi. Giant naevi may cover a significant proportion of the trunk or limbs taking on the shape of a bathing trunk, cape or stocking etc.[10]. All forms of congenital naevi tend to be hairy and deeply pigmented.

Histological appearances of congenital naevi differ from acquired compound or intradermal naevi in that the congenital naevi extend more deeply into the reticular dermis or even the subcutaneous tissues (Figure 13.18).

The naevus cells also tend to surround skin adnexae more closely than in acquired naevi. Some congenital naevi are combined intradermal and blue naevi.

Melanomas may occur more commonly in congenital naevi than acquired naevi. The increased incidence is greatest in giant naevi. Melanoma usually arises at the dermo-epidermal junction, but can arise in the deeper, intradermal component.

Balloon-cell Naevus

Balloon-cell naevi are indistinguishable from common melanocytic naevi, apart from at histological examination[11]. 'Balloon-cell' is the term which has been coined to describe a peculiar degenerative change in the cytoplasm of the naevus cell. Although naevi consisting entirely of balloon cells are a great rarity, a minor component of balloon cell change is seen in about 2 per cent of melanocytic naevi. Balloon cells are greatly enlarged due to vacuolation of the cytoplasm (Figure 13.19) which ultrastructural studies have shown to be due to degeneration of melanosomes[12]. Balloon-cell change is also seen in some melanomas, and in the balloon cells it may be difficult to assess nuclear atypia. Accordingly, it is important to sample a lesion with balloon cells adequately and assess the benign or malignant nature of the lesion from the non-balloon-cell component. Fortunately, melanomas consisting entirely of balloon cells are very rare.

Halo Naevus

Halo naevus (sometimes termed Sutton's naevus) is the term used to describe a naevus surrounded by a characteristic area of depigmentation[13]. There is no evidence of inflammation and the naevus gradually atrophies over a period of months or years. The change is thought to be an immune phenomenon, because circulating antibodies to naevus cells, and not to other melanocytes, are seen in the serum of affected patients. Ultrastructural studies show degenerative changes in the melanocytes in the naevus and surrounding skin[14]. The ultrastructural changes in melanocytes are similar in halo naevus and vitiligo and the two conditions may be connected.

Histological sections of halo naevus show a dense lymphocytic infiltrate in the distribution of a melanocytic naevus. The infiltrate may be so dense that it is difficult to see the underlying naevus cells (Figures 13.20 and 13.21). These must be sought and assessed carefully for the presence of cytological atypia, for melanomas may rarely contain a well-marked inflammatory infiltrate simulating halo naevus. There have been reports of the development of multiple halo naevi in patients from whom a malignant melanoma has recently been excised.

Dysplastic Naevus Syndrome

Also known as the B-K mole syndrome[15], this entity has recently been delineated as a familial type of precancerous melanosis. However, sporadic cases of the 'dysplastic mole syndrome' are also recognized. Dysplastic naevi are larger than ordinary naevi and may be more than 1 cm in diameter. They are usually numerous on the skin of an affected individual.

Histologically, the naevi are usually compound with a prominent junctional component. There may be inflammation at the base of the naevus. The junctional nests contain atypical naevus cells which may be spindle-shaped, the long axis of the cell being parallel to the skin surface. Although dysplastic naevi have the appearance just described, not every such naevus signifies the *familial* dysplastic naevus syndrome[16]. Such a diagnosis relies on clinical assessment of the patient and his or her relatives.

Lentigo Maligna[17]

These lesions often appear to be related to sun exposure. They are most common on the face but are also found on the trunk and are usually found in elderly patients. Clinically, the lesions are flat dark-brown macules which steadily grow in extent. Although there is continuous extension of the lesions, growth is usually slow and may be associated with areas of regression and depigmentation. Lentigo maligna is characteristically flat; any development of nodularity raises a suspicion of the development of lentigo maligna melanoma.

In histological sections there are three characteristic features (Figure 13.22):
(1) Solar elastosis of the dermis.
(2) Atrophy of the epidermis.
(3) Band-like hyperplasia of large, atypical melanocytes at the junctional zone of the epidermis. This band of atypical naevus cells may extend down the pilosebaceous follicles and eccrine ducts.

Nests of atypical melanocytes are not a feature of lentigo maligna and pagetoid infiltration of the epidermis is only an occasional feature. Mononuclear inflammatory-cell infiltration can be seen in lentigo maligna, but it is usually only mild in degree. Pagetoid infiltration of the epidermis and nesting of the naevus cells are the earliest manifestations of the development of melanoma and the presence of invasion of the papillary dermis may be masked by the well-marked lymphocytic infiltrate (Figure 13.23). Although there has been some suggestion that lentigo maligna melanoma has a better prognosis than melanoma elsewhere[18], recent studies suggest that if tumours of equal thickness are compared then there is little difference in behaviour.

Malignant Melanoma[19]

Four types of malignant melanoma are described. Most common, and probably as frequent as all the other types put together, is superficial spreading melanoma. The second most frequent type is nodular melanoma, and the combined incidence of the remaining types, acral lentiginous and lentigo maligna melanoma is less than 10 per cent of cases.

Although the classification of melanoma into these four types is useful in indicating their prognosis, probably more important than the type of melanoma is the depth of invasion of the tumour. The simplest and most effective method of assessing depth of invasion is the measurement by stage micrometry of the distance between the granular layer of the epidermis and the deepest extent of the infiltrating tumour. Breslow showed that tumours less than 0.76 mm in thickness had a good prognosis whereas those tumours more than 1.5 mm in thickness were so likely to have metastasized that prophylactic excision of draining lymph nodes produced an improval in survival[20]. When using Breslow's method it is important to ignore tongues of atypical melanocytes extending along the junctional zone of pilosebaceous follicles. In ulcerated lesions, Breslow recommended that measurement should be from the surface of the ulcer rather than the granular layer of the epidermis. Other features which signify a poor prognosis are sparse or absent melanin, absence of lymphocytic response and presence of vascular invasion. Lentigo maligna melanoma has been described above, the remaining three types of melanoma will now be discussed.

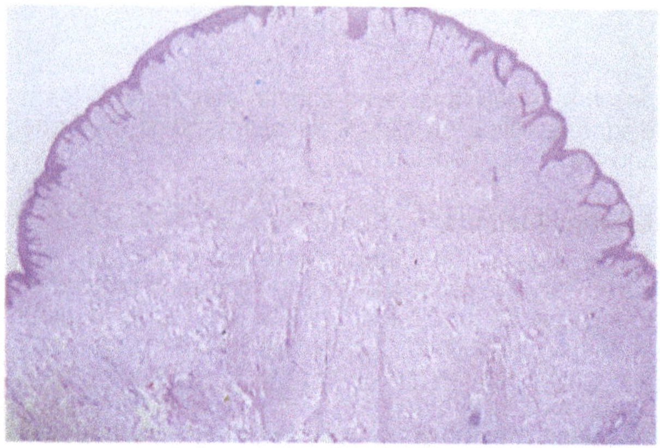

Figure 13.13 Desmoplastic naevus. At low magnification, the naevus cells are difficult to identify amongst the fibrous stroma.   H & E (A)

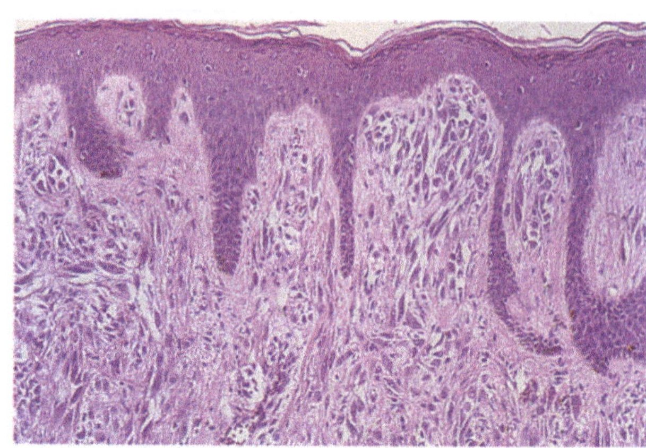

Figure 13.14 Desmoplastic naevus. At higher magnification, spindle-shaped naevus cells are seen amongst a well-marked fibroblastic stroma.   H & E (B)

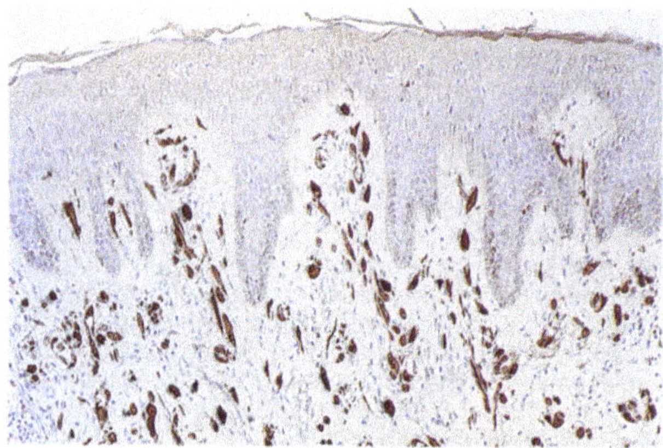

Figure 13.15 Desmoplastic naevus. The naevocytic nature of the spindle cells is confirmed by immunocytochemical staining with an antibody to S-100 protein. S-100 immunostain   (B)

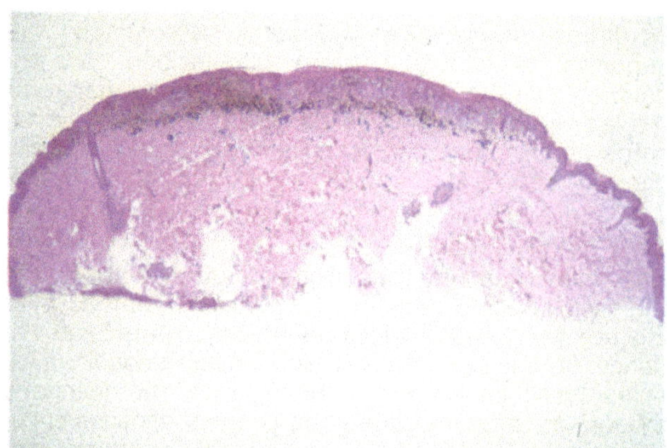

Figure 13.16 Pigmented spindle-cell naevus. The lesion is typically thin and bounded at its lower margin by a dense band of melanin pigment. This lesion was removed from a child aged 3 years.   H & E (A)

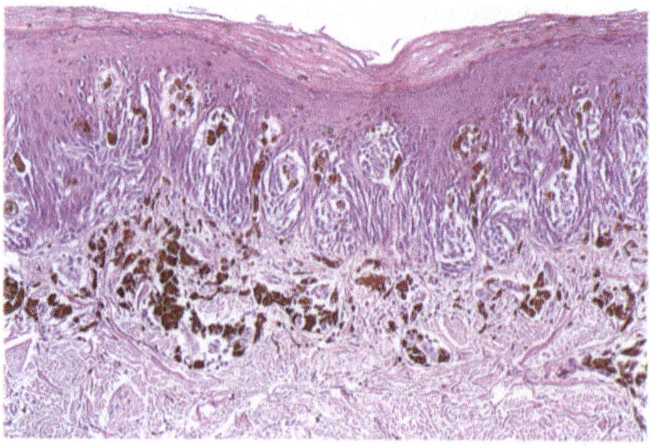

Figure 13.17 Pigmented spindle-cell naevus, showing the nests of junctional spindle-shaped naevus cells. H & E (A)

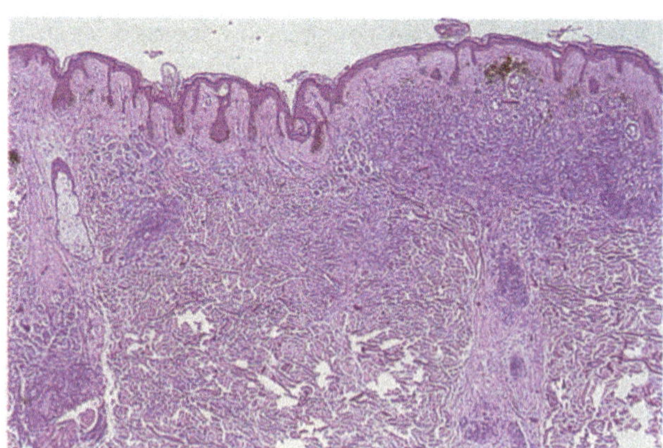

Figure 13.18 Congenital melanocytic naevus. An intradermal naevus with deep extension around hair follicles.   H & E (B)

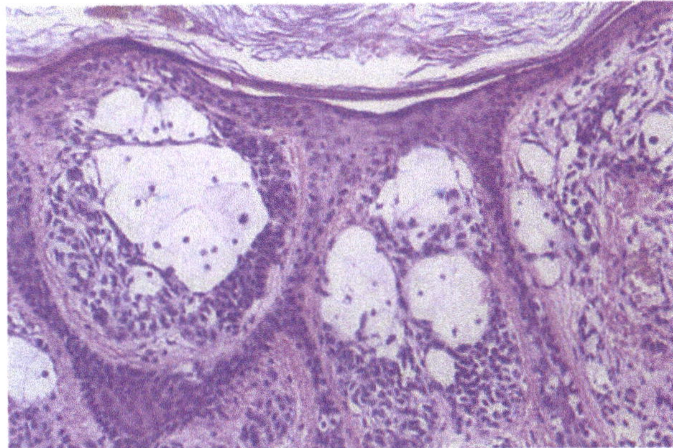

Figure 13.19 Balloon-cell change, compound naevus. The balloon cells are up to 10 times the diameter of the adjacent ordinary naevus cells, and are characterised by clear cytoplasm and a small central or slightly eccentric nucleus. H & E (B)

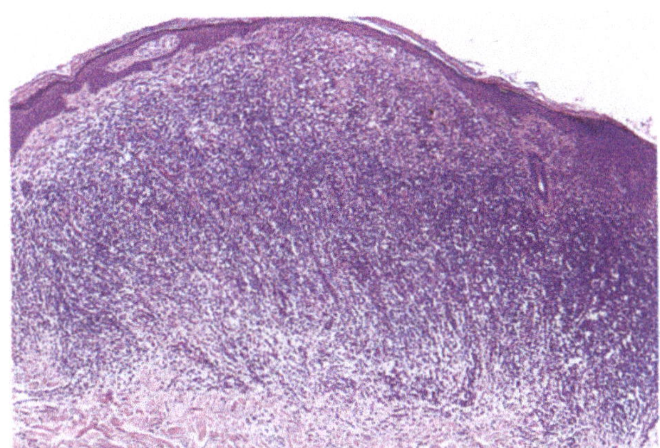

Figure 13.20 Halo naevus. A dense lymphocytic infiltrate obscures the underlying naevus. H & E (A)

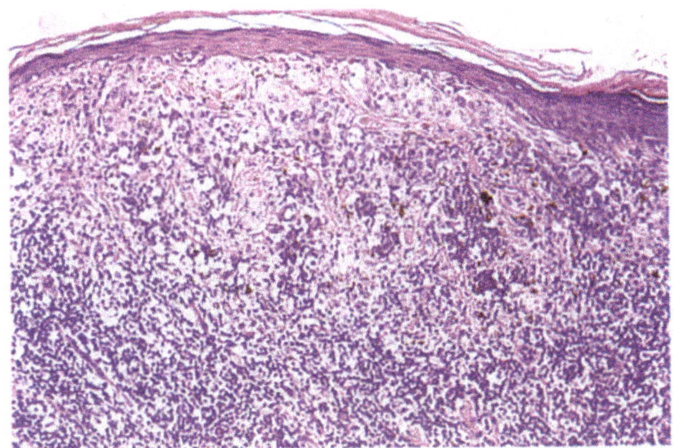

Figure 13.21 Halo naevus. At higher magnification, small numbers of residual junctional naevus cells can be identified. (B)

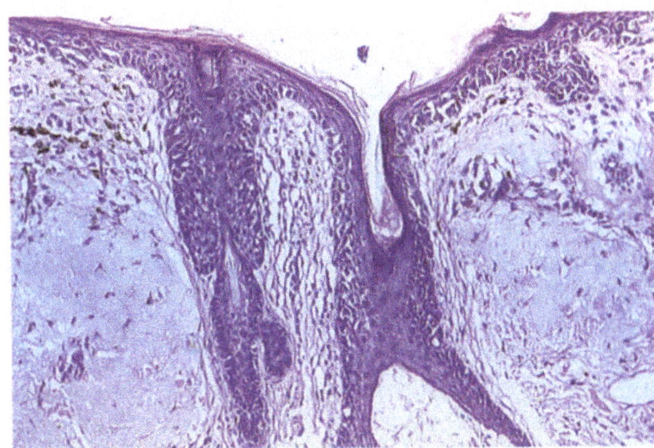

Figure 13.22 Lentigo maligna, characterised by epidermal atrophy, band-like proliferation of atypical junctional melanocytes extending into hair follicles and solar elastosis of dermal collagen. H & E (B)

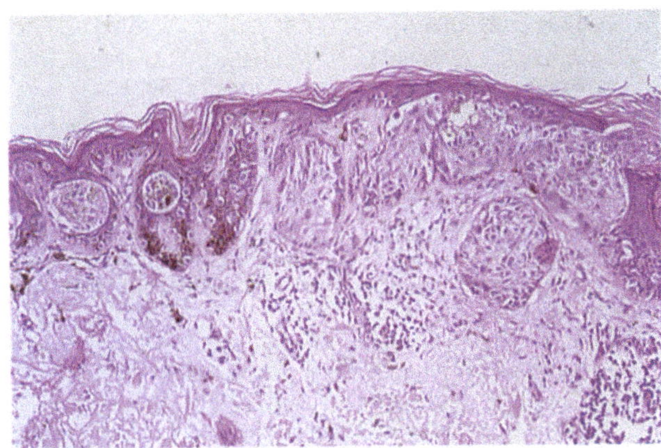

Figure 13.23 Lentigo maligna melanoma. Junctional nests of atypical melanocytes are evoking a zone of inflammatory response within the dermis. H & E (B)

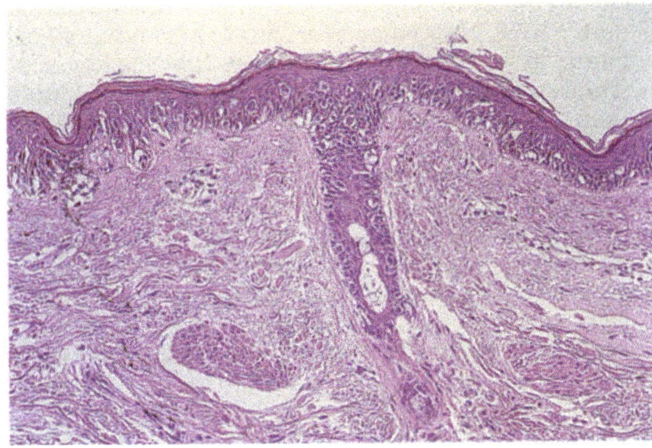

Figure 13.24 Superficial-spreading melanoma, showing 'Pagetoid' invasion of the epidermis. H & E (A)

Superficial-spreading Melanoma

These are tumours of the skin chiefly in young or middle-aged individuals. In many series of melanomas they are the commonest type, accounting for over half the cases. The lesion is a flat or slightly raised macule which characteristically shows variation in the amount of pigment present.

The principal histological feature of superficial-spreading melanoma is the lateral extension of cytologically atypical melanocytes along the junctional zone of the epidermis (Figures 13.24–13.26). There is almost always a junctional component in all forms of melanoma, but in the superficial-spreading type the atypical melanocytes extend for more than three rete ridges beyond the edge of the invasive component of the tumour.

A second important distinguishing feature of superficial spreading melanoma is the presence of pagetoid invasion of the epidermis. Single atypical melanocytes become distributed throughout the epidermis. In some areas these single cells coalesce to form nests of tumour cells.

Other features are less useful diagnostically. Melanin pigmentation may be very variable and is often to be found in melanophages rather than tumour melanocytes. The tumour cells are usually epithelioid. Mitotic activity may be seen within the tumour, but can be absent. Regression is common in superficial-spreading melanomas. It is characterized histologically by a sparse lymphocytic infiltration of the dermis, atrophy of the epidermis and lamellar fibrosis of the papillary dermis. When regression has occurred it is difficult to assess the thickness of the tumour by Breslow's method.

Nodular Melanoma

Except in some cases of melanoma arising in congenital naevi, nodular melanomas (like superficial-spreading melanomas) arise at the dermo-epidermal junction[21]. Unlike superficial-spreading melanoma, the nodular type has an early vertical growth phase. Growth also tends to be more rapid than in superficial-spreading lesions, and the tumour is grossly nodular or even polypoid in shape (Figure 13.27). Ulceration of the epidermis is most common in the nodular type of melanoma.

The characteristic histological feature of nodular melanoma is the presence of atypical, usually epithelioid naevoid cells extending upwards from the junctional zone into the epidermis and downwards into the dermis (Figure 13.28). There may be a chronic inflammatory cell infiltrate at the base of the lesion, which shows no evidence of the maturation seen in benign naevi. Mitotic figures are usually seen in melanomas, but may be very sparse and are not an absolutely diagnostic feature in that they may be seen in Spitz naevi. Melanin pigmentation is very variable in amount. If completely absent, it may be difficult to characterize the lesion as a melanoma rather than some other anaplastic neoplasm of skin. In such cases immunocytochemical staining of the tumour cells by antigens to S-100 protein and neurone-specific enolase may help to confirm that the lesion is a melanoma.

Acral Lentiginous Melanoma

Acral lentiginous melanoma occurs on the palms, soles and nail beds of the extremities. There are some features reminiscent of lentigo maligna, but the lesion appears to have a distinctive morphology and biological behaviour[22,23]. The characteristic feature of acral melanomas is the presence of an extensive band of junctional atypical melanocytes similar to that which characterizes lentigo maligna (Figure 13.29). However, in acral lesions the rete ridges of the skin are elongated rather than atrophied and the atypical melanocytes are spindle shaped and show frequent nesting. Melanin pigmentation is marked and spills out of the naevus cells into the overlying plantar or palmar skin. These features make it difficult to gain any clinical impression of the thickness of the lesion. The invasive component of acral lentiginous melanoma is very similar in appearance to that seen in other types of melanoma, apart from the preponderance of spindle cells.

References

1. Birbeck, M. S., Breathnach, A. S. and Everall, J. D. (1961). An electron microscope study of basal melanocytes and high-level clear cells (Langerhans cells) in vitiligo. *J. Invest. Dermatol.*, **37**, 51

2. Bhawan, J. (1979). Melanocytic nevi. A review. *J. Cutan. Pathol.*, **6**, 153

3. Levene, A. (1980). On the natural history and comparative pathology of the blue naevus. *Ann. R. Coll. Surg. Engl.*, **62**, 327

4. Rodriquez, H. A. and Ackerman, L. V. (1968). Cellular blue naevus. *Cancer*, **21**, 393

5. Leopold, J. G. and Richards, D. B. (1968). The interrelationship of blue and common naevi. *J. Pathol.*, **95**, 37

6. Paniago-Pereira, C., Maize, J. C. and Ackerman, A. B. (1978). Nevus of large spindle and/or epithelioid cells (Spitz's nevus). *Arch. Dermatol.*, **114**, 1811

7. Kamino, H., Flotte, T. J., Misheloff, E., Greco, M. A. and Ackerman, A. B. (1979). Eosinophilic globules in Spitz's nevi. New findings and a diagnostic sign. *Am. J. Dermatopathol.*, **1**, 319

8. Barr, R. J., Morales, R. V. and Graham, J. H. (1980). Desmoplastic nevus: a distinct histologic variant of mixed spindle cell and epithelioid cell nevus. *Cancer*, **46**, 557

9. Sagebiel, R. W., Chinn, E. K. and Egbert, B. M. (1984). Pigmented spindle cell nevus. Clinical and histologic review of 90 cases. *Am. J. Surg. Pathol.*, **8**, 645

10. Mark, G. J., Mihm, M. C. and Liteplo, M. G. (1973). Congenital melanocytic nevi of the small garment type. Clinical, histologic and ultrastructural studies. *Hum. Pathol.*, **4**, 395

11. Wilson-Jones, E., and Sanderson, K. V. (1963). Cellular naevi with peculiar foam cells. *Br. J. Dermatol.*, **75**, 47

12. Hashimoto, K. and Bale, G. F. (1972). An electron microscopic study of balloon cell naevus. *Cancer*, **30**, 530

13. Findley, G. H. (1957). The history of Sutton's naevus. *Br. J. Dermatol.*, **69**, 389

14. Swanson, J. L., Wayte, D. M. and Helwig, E. B. (1968). Ultrastructure of halo nevi. *J. Invest. Dermatol.*, **50**, 434

15. Clark, W. H. Jr, Reimer, R. R., Greene, M., Ainsworth, A. M. and Mastrangelo, M. J. (1978). Origin of familial malignant melanomas from heritable melanocytic lesions. 'The B-K mole syndrome.' *Arch. Dermatol.*, **114**, 732

16. Elder, D. E., Goldman, L. I., Goldman, S. C., Green, M. H. and Clark, W. H. Jr (1980). Dysplastic nevus syndrome: a phenotypic association of sporadic cutaneous melanoma. *Cancer*, **46**, 1787

17. Clark, W. H. Jr and Mihm, M. C. Jr (1969). Lentigo maligna and lentigo-maligna melanoma. *Am. J. Pathol.*, **55**, 39

18. McGovern, V. J., Shaw, H. M., Milton, G. W. and Farago, G. A. (1980). Is malignant melanoma arising in Hutchinson's melanotic freckle a separate disease entity? *Histopathology*, **4**, 235

19. Maize, J. C. (1983). Primary cutaneous malignant melanoma. *J. Am. Acad. Dermatol.*, **8**, 857

20. Breslow, A. (1975). Tumor thickness, level of invasion and node dissection in stage I cutaneous melanoma. *Ann. Surg.*, **182**, 572

21. Ackerman, A. B. (1980). Malignant melanoma: a unifying concept. *Hum. Pathol.*, **11**, 591

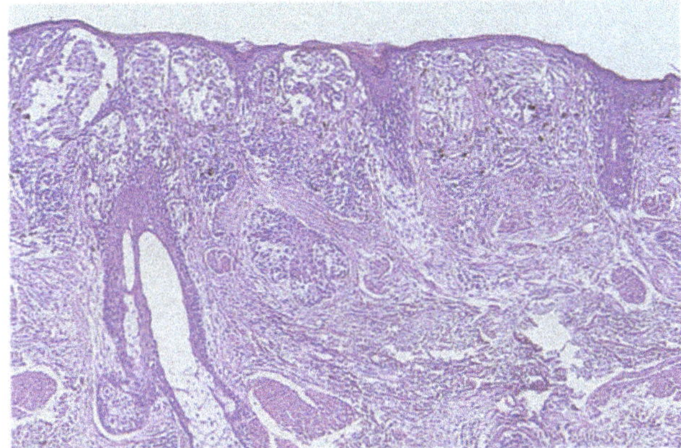

Figure 13.25 Superficial-spreading melanoma. Irregular nests of atypical naevus cells are invading the epidermis. H & E (B)

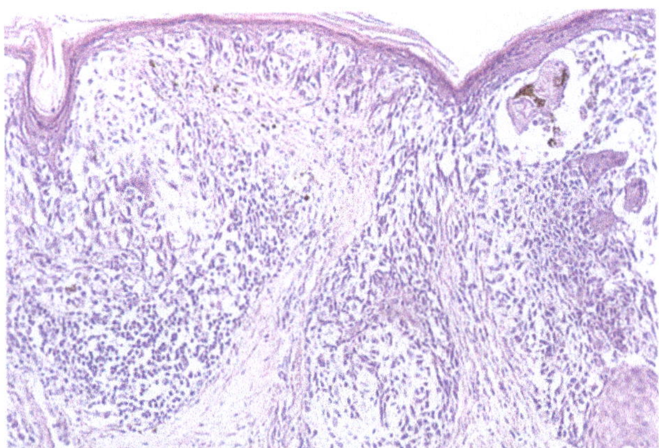

Figure 13.26 Superficial-spreading melanoma. Early invasion of the papillary dermis is seen on the right of the photomicrograph. H & E (B)

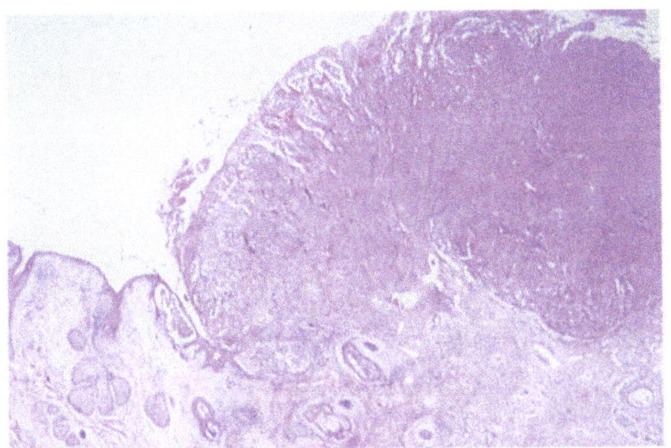

Figure 13.27 Polypoid nodular melanoma. H & E (A)

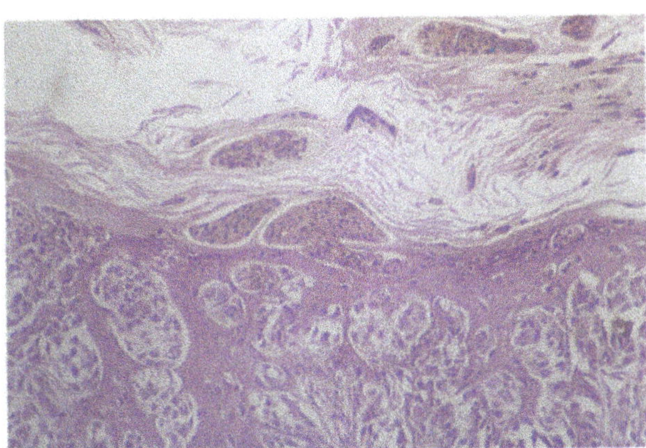

Figure 13.28 Nodular melanoma, showing ulcerating invasion of the overlying epidermis by nests of atypical melanoma cells. H & E (B)

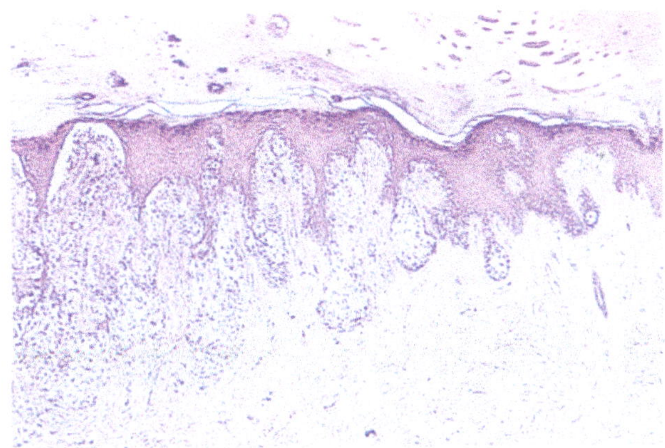

Figure 13.29 Acral lentiginous melanoma. The hyperkeratosis is typical of plantar skin. Nests of atypical junctional melanocytes show both an epidermal and a dermal invasive component. H & E (B).

22. Paladugu, R. R., Winberg, C. D. and Yonemoto, R. H. (1983). Acral lentiginous melanoma. A clinicopathologic study of 36 patients. *Cancer*, **52**, 161

23. Krementz, E. T., Feed, R. J., Coleman, W. P. 3rd, Sutherland, C. M., Carter, R. D. and Campbell, M. (1982). Acral lentiginous melanoma. A clinicopathologic entity. *Ann. Surg.*, **195**, 632

Seborrhoeic Warts (Basal cell papilloma)

Seborrhoeic warts are extremely common, benign, warty nodules and plaques consisting of thickened and hyperkeratotic epidermal tissue. They become more common with increasing age. Although more frequently found on the head, upper trunk and backs of the hands, they may occur anywhere. Usually they have a light brown or yellowish-brown discolouration. When more deeply pigmented they are frequently mistaken for malignant melanoma. Virtually nothing is known of their aetiology.

Histopathology

The lesion appears stuck on to the skin surface, i.e. above the general level of the skin surface. Overall it is seen to consist of irregularly thickened epidermis and hyperkeratosis (Figure 14.1). It is of variable size but has sharply defined margins with normal epidermis either side. The cells in the lesions are 'basaloid', that is, they are basophilic and cuboidal, but are slightly larger than ordinary basal cells or the cells of a basal cell carcinoma (Figure 14.2). The dermo-epidermal junction beneath the lesion is very irregular, and slices of dermal papillae often appear within the substance of the lesion due to their projecting irregularly upwards and then being cut in the plane of the section. It is also usual to notice small horn cysts within the substance of the tumour (Figure 14.3) and it is thought that these arise by a process of squamous metaplasia. In 'flat' seborrhoeic warts there is often a 'church steeple' configuration to surface epidermis and thickened hyperkeratotic stratum corneum (Figure 14.4). Degenerative changes are also commonly found, especially in the larger lesions – cells appear to lose contact with each other and individual cells become vacuolated and eventually fragmented. For reasons that are unclear, seborrhoeic warts often become inflamed, and it is commonplace to observe a moderately dense cellular infiltrate of lymphocytes and histiocytes immediately beneath the lesion, frequently invading its substance.

Differential Diagnosis

The differential diagnosis is that of a localized warty nodule or plaque and includes viral wart, solar keratosis and Bowen's disease (see Table 14.1).

Variants of Seborrhoeic Wart

Borst–Jadassohn intraepidermal epithelioma. Whatever Borst and Jadassohn originally described[1,2], this term (BJIE) has now become attached to a particular histopathological picture possessing both features of seborrhoeic warts and features of an intraepidermal epithelioma. Clinically the lesion appears to be an ordinary seborrhoeic wart. Histopathologically BJIE has the overall architecture of a seborrhoeic wart. In addition to the usual features there are areas in which the keratinocytes are larger and flatter in profile than usual and are arranged in swirls and eddies at the centre of which there is squamous metaplasia or horn cysts (Figure 14.5). There are also clusters of irregular small dark cells containing several mitotic figures (Figure 14.6). It has been suggested that the BJIE lesion results from 'irritation' of a seborrhoeic wart. As some lesions of Bowen's disease (see pages 111, 114) and squamous cell carcinoma may have superficially similar appearances, great care must be taken to distinguish these malignant epidermal lesions from BJIE which is essentially benign. Pointers to BJIE include the overall seborrhoeic wart-like arrangement, the lack of any tendency to invade surrounding tissues and absence of bizarre nuclear figures.

Inverted follicular keratosis (IFK). Clinically this lesion invariably occurs on the face as a skin-coloured smooth or sometimes warty nodule. The microscopic appearance has similarities to the BJIE in that squamous eddies and clusters of small dark cells are often present. However, unlike other types of seborrhoeic wart the bulk of the tumour is below the general level of the skin surface (Figure 14.7). In most cases it may be seen that there is close association of the lesion with the pilosebaceous apparatus – the significance of this is uncertain. How-

Table 14.1 Differential diagnosis of seborrhoeic warts

Lesion	Predominant sites	Major differentiating features
Seborrhoeic wart	face, scalp, trunk, upper limbs	regular small basaloid cells, stuck on appearance, horn cysts
Solar keratosis	face, scalp, backs of hands and forearms	irregular epidermal thickening and epidermal dysplasia with parakeratosis
Squamous cell carcinoma	as above	as above but more pronounced, clumps and sheets of abnormal epidermal cells within dermis
Viral wart	hands, feet, limbs, face	normal epidermal differentiation, marked hypergranulosis with basophilic stippling and perinuclear vacuolation
Epidermal naevus	any site	regular epidermal thickening with normal differentiation and 'church steeple' hyperkeratosis

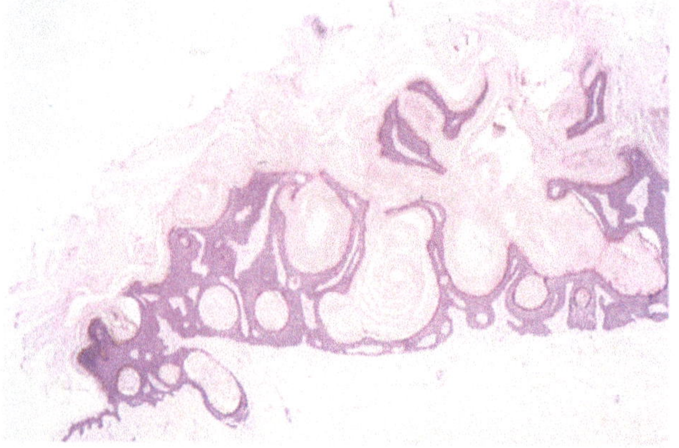

Figure 14.1   Seborrhoeic wart. Note the 'stuck on' appearance.   H & E (A)

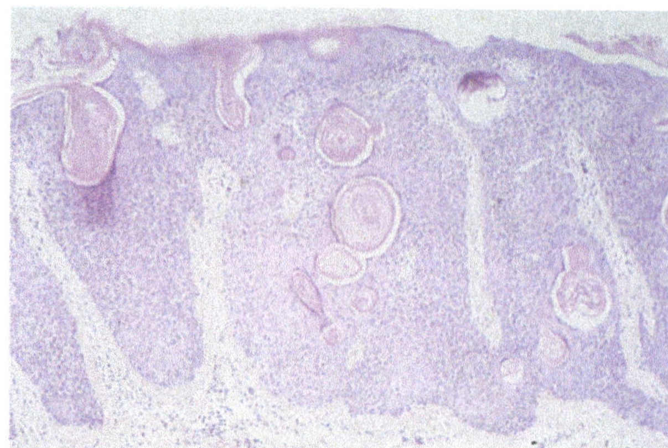

Figure 14.2   Seborrhoeic wart showing basaloid type of cells slightly larger than seen in basal cell carcinoma.   H & E (C)

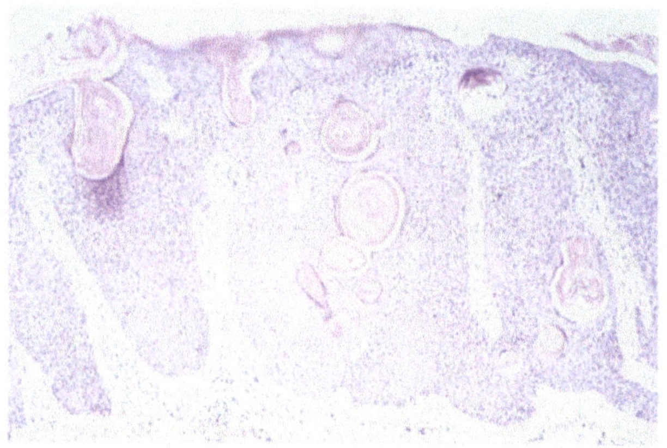

Figure 14.3   Seborrhoeic wart showing numerous horn cysts.   H & E (B)

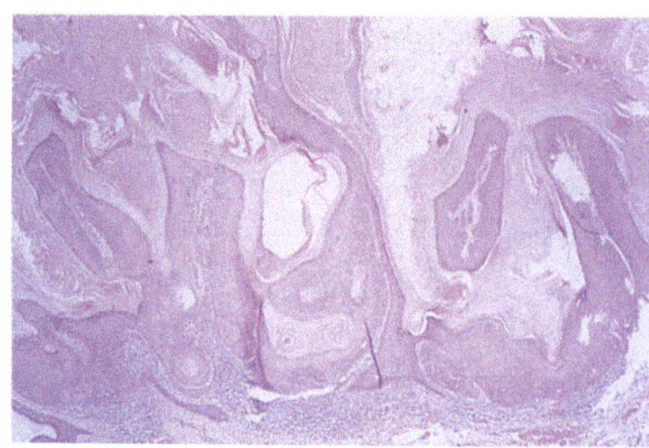

Figure 14.4   Seborrhoeic wart with peaked epidermal hypertrophy.   H & E (B)

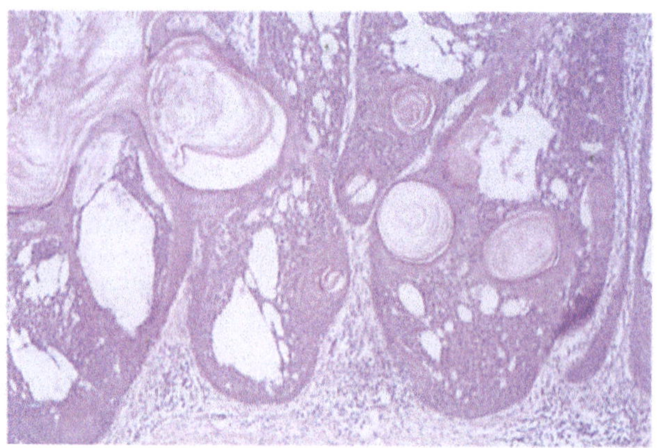

Figure 14.5   Irritated seborrhoeic wart showing horn cysts and squamous metaplasia.   H & E (B)

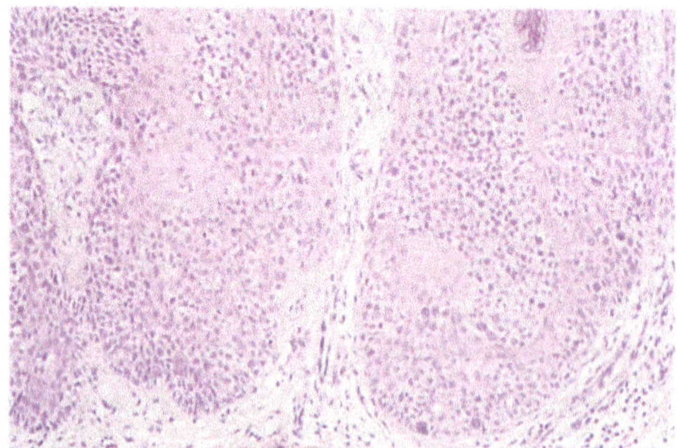

Figure 14.6   Irritated seborrhoeic wart showing areas of squamous metaplasia and other areas with small dark cells some of which are in mitosis. H & E (C)

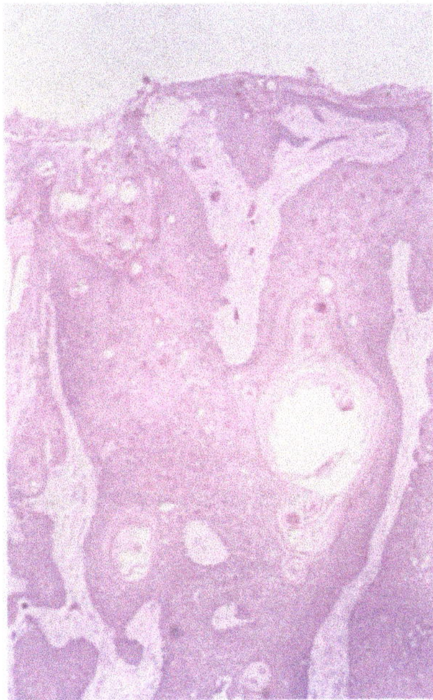

Figure 14.7a Inverted follicular keratosis. There is a follicle-like mass of epithelium within the dermis. H & E (B)

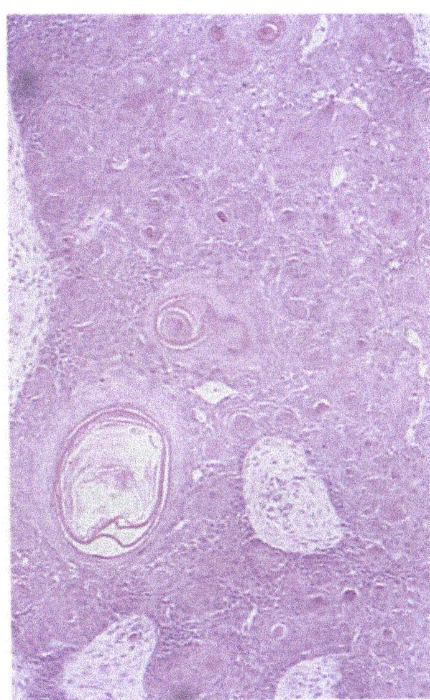

Figure 14.7b Inverted follicular keratosis. Detail of Figure 14.7a to show squamous metaplasia and appearance of cellular pleomorphism. H & E (C)

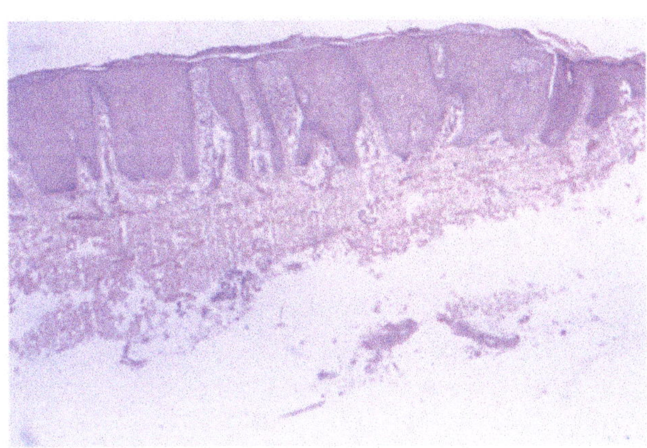

Figure 14.8 Degos' acanthoma. There is an area of regular epidermal hypertrophy in which the epidermal cells are paler than usual. H & E (A)

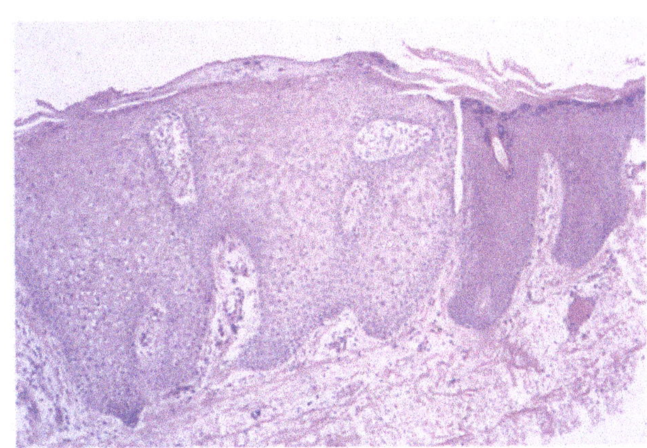

Figure 14.9 Degos' acanthoma. Junction with normal epidermis. H & E (B)

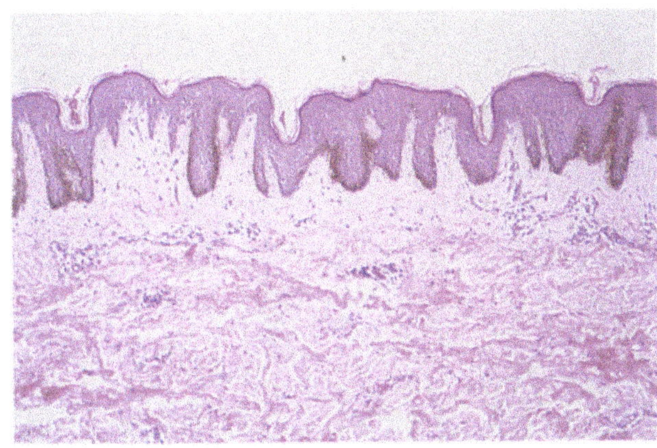

Figure 14.10 Warty epidermal naevus. H & E (B)

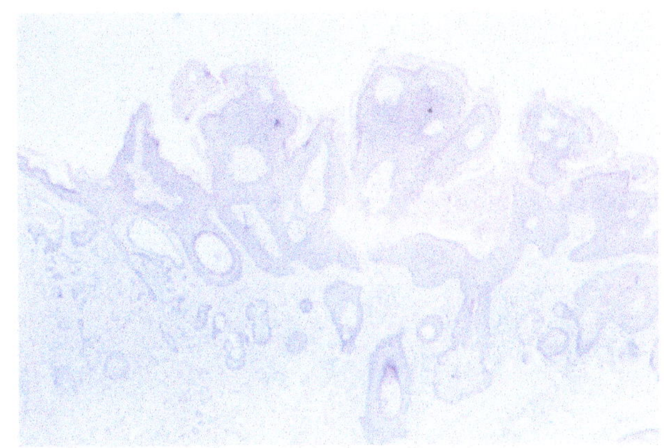

Figure 14.11 Beckers naevus. Epidermal and melanocytic hypertrophy. H & E (B)

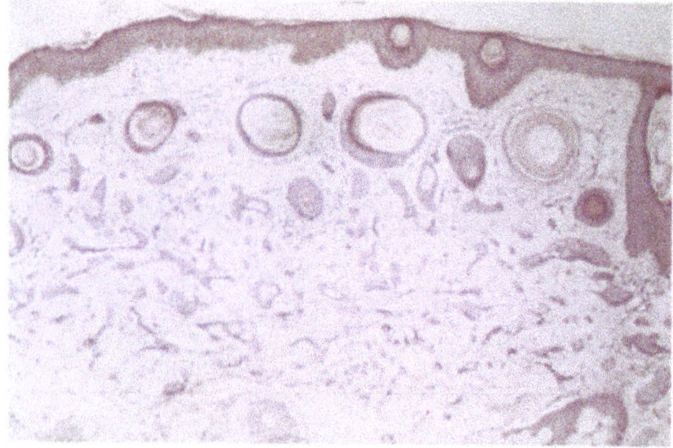

Figure 14.12   Syringoma. There are numerous strands of epithelium some of which contain ductular structures and small cysts.   H & E (A)

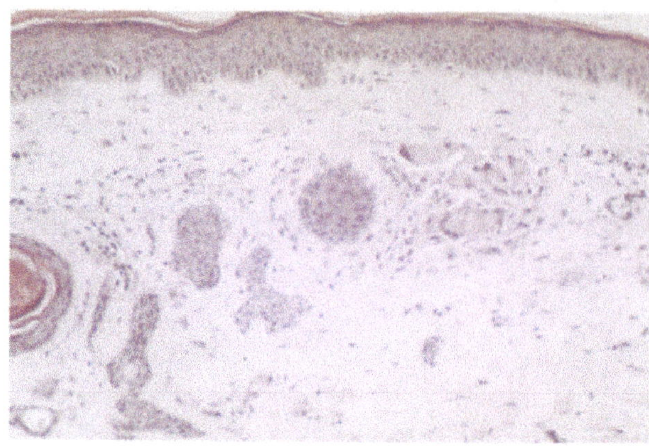

Figure 14.13   Syringoma to show small area of granulomatous inflammation at site of cyst.   H & E (B)

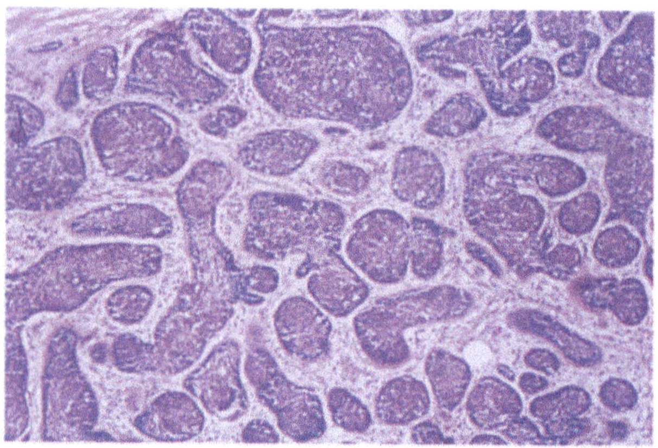

Figure 14.14   Cylindroma. Rounded and irregular masses of epithelium which contain predominantly basaloid cells and a lesser component of clear cells.   H & E (B)

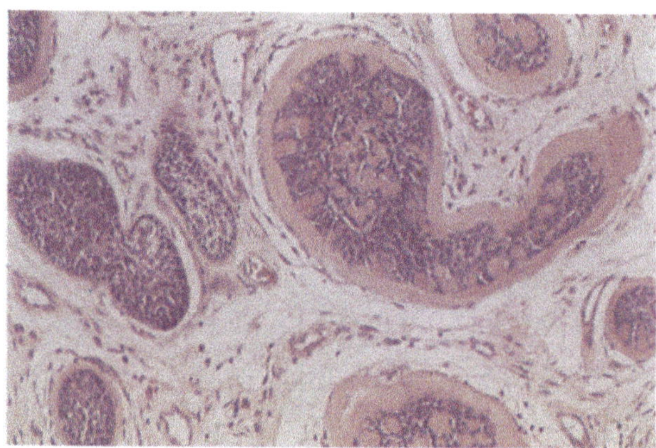

Figure 14.15   Cylindroma. A pink homogenous band of colloid like material can be seen around a basaloid mass.   H & E (C)

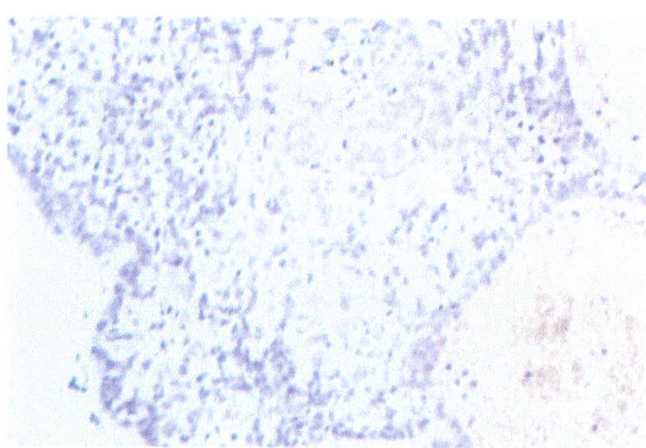

Figure 14.16   Eccrine spiradenoma. Epithelium containing tiny sweat ducts and dilated vascular spaces.   H & E (C)

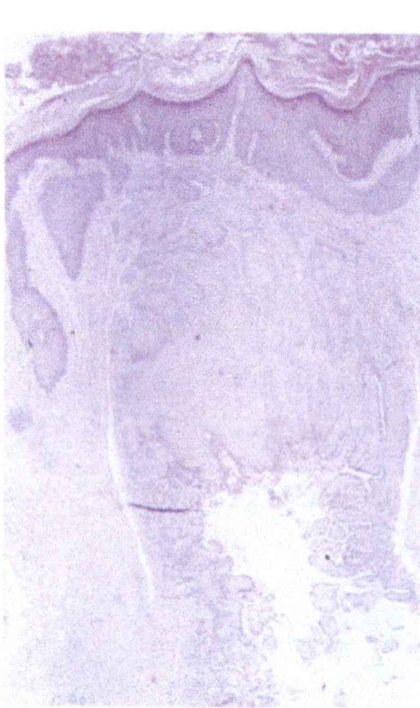

Figure 14.17
Syringocystadenoma papilliferum. An epithelial mass containing a cavity lined by villus projections.   H & E (B)

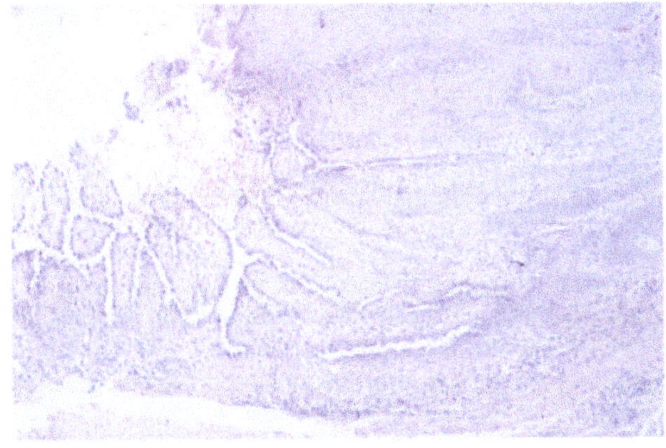

Figure 14.18 Syringocystadenoma papilliferum. Detail of Figure 14.17. H & E (C)

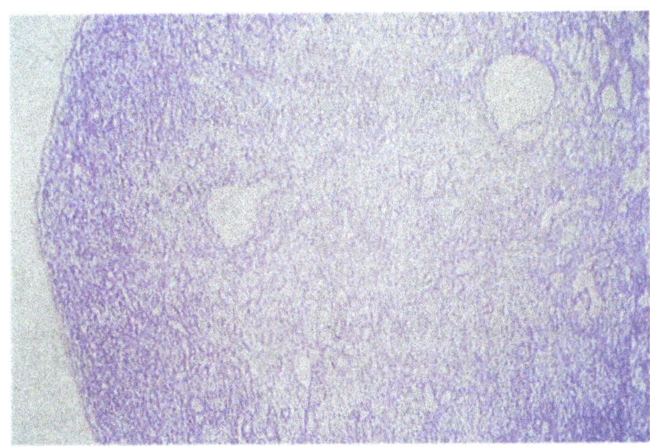

Figure 14.19 Nodular hidradenoma. Epithelial mass consisting predominantly of clear cells and containing many duct-like structures. H & E (B)

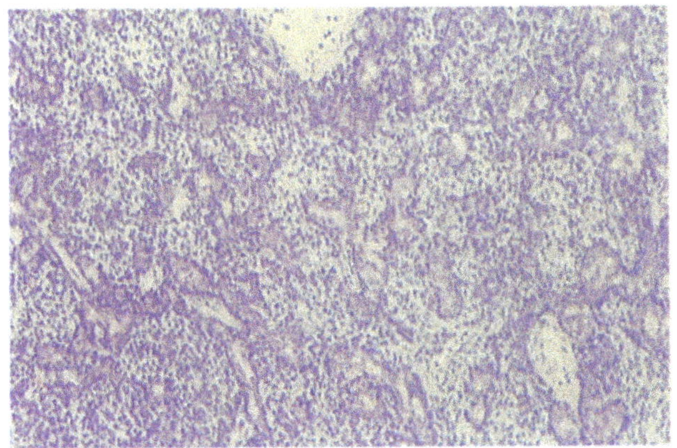

Figure 14.20 Detail of Figure 14.19. H & E (C)

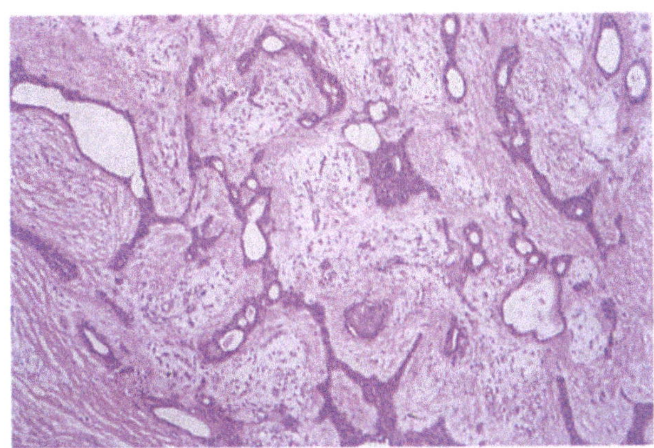

Figure 14.21 Chondroid syringoma. Duct containing strands of epithelial cells in myxoid stroma. H & E (B)

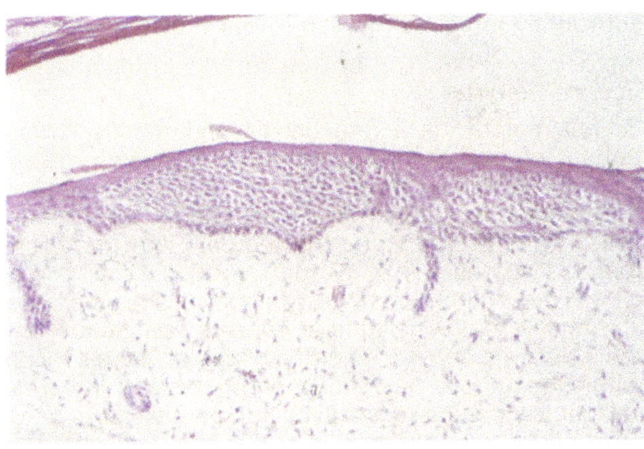

Figure 14.22 Hidroacanthoma simplex. Clusters of uniform clear cells within the epidermis. H & E (C)

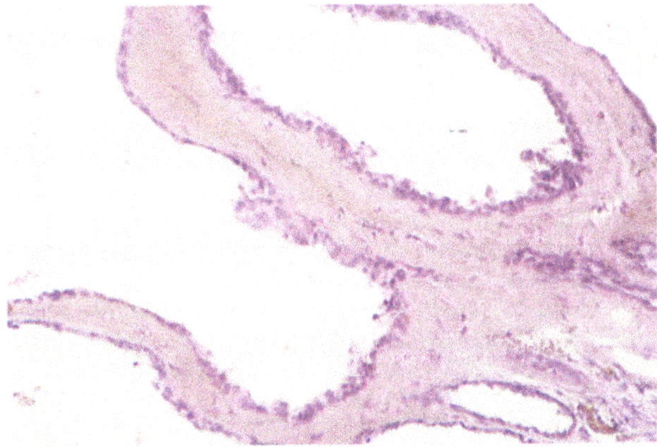

Figure 14.23 Apocrine hidrocystoma. Many dilated aprocrine sweat ducts. H & E (A)

ever, some authorities believe that the lesion is in fact a hair follicle tumour.

Clear cell acanthoma[3] (syn. Degos acanthoma). There is no evidence that this benign neoplasm is a variant of seborrhoeic wart. However, as it is composed of hypertrophied benign epidermal tissue and is 'stuck on' to the skin surface in a similar way to seborrhoeic warts, it seems reasonable to describe it here. Clinically it presents as a red, exudative, sessile nodule measuring some 0.5–2 cm in diameter. Often the story is that it has been present and static in size for several years causing no symptoms. Histologically there is often a striking similarity to psoriasis. There is focal, well-delimited, marked epidermal thickening with psoriasiform elongation of the rete pegs (Figure 14.8). The cells are usually larger than those in a seborrhoeic wart and there are no horn cysts[3]. An interesting finding noted in all clear cell acanthomas is the presence of glycogen in the abnormal epidermis, as demonstrated by the PAS stain and diastase treatment (Figure 14.9). Neutrophilic polymorphonuclear leukocytes are usually present both in the dermal papillae and in the body of the lesion.

Pedunculated fleshy skin tags. Many benign skin tumours may be extruded, resulting in a similar clinical appearance. Benign melanocytic naevi, naevus superficialis lipomatosis and neurofibromata are examples of lesions that may become pedunculated. It appears that seborrhoeic warts may also occasionally be involved in a similar process.

Epidermal Naevus

Epidermal naevus may be a small and localized warty plaque or a large linear or zosteriform lesion. They are generally present at birth and persist and become wartier as the patient ages. They are sometimes scaling and psoriasiform in appearance. The histological appearance is essentially that of epidermal hypertrophy. Often the hypertrophy is of the regular 'church steeple' type with marked hyperkeratosis (this is also seen in some seborrhoeic warts) (Figure 14.10). It may also simulate psoriasis with regular bulbous enlargement of the epidermal rete pegs and parakeratosis. Becker's naevus is a special variety of epidermal naevus often seen over the shoulder or upper arm. It is often pigmented and hairy as all epidermal elements may be hypertrophied (Figure 14.11).

Sweat Gland Tumours

Sweat gland tumours are not uncommon lesions which frequently cause difficulty in histopathological diagnosis. Many are often regarded as hamartomata rather than true tumours. It is often the case that all the pathologist can say after detailed inspection is that the section represents a 'benign adnexal tumour', or slightly more precisely, 'a benign adnexal tumour of sweat gland origin'. Table 14.2 summarizes the main features of the most commonly encountered lesions. Sweat gland tumours seem to stimulate the formation of a particular type of surrounding connective tissue with a preponderance of amorphous proteoglycan-containing material. This feature, once recognized, may be extremely helpful in diagnosis. It should be noted that some basal cell carcinomata may show areas that seem to have differentiated towards sweat gland tissue. These usually do not cause difficulty in diagnosis once the propensity for this to occur is realized.

Syringoma

This not uncommon disorder usually presents as multiple small skin-coloured papules in young adults on the upper part of the cheeks and beneath the eyes. Occasionally numerous lesions appear very quickly and develop on the trunk and limbs as well. The condition then simulates an inflammatory dermatosis such as lichen planus, and has come to be known as 'Eruptive Hidradenoma'.

Histopathology. Numerous small rounded, angulate or comma-shaped epithelial structures can be seen in the upper and mid dermis. These usually contain either lamellated horn or ductular structures (Figure 14.12). Occasionally larger, cyst-like structures are found, some of which have burst, causing an area of granulomatous inflammation (Figure 14.13). Morphoeic basal cell carcinoma has to be considered in differential diagnosis (see page 115). The quality of the surrounding dermal connective tissue should assist in the differentiation as it is usually dense and scar-like in the morphoeic basal cell carcinoma and of a distinctive quality in syringoma.

Cylindroma

Cylindroma may be solitary or multiple and present clinically as smooth, skin-coloured nodules.

Pathology. The appearance is quite distinctive. The dermis is occupied by irregularly rounded masses of epithelial cells, each surrounded by a broad band of pinkish homogenous-looking material (Figure 14.14). The epithelial cells are of two main types – small dark cells with densely basophilic nuclei and large cells with more vesicular nuclei. Some of the cells in the masses undergo necrosis, so that there are small eosinophilic blobs within the tumour masses (Figure 14.15).

Eccrine Spiradenoma

This uncommon tumour is usually solitary and sometimes tender and painful.

Histopathology. There are several quite large, rounded tumour masses in the dermis which contain basophilic epithelial cells at the periphery of the lobules, and many clearer appearing cells around the lumina of ducts. There are also large numbers of irregular thin-walled vascular channels in the lobules (Figure 14.16). The latter may be sufficiently prominent to simulate a vascular tumour.

Eccrine Poroma[5]

Eccrine poroma is a rare benign and mostly solitary tumour of eccrine origin that not infrequently occurs on the palms and soles. When it does, the resulting intracutaneous nodule may be surrounded by a narrow collarette of thicker stratum corneum. Large, irregularly rounded aggregates of uniform small cells with dark central nuclei and clear cytoplasm may occupy the upper and mid dermis. The tumour appears continuous with the upper epidermis. There are sparse sweat ducts within the tumour masses. Glycogen is found within the cells of the tumour by staining with periodic acid–Schiff reagent. The dermal duct tumour is a similar benign neoplasm, but occurs lower in the dermis, and the lobules of which it is composed are somewhat smaller[6].

Syringocystadenoma Papilliferum

This uncommon tumour is supposedly of apocrine origin. It arises usually on a pre-existing naevus sebaceous of the scalp but uncommonly occurs as a solitary lesion on

Table 14.2 Main features of common sweat gland tumours

Type of Lesion	Main Histological Features	Main Clinical Features
Syringoma	Small comma-shaped duct containing structures and small horn cysts.	Small white papules beneath eyes and uncommonly over trunk and limbs.
Cylindroma	Nodules of small basophilic cells and smaller number of larger paler cells. Often surrounded by homogeneous eosinophilic colloid-like material.	Solitary or multiple nodules on face and scalp.
Eccrine spiradenoma	Lobules of interlacing basophilic cells with many blood-filled spaces. May contain duct-like structures.	Solitary nodule.
Eccrine poroma	Lobule of small uniform basophilic cells attached to or near to epidermis.	Nodule often on palm or sole when surrounded by horny collar.
Syringocystadenoma papilliferum	Crypt-like invagination lined by villous structures with clefting between two types of epithelium.	Deep nodule with central punctum oozing serous fluid.
Nodular hidradenoma	Nodular masses of small epithelial cells which may have clear cytoplasm (clear cell hidradenoma). Rarely is pigmented.	Solitary nodule.
Chondroid syringoma	Lobules of myxomatous degeneration and small groups basophilic epithelial cells, some with ducts.	Solitary nodule.
Hidroacanthoma simplex	Intraepidermal, well defined collection of larger clear cells.	Solitary plaque

the vulva. There is usually a central pore on the lesion. Histologically the tumour mass can be seen to consist of an invagination or a series of sinuses opening at the skin surface, the walls of which are irregular and thrown up into folds or villi (Figure 14.17). The cells lining the folds are cuboidal and the cells on which they rest are flattened in shape. Numerous plasma cells in the stroma are also typical (Figure 14.18).

Nodular Hidradenoma

This is really a collective term for a group of similar solid benign sweat gland tumours that have received a variety of names in the past. They are generally solitary, smooth, skin-coloured nodules. Histologically they consist of small rounded and angulated cellular masses in the mid or deep dermis (Figure 14.19). The cellular composition of the lesions varies from those that have a predominance of cells with pale cytoplasm (clear cell hidradenoma) to those that consist mainly of smaller dark cells. Sweat ducts are found within the tumour nodules (Figure 14.20).

Chondroid Syringoma (Mixed tumour of the skin)

These uncommon, benign sweat gland tumours are not dissimilar morphologically from mixed salivary tumours. They contain small epithelial elements fading into a homogenous pale cartilage-like stroma. The small epithelial aggregates contain prominent duct-like structures (Figure 14.21).

Hidroacanthoma Simplex

This lesion has some similarity to a seborrhoeic wart both clinically and histologically. It is a flat warty plaque lesion clinically. Inspection of a biopsy shows collections of clear cells within the substance of a thickened epidermis giving rise to an appearance quite like that of what has come to be known as Borst–Jadassohn intraepidermal epithelioma and assumed to be due to 'irritation' of a seborrhoeic wart (Figure 14.22). The clear cells contain glycogen and it is thought that they have an eccrine origin.

Hidrocystoma

These are cystic lesions that may be of either eccrine or apocrine origin. The cystic spaces are often irregular in outline and there are two cell layers in the cyst wall lining (Figure 14.23).

Tumours with Hair Follicle and Sebaceous Gland Differentiation

Trichoepithelioma (Epithelioma Adenoides Cysticum)

Trichoepithelioma mostly occurs on the face or scalp. The lesions are smooth intracutaneous nodules. The appearance of multiple lesions on the face is referred to as epithelioma adenoides cysticum and is inherited as a dominant trait (Brooks' tumours). Solitary lesions on the face also occur and tend to be larger than the multiple lesions and enlarge slowly. Quite understandably they are often mistaken for basal cell carcinoma.

Histopathology. In the upper and mid dermis there are many aggregates of small basaloid epithelial cells, but with a few larger paler cells centrally. Horn-filled cysts of different sizes within the tumour lobules are a consistent feature and helpful in distinguishing the lesion (Figure 14.24). It will be evident that the lesion is often difficult to distinguish from basal cell carcinoma histologically (and sometimes clinically). Indeed in some instances it is unjustifiable to make a firm differentiation.

Desmoplastic Trichoepithelioma

Small epithelial cysts and antler-shaped epithelial structures are embedded in a fibrous stroma in this uncommon lesion (Figure 14.25). The lesion should be carefully distinguished from syringoma and morphoeic basal cell carcinoma.

Trichofolliculoma

There is often a central dell or even a pit representing an attempt at formation of a central hair canal in this uncommon solitary nodular tumour. There are numerous tumour lobules and sinuses consisting of basaloid cells. The lobules resemble distorted hair follicle structures (Figure 14.26). Trichofolliculoma must be distinguished from trichoepithelioma and basal cell carcinoma.

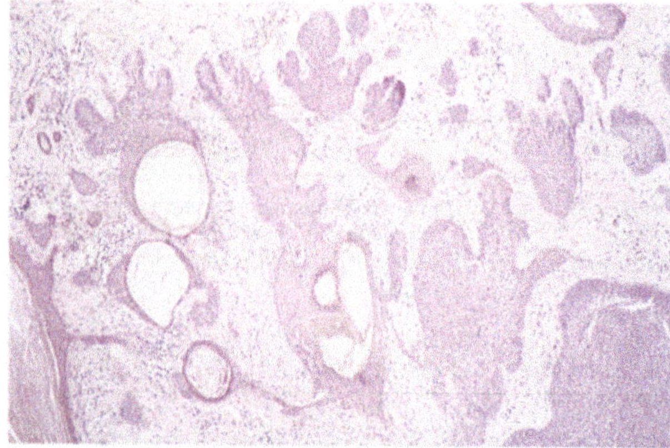

Figure 14.24 Trichoepithelioma. Many epithelial masses and horn-filled cysts. H & E (A)

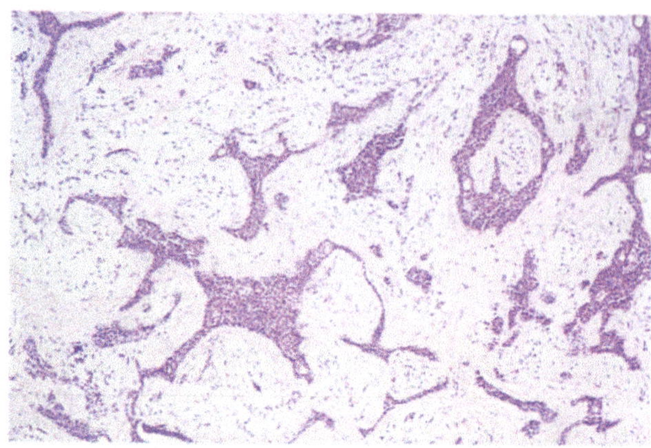

Figure 14.25 Desmoplastic trichoepithelioma. Irregular epithelial masses in a fibrous stoma. H & E (B)

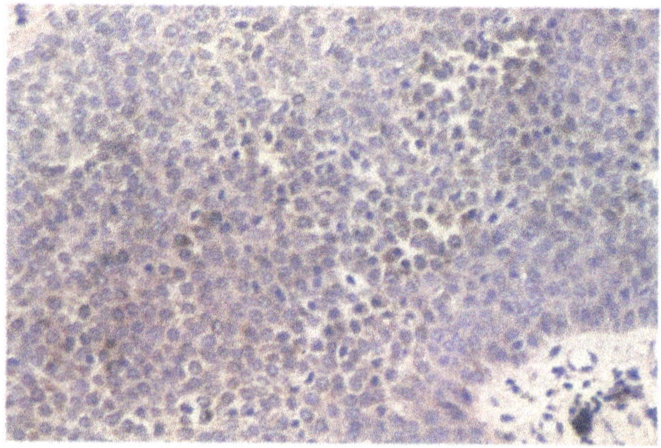

Figure 14.26 Trichofolliculoma. Irregular epidermal hypertrophy with follicular differentiation. H & E (B)

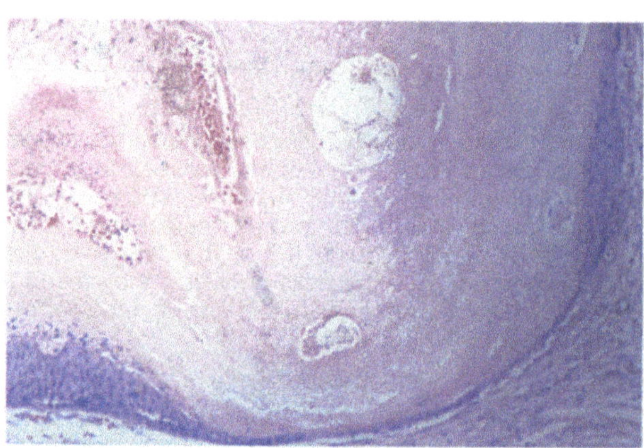

Figure 14.27 Pilomatrixoma. Basaloid cells can be seen to be transforming into a mummified mass. H & E (B)

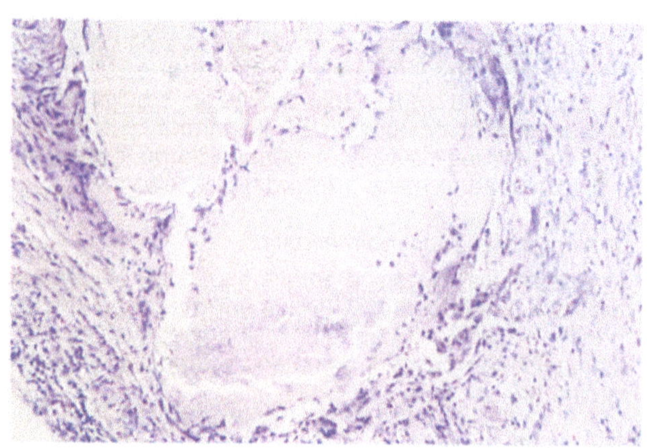

Figure 14.28 Pilomatrixoma. Ghost cells can be seen. H & E (C)

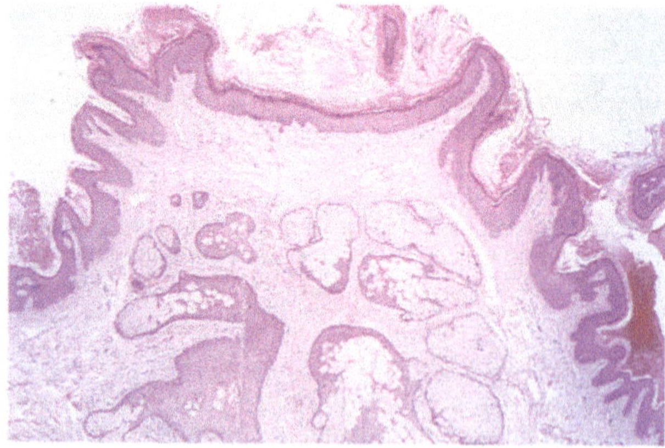

Figure 14.29 Naevus sebaceous. Irregular abnormal sebaceous glands are evident near the surface. H & E (B)

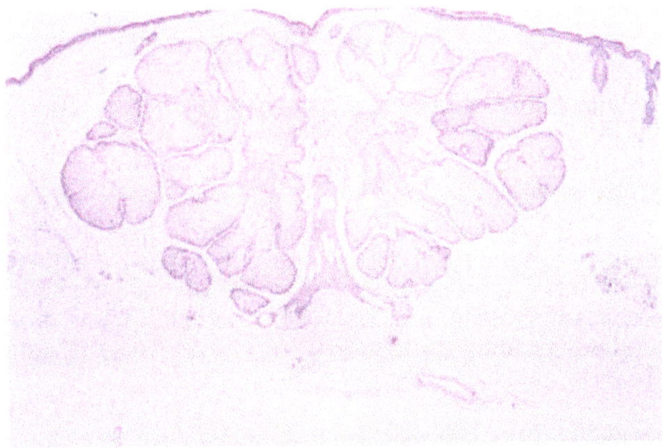

Figure 14.30 Senile sebaceous hypertrophy. Massive hypertrophy of sebaceous gland elements near the surface. H & E (A)

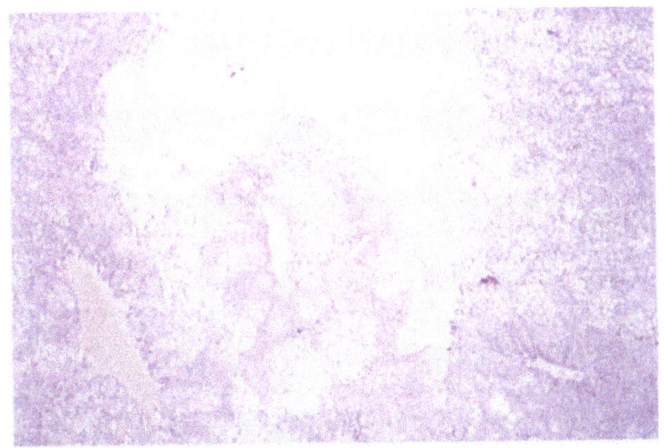

Figure 14.31 Sebaceous adenoma. H & E (B)

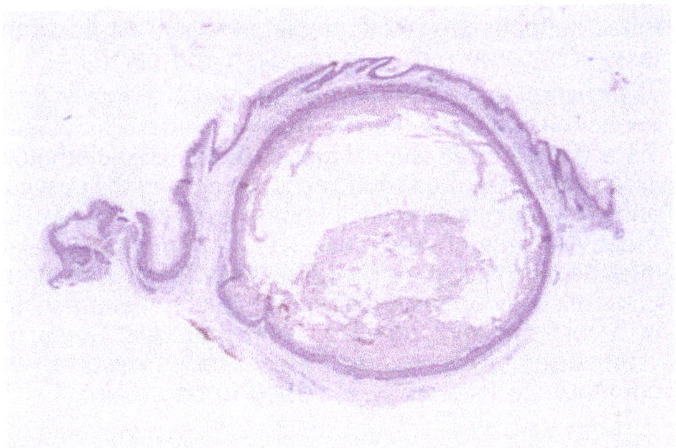

Figure 14.32 Epidermoid cyst. H & E (A)

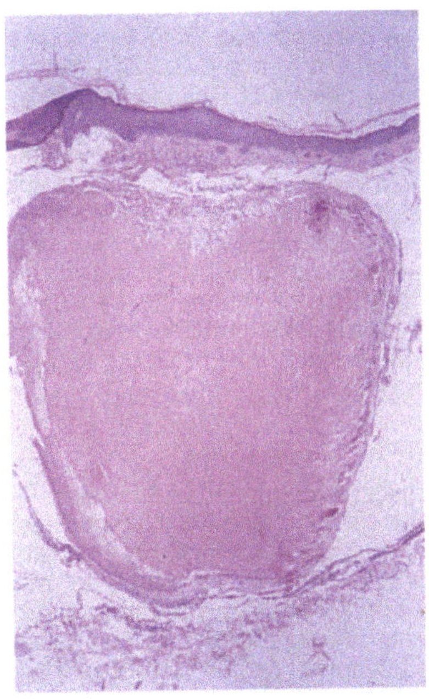

Figure 14.33 Pilar cyst with granulomatous inflammation around it. H & E (A)

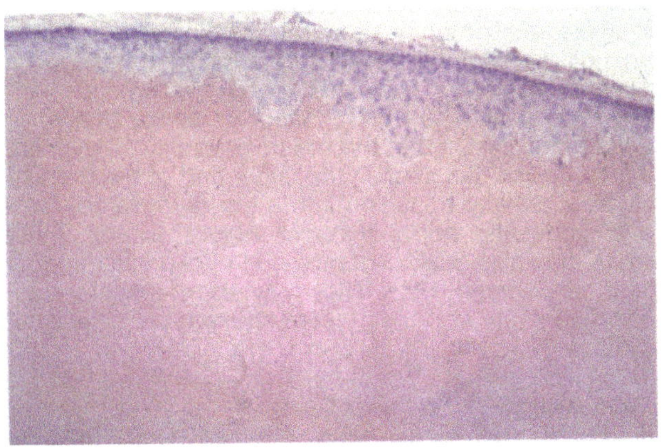

Figure 14.34 Wall of pilar cyst showing trichilemmal keratinization. H & E (C)

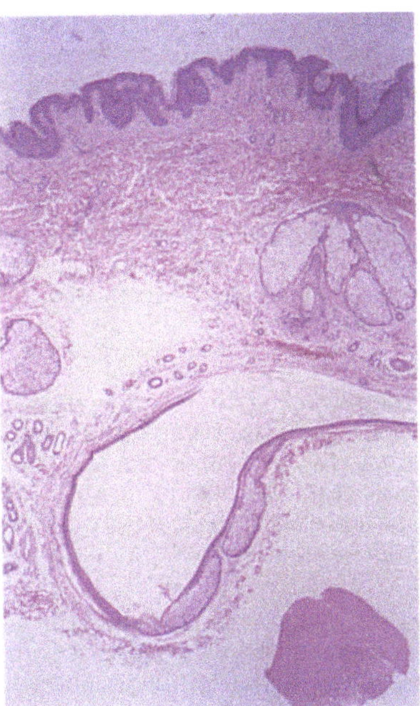

Figure 14.35 Sebocystoma multiplex. Sebaceous glands can be seen attached to the cyst wall. H & E (A)

Lesions with even greater differentiation towards hair follicles are also found. A lesion of this latter type may justifiably be termed a hair follicle naevus. The histological appearance is variable but the section will contain hair follicle-like tissue which may or may not be differentiated into a hair shaft and may or may not possess a hair papilla.

Comedone Naevus

Persistent clusters of prominent comedones on the trunk or limbs in zosteriform or linear arrangements are occasionally encountered. These appear to result from a developmental (naevoid) abnormality of hair follicles and are not neoplastic in origin. Horny plugs are found in the centre of dilated follicles histologically. Acneiform inflammation may also be seen.

Pilomatrixoma (Calcifying Epithelioma of Malherbe)

This tumour usually arises as a single hard intracutaneous nodule on the face or scalp, though multiple lesions sometimes occur. The lesion is believed to develop from hair follicle matrix tissue. The histological appearance is quite characteristic and is easily recognized. There are irregular masses of what appears to be cartilage on first inspection within the dermis (Figure 14.27). Throughout the homogenous substance of these masses there are 'ghost-like' outlines of small cells and at the rim of the masses or in clusters elsewhere there are small basophilic epithelial cells (Figure 14.28). There is a variable amount of calcification throughout the lesion. It is presumed that there is a continuous transformation of the small epithelial cells into the mummified ghost-like cells. Granulomatous inflammation is often observed around the tumour.

Naevus Sebaceous (Organoid Naevus)

The most frequent clinical presentation of this relatively common lesion is that of an orange–yellow, hairless plaque which later develops into a nodule on the scalp, face or occasionally elsewhere in an infant. In later life naevus sebaceous becomes more warty and may develop other epithelial tumours within its substance, including syringocystadenoma papilliferum (see page 105) and basal cell carcinoma[7].

Pathology. There may be changes in all epithelial structures but the abnormality may also be confined to the sebaceous glands. The sebaceous glands are increased in number and size and are nearer the skin surface than usual (Figure 14.29). In addition there is thickening of the peripheral germinative cells and irregularities in the degree of lipidization of the sebaceous cells. Occasionally 'holes' are present within the abnormal sebaceous gland lobules. Hyperplasia and dilatation of eccrine and apocrine glands may be noted, as may papillary hyperplasia and thickening and wartiness of the epidermis.

Senile Sebaceous Hypertrophy

This is an extremely common disorder that may present *per se* or be noted incidentally. It is characterized by the appearance of orange–yellow nodules on the forehead, temples or central facial areas. The nodules are 1–3 mm in diameter and smooth, and may have a central punctum or dell. They are frequently misdiagnosed as basal cell carcinoma.

Histopathology. There is massive sebaceous gland enlargement. The enlarged lobules are embedded abnormally high within a loose dermal stroma showing telangiectasia and solar elastotic degeneration (Figure 14.30).

Sebaceous Adenoma

This is a rare benign lesion which mostly presents as a solitary expanding nodule on the face or scalp. Histologically there is irregular enlargement of one or several sebaceous gland lobules which contain many more undifferentiated germinative cells than usual (Figure 14.31).

Cysts

A true cyst is an epithelium-lined cavity that does not communicate with other structures. Unfortunately the term is often loosely used to describe any abnormal fluid-filled cavity (e.g. 'acne cyst' or 'cystic degeneration' in basal cell carcinoma).

Epidermoid Cyst

This lesion is extremely common and found almost anywhere as a variably sized, firm but fluctuant, mobile intracutaneous smooth-surfaced swelling. At times the lesions become red, more swollen and painful.

Histopathology. The lining of the cyst is 2–4 cells thick, appearing to differentiate normally into stratum corneum via a granular cell layer (Figure 14.32). Granulomatous inflammation is often found at points around the cyst wall and in old lesions there is fibrosis in addition. Presumably these are sites at which the cyst contents have leaked into the dermis (Figure 14.33). In older lesions the horny contents may undergo degenerative changes, resulting in a foul-smelling, greyish viscid material. These are often erroneously known as sebaceous cysts as the contents are incorrectly assumed to be sebum.

Milial Cysts

Milia are tiny epidermoid cysts occurring high up within the dermis. They are apparent as small white horny papules on the face, where they arise spontaneously, or elsewhere after blistering (common in epidermolysis bullosa and in porphyria cutanea tarda).

Pilar Cysts (trichilemmal cysts)[8]

Pilar cysts are common and typically on the scalp and scrotum, but may occur elsewhere too. They are often multiple and sometimes familial. Histologically the lining epithelium resembles that of external root sheath. It is several cell layers thick and stains for glycogen with the PAS stain. The differentiation is unlike that of an epidermoid cyst in that there is no granular cell layer and it is more like that seen in the upper part of the follicular canal, a gradual transition into a less lamellated, more even-appearing horny material (Figure 14.34). These cysts may also 'leak contents' and evoke inflammation as in epidermoid cysts. They may also degenerate and liquefy and are also then incorrectly termed 'sebaceous cysts'.

Proliferating Trichilemmal Cysts

These unusual lesions present as enlarging nodules or cysts on the scalp, often in elderly women. The trichilemmal cyst is lobulated and hypertrophied. The epithelial lining shows marked hyperplasia in places.

Sebocystoma Multiplex (steatocystoma)

These are the only cysts that may contain true sebaceous gland elements in their walls. They are often multiple and may occur anywhere on hair-bearing skin as variably sized cystic structures. They are sometimes familial and occasionally part of a more generalized complex syndrome[9].

Pathology. There are irregular cystic spaces lined by epithelia which sometimes show differentiation as in an epidermoid cyst and sometimes a sebaceous type of differentiation with the production of sebum (Figure 14.35). In the latter type there may be nodules of sebaceous gland tissue embedded in the walls of the cyst. As with the other types of cyst, inflammation can occur around the cyst wall.

References

1. Mehregan, A. H. and Pinkus, H. (1964). Intraepidermal epithelioma: a critical study. *Cancer*, **17**, 609

2. Steffen, C. and Ackerman, B. (1985). Intraepidermal epithelioma of Borst–Jadassohn. *Am. J. Dermatopathol.*, **7**, 5

3. Brownstein, M. H., Fernando, S. and Shapiro, L. (1973). Clear cell acanthoma. Clinicopathologic analysis of 37 new cases. *Am. J. Clin. Pathol.*, **59**, 306

4. Hashimoto, K. and Lever, W. F. (1969). Histogenesis of skin appendage tumours. *Arch. Dermatol.*, **100**, 356

5. Pinkus, H., Rogin, J. R. and Goldman, P. (1956). Eccrine poroma: Tumours exhibiting features of the epidermal sweat duct unit. *Arch. Dermatol.*, **74**, 511

6. Winkelmann, R. K. and McLeod, W. A. (1966). The dermal duct tumour. *Arch. Dermatol.*, **94**, 50

7. Wilson-Jones, E. and Heyl, T. (1970). Naevus sebaceous. A report of 140 cases with special regard to the development of secondary malignant tumours. *Br. J. Dermatol.*, **82**, 99

8. Rulon, D. and Hewig, E. B. (1974). Cutaneous sebaceous neoplasms. *Cancer*, **33**, 82

9. Leonard, D. D. and Deaton, R. (1974). Multiple sebaceous gland tumours and visceral carcinomas. *Arch. Dermatol.*, **110**, 917

Actinic (Solar, Senile) Keratoses

Actinic keratoses are small warty nodules or scaling plaques that occur mostly in the light exposed sites of the skin but are also occasionally observed in areas that have been exposed to X-irradiation or to chronic heat injury. They should be regarded as precancerous lesions[1], but their transformation to frankly malignant squamous cell carcinoma appears uncommon. Although they occur focally, the surrounding areas of epidermis also show abnormalities of cell size, shape and arrangement, suggesting early dysplastic change[2].

Histopathology

Histologically they are distinguished by cytological abnormalities and by irregularities of epidermal differentiation. Along the basal layer of the affected epidermis there are foci of abnormal cells with larger hyperchromatic nuclei which may also appear irregular in shape. At times these foci are prominent and appear to 'bud' into the dermis (Figure 15.1). Cell kinetic studies using tritiated thymidine indicate that there is an increased rate of epidermal cell production in the lesions. The abnormal area of epidermis is often slightly thickened and surmounted by a parakeratotic scale (Figure 15.2) but in some lesions (atrophic keratosis) the changes are more subtle, the epidermis is, if anything, thinner than usual and the stratum corneum is orthokeratotic (Figure 15.3). In most solar keratoses there is some evidence of disturbed keratinization and loss of the normal epidermal organization. Premature (and maybe abnormal) keratinization results in the appearance of eosinophilic hyalinized cellular remnants within the epidermis.

Often segments of abnormal basal epidermis fail to make or lose contact with nearby normal epidermis so that there appears to be a cleft between the two types of epithelium. This may be particularly noticeable around hair follicles. This appearance with sheets of abnormal cells close by but not contacting the normal epidermis, is known as carcinoma segregans (Figure 15.4).

Although quite large areas of epidermis may be affected by the preneoplastic process, adnexal epithelium seems to be protected from the process in that these structures stay uninvolved while surrounded by the abnormal tissue. When the normal eccrine duct is seen to be surrounded by parakeratotic stratum corneum the appearance is known as 'Freudenthal's funnel' (Figure 15.5).

There is a variable amount of inflammatory cell infiltrate associated with solar keratoses. Lymphocytes and histiocytes are the predominant cell types. Occasionally the inflammation is marked and associated with vacuolation and esoinophilic hyalinization of basal epidermal cells. The histological picture then has an overall similiarity to lichen planus and the lesions are termed lichenoid keratoses (Figure 15.6). This may be an attempt at immune rejection of the lesion[3].

Cutaneous Horn

Any projecting horny accretion may be called a cutaneous horn. The majority of such lesions are caused by an underlying solar keratosis (Figure 15.7). Other causes include squamous cell carcinoma, seborrhoeic warts and even viral warts. The reason for the focal failure of desquamation in this rather dramatic fashion in unknown.

Pitfalls in Diagnosis of Solar Keratosis

(1) When there is but minimal cytological abnormality and minimal epidermal thickening without parakeratosis it takes an experienced eye to diagnose a solar keratosis with confidence. Such minor degrees of dysplasia are common in sun-damaged sites.

(2) When there is marked basal cell erosion and a heavy band-like inflammatory cell infiltrate immediately subepidermally there is sometimes difficulty in distinguishing the condition from lichen planus (see page 53) or even lupus erythematosus. However, the cytological abnormalities should allow the correct diagnosis.

(3) Care should be taken to distinguish solar keratosis from a superficial basal cell carcinoma. This may be more difficult than it sounds because basal cell carcinomas can develop areas of squamous metaplasia and solar keratoses can produce 'buds' of basaloid-appearing cells.

Bowen's Disease (syn: Intraepidermal epithelioma)

Bowen's disease is a localized area in which the epidermis demonstrates the characteristics of neoplastic transformation within the confines of the basal lamina, i.e. there is no local invasion or metastasis. Clinically the lesions appear as thickened, red, scaling patches which may resemble psoriasis or patches of eczema. This type of lesion has been associated especially with the ingestion of arsenic and X-irradiation. They also occur after chronic solar exposure but less frequently than either solar keratosis or squamous cell epithelioma.

Histopathology

Histologically the epidermis is thickened and parakeratotic. There is often a psoriasiform profile in that there is regular prolongation of the epidermal rete pegs but this is by no means invariable (Figure 15.8). Keratinocytes within the lesion are irregularly enlarged. Their nuclei show great irregularity in size, shape and degree of

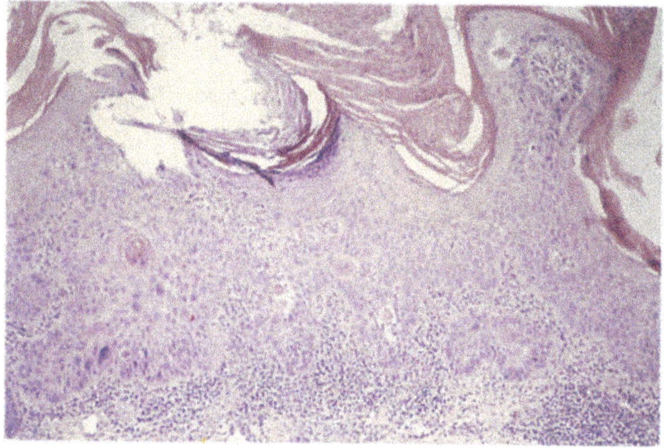

Figure 15.1 Solar keratosis with buds of dysplastic cells beneath the epidermis. H & E (B)

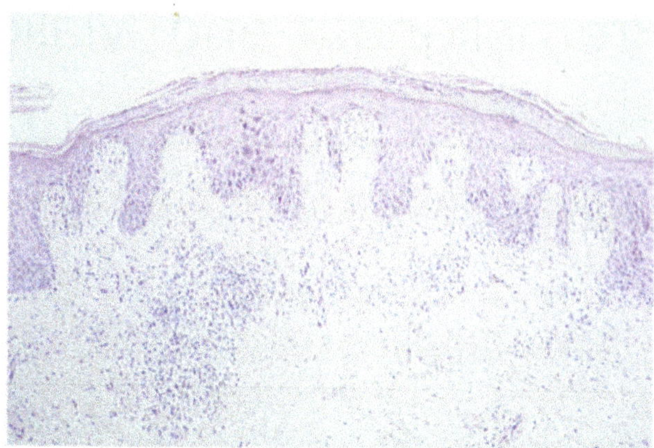

Figure 15.2 Solar keratosis showing large basophilic irregular nuclei and irregular thickening and a parakeratotic scale. H & E (B)

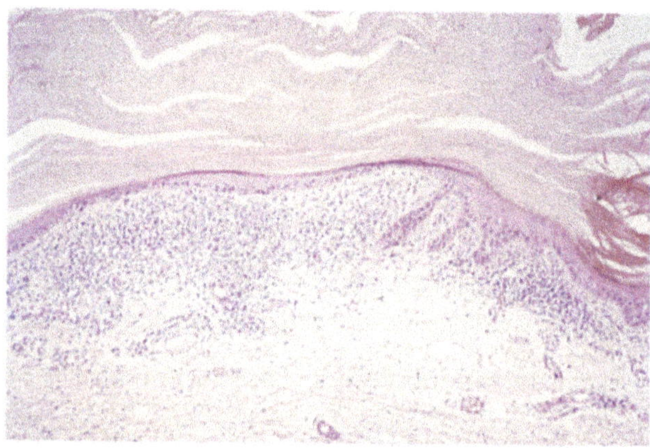

Figure 15.3 Solar keratosis. The epidermis is thinner than usual in places and there is a heavy subepidermal inflammatory cell infiltrate. There is also massive hyperkeratotic and parakeratotic scale. H & E (B)

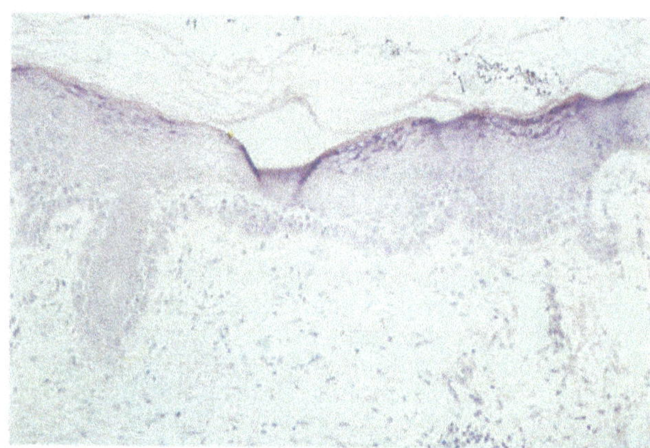

Figure 15.4a Carcinoma segregans change in a solar keratosis. There is a sheet of abnormal cells at the base of the epidermis but slightly separated from it. H & E (B)

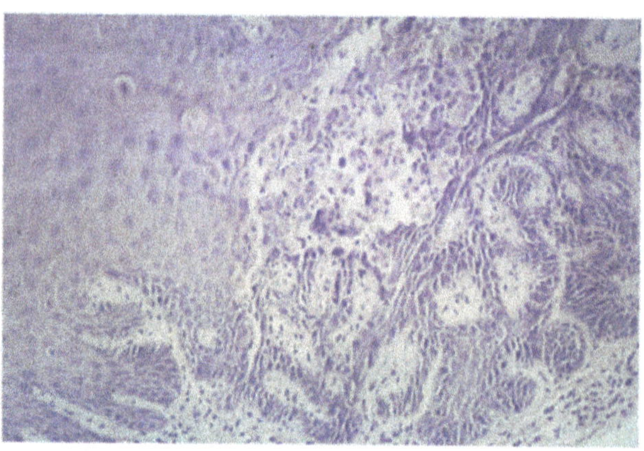

Figure 15.4b Carcinoma segregans change. The abnormal cells are arranged in an interlacing pattern beneath the epidermis. H & E (C)

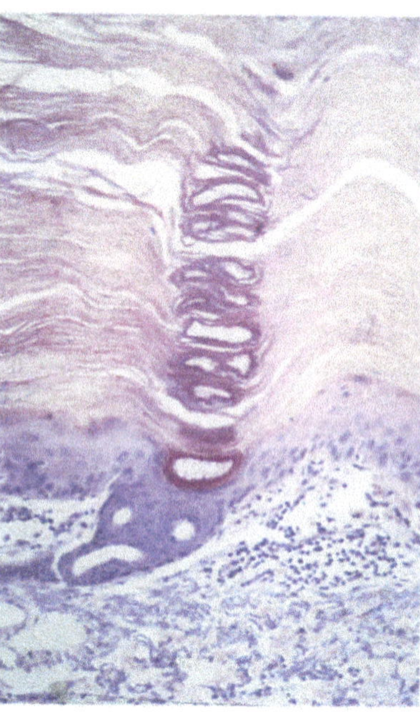

Figure 15.5 Freudenthal's funnel. The epidermal sweat duct and surrounding eccrine duct cells are uninvolved by the solar keratosis on either side. H & E (B)

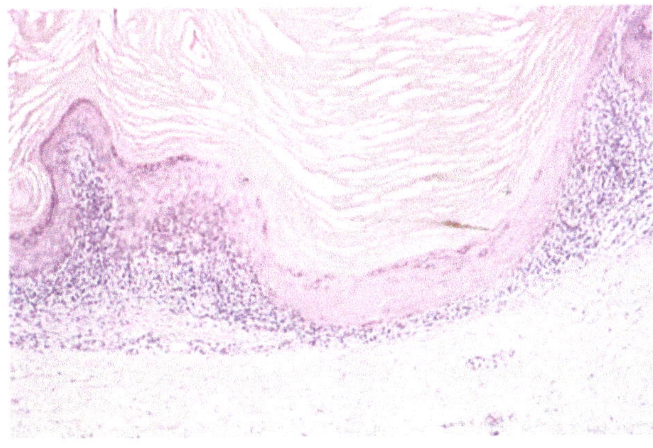

Figure 15.6a   Lichenoid solar keratosis. There is a heavy inflammatory cell infiltrate at the base of the epidermis that is involving it in places.   H & E (B)

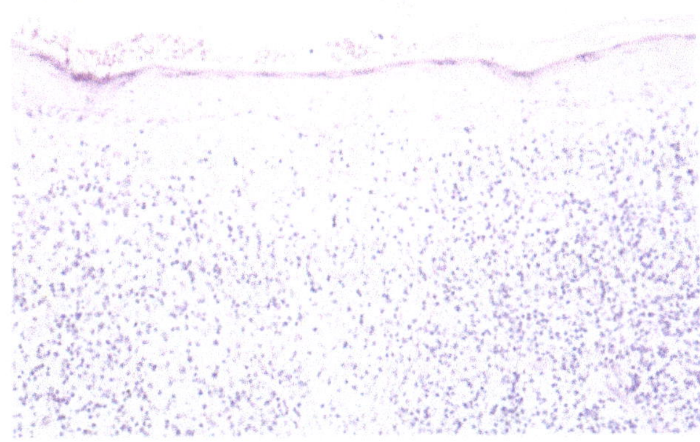

Figure 15.6b   Lichenoid solar keratosis. Many cytoid bodies are present at the base of the epidermis. There is also a heavy inflammatory cell infiltrate.   H & E (B)

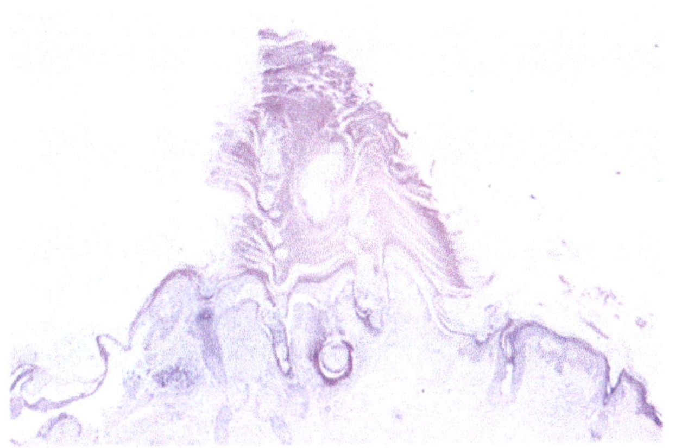

Figure 15.7   Solar keratosis with cutaneous horn.   H & E (A)

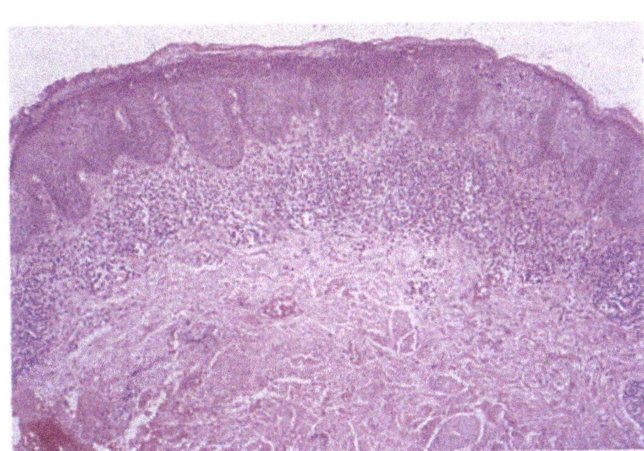

Figure 15.8a   Bowen's disease. There is a psoriasiform thickening of the epidermis.   H & E (A)

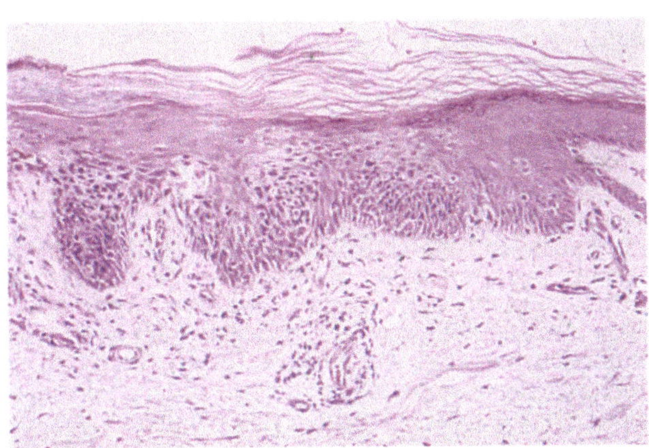

Figure 15.8b   Bowen's disease. Irregular thickening of the epidermis. The epidermis contains many abnormal hyperchromatic cells.   H & E (B)

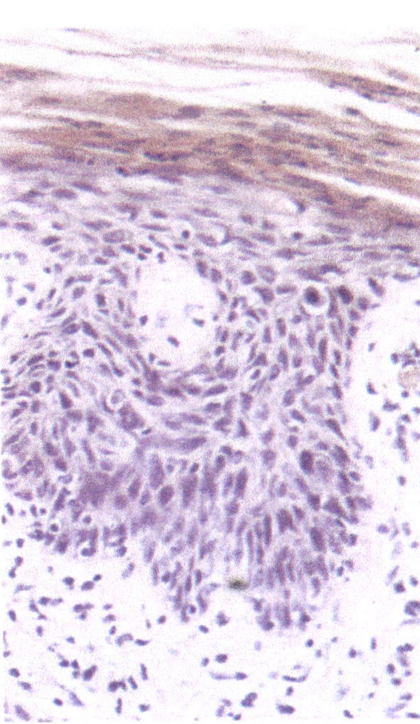

Figure 15.9   Bowen's disease. Many abnormal cells in the epidermis, some of which are in mitosis.   H & E (C)

basophilia. Numerous mitoses are often evident and sometimes abnormal nuclei (e.g. tripolar mitoses are seen (Figure 15.9)). A variably dense inflammatory cell infiltrate composed of lymphocytes and histiocytes is usually present in the upper dermis beneath the lesion.

Differential Diagnosis

Histological diagnosis usually presents no difficulty. However, Bowen's disease is occasionally confused (a) with psoriasis, although this does not possess the cytological abnormalities of Bowen's disease and shows regular hyperplasia, (b) solar keratosis, from which it can be distinguished by the absence of any normal epidermis in the lesion, (c) squamous cell carcinoma – the distinction is made by the detection of invading epidermal tissue within the dermis (see later), and (d) Paget's disease (see next column) where there are nests of large pale cells within the epidermis which although obviously abnormal are not often as frankly abnormal as are the epidermal cells in Bowen's disease.

Erythroplasia of Queyrat

This condition should be regarded as Bowen's disease of the penis. Clinically the condition presents as a glazed, velvety red plaque which may involve the glans or the shaft of the penis. The degree of cellular abnormality is less pronounced than in Bowen's disease and there is little overlying parakeratotic horn. There is pronounced infiltrate composed predominantly of plasma cells and lymphocytes (Figure 15.10).

Bowenoid Papulosis[4]

It is only in the past few years that this disorder has been clinically characterized and only in the past 2–3 years that its cause pinpointed. It presents as brownish pink macules or maculopapules on the penis or vulva or elsewhere on the genitalia. The histological appearance is that of Bowen's disease (Figure 15.11) but it does not behave as such as many cases remit spontaneously. Immunocytochemical and DNA hybridization studies have located the human papilloma virus (wart virus) of antigenic strain type 16 in the lesion and it must be presumed that this is the cause of the disorder.

Squamous Cell Carcinoma

This lesion takes the form of warty plaques, nodules or ulcers that mostly occur on light-exposed sites but also on chronically scarred or ulcerated areas, on the genitalia and on the lips. Other sites may rarely be affected. They are frankly malignant lesions of differentiating epidermis.

Histopathology

Histologically they are distinguished by the presence of an irregular, thickened mass of abnormal epidermis which demonstrates abnormal differentiation. Often the lesion is cup shaped with a central horny mass in the cavity which projects from the skin surface (Figure 15.12), when it may be confused with a keratoacanthoma. Other types of lesion include those with a warty and/or plaque-like configuration, and nodular and ulcerated tumorous lesions. Typically thickened areas of epidermal cells at various stages of differentiation invade the surrounding dermis (Figure 15.13). Separated islands of this abnormal epidermis can also be detected at various distances from the main bulk of the tumour. Cytologically the epidermal cells often show great irregularity of size, shape and staining properties. However, many lesions show much less obvious cellular abnormality.

The nuclei are irregular and several abnormal mitotic figures may be evident in one high power field. Horn pearls are evidence of ectopic and abnormal differentiation (Figure 15.14). There is often a considerable inflammatory response in the underlying dermis in which a wide variety of cell types may be represented.

Paget's Disease[5]

Paget's disease is a type of intraepidermal epithelioma affecting the skin of the nipple and areola and is due to the spread of an intraduct carcinoma of the breast along the duct and into the epidermis. Clinically the condition is difficult to distinguish from an eczematous rash.

Histopathology

The histological appearance is quite distinctive. There are nests of variable size consisting of larger, paler cells and the surrounding normal epidermal cells (Figure 15.15). Serial sectioning will sometimes demonstrate the intraduct carcinoma as the abnormal duct rises to meet the epidermis. The abnormal cells stain strongly for mucosubstances with periodic acid and Schiff reagent.

Differential Diagnosis

Although the histological appearance is quite distinctive it can be mimicked by Bowen's disease from which it can be differentiated by the greater irregularity of cells in the latter disorder.

Extramammary Paget's disease[6]

A very similar disorder can affect the skin of the groin, lower abdomen or perineum. In about half such cases the condition is the result of spread from an apocrine carcinoma but in the remainder no such underlying neoplastic lesion can be identified.

Keratoacanthoma[7]

This lesion is in reality a self-limiting localized squamous cell carcinoma with the propensity rapidly to form a cup-shaped protuberance the centre of which is filled with a mass of stratum corneum. It usually arises rapidly – frequently on the face – forming a steep sided nodule that may reach 2 cm in diameter or occasionally even more. If left untreated it begins to decrease in size after several weeks and then disappears finally to leave a scar.

Histopathology

The hallmark of this lesion is the symmetrical configuration of a protruding epidermal nodule containing a central horn-filled crypt (Figure 15.16). Overall the lesion has some similarity to a monstrous deformed hair follicle, and indeed there is evidence that keratoacanthomas are derived from hair follicles. The dermo-epidermal interface at the inferior pole of the lesion tends to be very irregular and may be difficult to distinguish from squamous cell carcinoma (Figure 15.17). There may be individual cell keratinization with scattered eosinophilic homogenous looking keratinocytes but little in the way of true horn pearl formation (Figure 15.18). In general the degree of cell atypia is low and if large numbers of abnormal nuclei and mitoses are seen it is more likely that the lesion is in fact a squamous cell carcinoma. There is usually a quite marked inflammatory cell infiltrate. At the sides of the lesion there is often an apparent hyperplasia of the hair follicles flanking the main tumour mass.

The aetiology of keratoacanthoma is unclear but as they can be induced experimentally by the same stimuli that cause squamous cell carcinoma, and as they appear in light-exposed areas, they should be considered as 'self healing neoplasms'. It cannot be emphasized too strongly that it may be difficult to distinguish keratoacanthoma from squamous cell carcinoma and that it is probably better to err on the side of caution and overdiagnose squamous cell carcinoma than make a potentially tragic mistake.

Familial Self-healing Epithelioma[8] (Ferguson-Smith disease)

This condition is a rare familial disorder in which proliferative irregular masses occur on the upper limbs and face which eventually heal with considerable scarring. Histologically they may bear little resemblance to keratoacanthoma in overall structure as they seem to consist of ramifying epithelial channels. However, it seems that they do represent a particular variety of keratoacanthoma.

Basal Cell Carcinoma

This is a common locally invasive tumour of small basophilic epidermal cells that are thought to be derived from basal cells. Basal cell carcinoma (BCC) presents as either a pearly (or sometimes pigmented) nodule or an ulcer with a raised rounded edge or a scaly pink (superficial) plaque with a fine raised margin, or more rarely as a sclerotic (morphoea-like) plaque. Although they mostly occur on light-exposed skin they are by no means restricted to such areas and lesions may occur on the trunk or upper limbs.

Histological Description

The histological appearances parallel the clinical types mentioned above.

Nodulo-ulcerative type. In this type of BCC, rounded masses of basophilic epidermal cells occupy the upper and mid dermis (Figure 15.19) Although the outline of the lesion is typically rounded, strands of tumour tissue may also invade the surrounding dermis (Figure 15.20). Many mitotic figures are obvious throughout the mass of tumour cells. Autoradiographs of BCC tissue after exposure to tritiated thymidine show large numbers of labelled cells. This does not signify rapid growth and there also appears to be a high rate of cell necrosis within the lesion. The cells at the margin of the tumour mass are visually 'palisaded' in that they are arranged

vertically to the main tumour mass (Figure 15.21). A variety of arrangements of the abnormal clumps of tissue are seen. Sometimes the tumour seems to consist of interlacing strands giving rise to an 'adenoidal' of 'pseudoglandular' arrangement (Figure 15.22). The margins of the lesions are often separated by a gap from the surrounding dermis. This appearance is artefactual and due to leaching out of mucosubstances by the processing technique. Mucoid degenerative change is also frequently seen within the main tumour mass (Figure 15.23) and is responsible for the 'pearly' appearance. Pigmentation is also commonly observed and due to the inclusion of melanocytes in the lesion. It may be so marked as to cause clinical confusion and a mistaken diagnosis of malignant melanoma (Figure 15.24). When the tumour mass is near the skin surface, ulceration may take place.

Occasionally areas within the tumour mass take on a different appearance and squamous differentiation with horn pearl formation is seen. This 'squamous metaplasia' can mislead the pathologist into believing that the lesion is in fact a squamous cell carcinoma. Basal cell carcinoma tissue may also show differentiation towards epidermal adnexal structures. Thus occasionally follicle-like tissue or sebaceous gland-like structures may be observed within the tumour mass.

Superficial basal cell carcinoma. The histological appearance of a superficial BCC is broadly similar to that of the nodulo-ulcerative type. The differences are in the much higher position of the tumour tissue within the skin and in the much smaller nodules of tumour tissue. Usually connections with the basal part of the epidermis can be identified and small collections of basophilic tumour are present at several points in the subepidermal zone.

Sclerotic (morphoeic) basal cell carcinoma. The distinguishing feature of this type of BCC is the admixture of dense fibrous stroma with strands and small clumps of tumour tissue. The density of fibrous tissue may be such as to make identification of BCC tissue quite difficult resulting in the misdiagnosis of morphoea or scar. Inspection of several sections may be required before the diagnosis can be established. Another difficulty arises when the strands of tumour tissue seem tubular consisting of two rows of cells only (Figure 15.25) as this picture can be mistaken for that of syringoma (see page 104).

Differential Diagnosis of BCC

Many of the pitfalls in diagnosis have already been mentioned. These and others were summarized in Table 15.1

Table 15.1 Differential diagnosis of basal cell carcinoma

Differential diagnosis	Cause of difficulty	Distinguishing features of BCC
Squamous cell carcinoma	Squamous metaplasia in body of tumour tissue	Typical overall appearance of BCC
Morphoea or scar	Paucity of tumour tissue in densely fibrous lesion of sclerotic (morphoeic) BCC	Strands or small clumps of BCC cells in some areas of lesion
Syringoma	Strands of BCC in pseudo-tubular arrangement	Larger typical clumps of BCC cells usually found. No typical comma-shaped structures of syringoma
Follicular hamartoma e.g. trichoepithelioma	Follicular arrangement of BCC tissue. Squamous metaplasia giving rise to horn cysts.	Overall arrangement of tumour and surrounding connective tissue is that of BCC – few horn cysts only
e.g. sebaceous gland tumour	Sebaceous differentiation	– typical BCC in some areas
Solar keratoses	Occasionally solar keratoses may show basaloid type of proliferative change and simulate superficial BCC	Small clumps of BCC tissue show palisading at periphery. No dysplasia of intervening epidermis

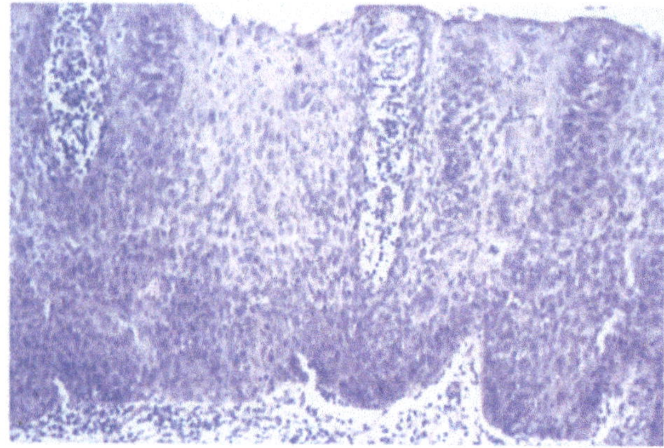

Figure 15.10 Erythroplasia of Queyrat (Bowen's disease affecting the glans penis).   H & E (B)

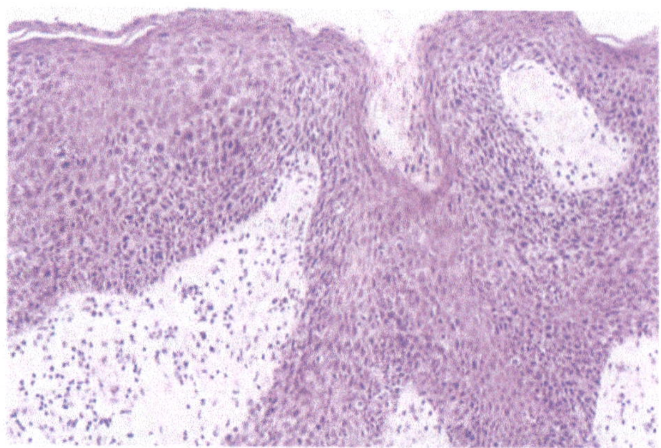

Figure 15.11 Bowenoid papulosis. Many irregularly staining dysplastic cells in the epidermis of the glans penis.   H & E (B)

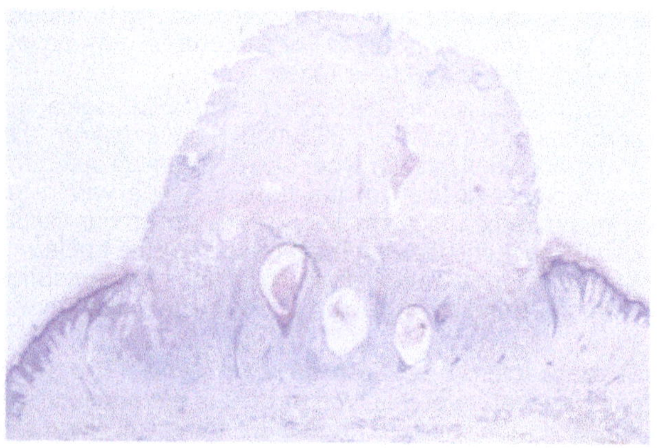

Figure 15.12a Squamous cell carcinoma. Gross epidermal thickening and horn formation was evident in this slowly growing squamous cell carcinoma.   H & E (A)

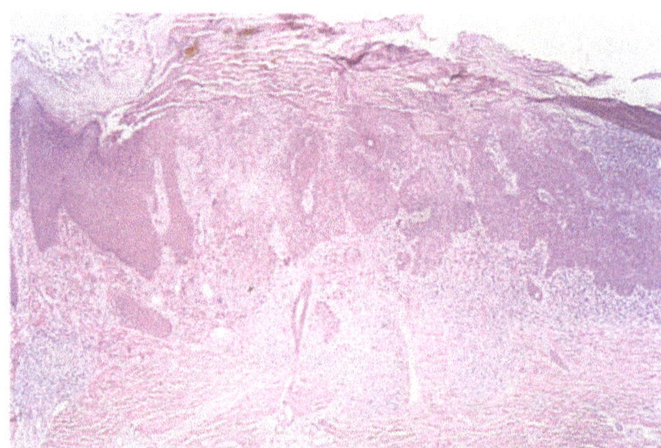

Figure 15.12b Squamous cell carcinoma showing marked thickening and irregularity of abnormal epidermis.   H & E (B)

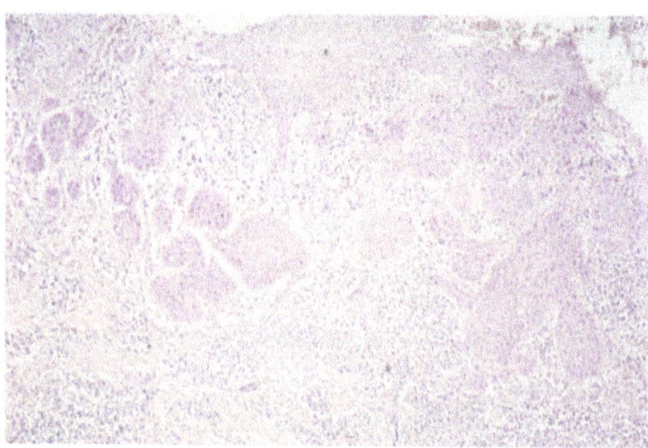

Figure 15.13a Clumps of abnormal squamous epithelium invading the dermis. There is a marked inflammatory cell infiltrate as well.   H & E (B)

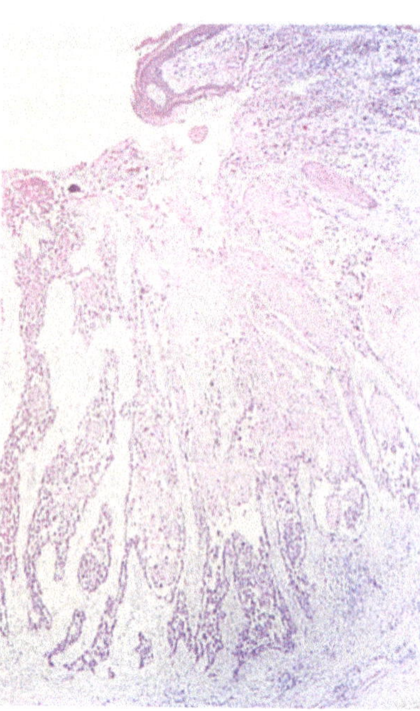

Figure 15.13b
Squamous cell carcinoma, showing adenoidal pattern and marked invasion into the dermis.   H & E (B)

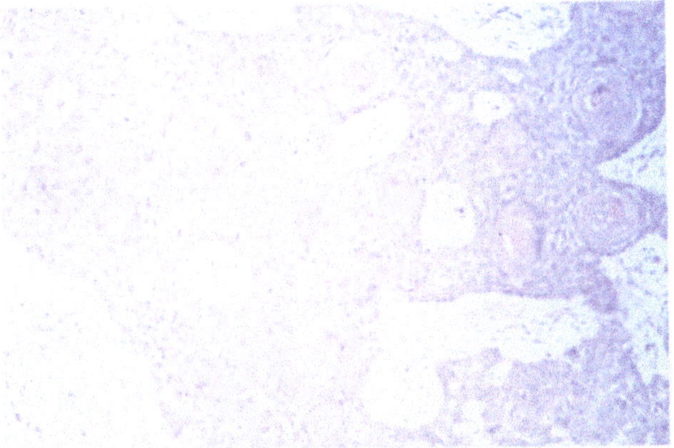

Figure 15.14 Squamous cell carcinoma showing foci of squamous differentiation.   H & E (B)

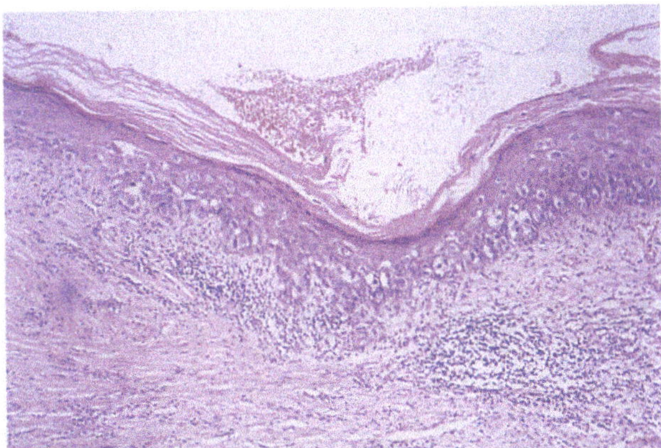

Figure 15.15 Paget's disease of the breast. The epidermis is invaded by many abnormal clear cells.   H & E (B)

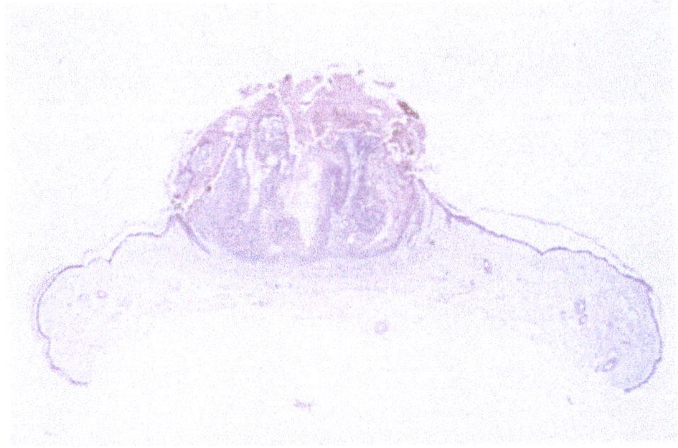

Figure 15.16a Keratoacanthoma showing cup-shaped depression filled with horny mass.   H & E (A)

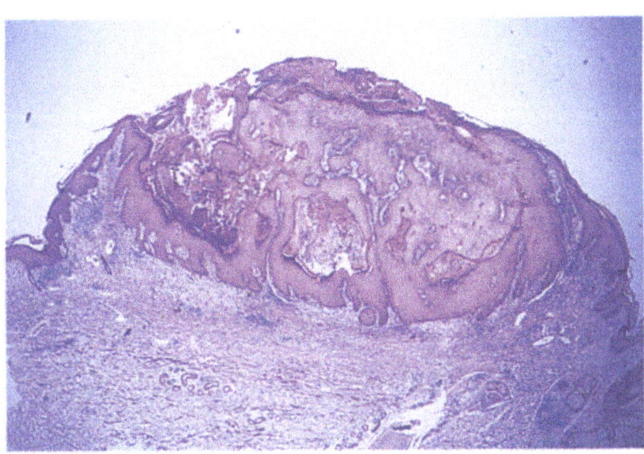

Figure 15.16b Keratoacanthoma. Cup-shaped invagination showing horn-filled crater.   H & E (A)

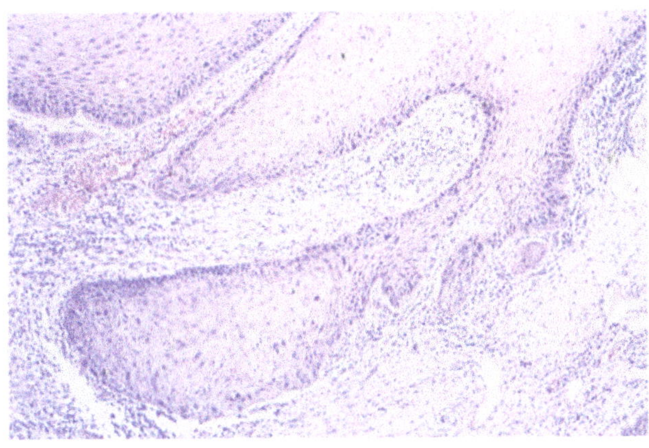

Figure 15.17 Base of keratoacanthoma showing irregular prolongations into the dermis.   H & E (B)

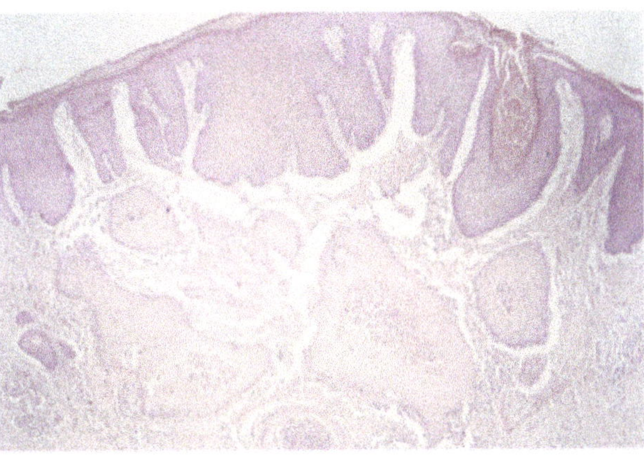

Figure 15.18 Keratoacanthoma. This lesion has been sectioned at the side of the invagination and its distinction from squamous cell carcinoma may be difficult.   H & E (B)

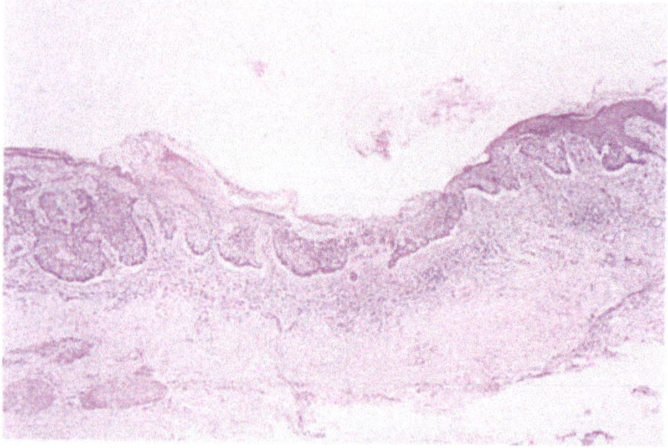

Figure 15.19 Basal cell carcinoma. Basophilic clumps of epithelial cells are present in the upper dermis. Note the apparent gap between the surrounding dermis and the abnormal masses of cells. H & E (A)

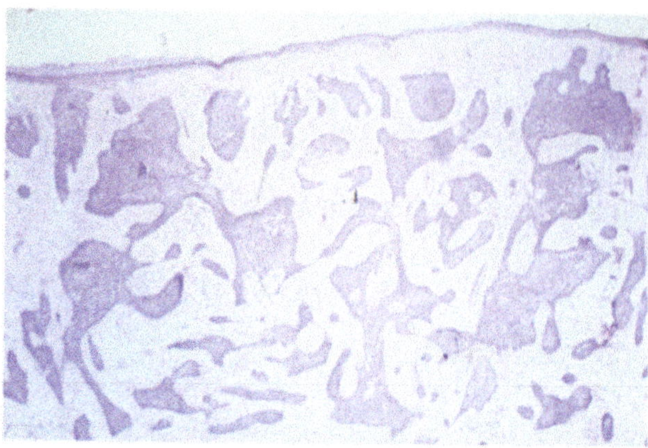

Figure 15.20 Basal cell carcinoma occupying most of the dermis. H & E (A)

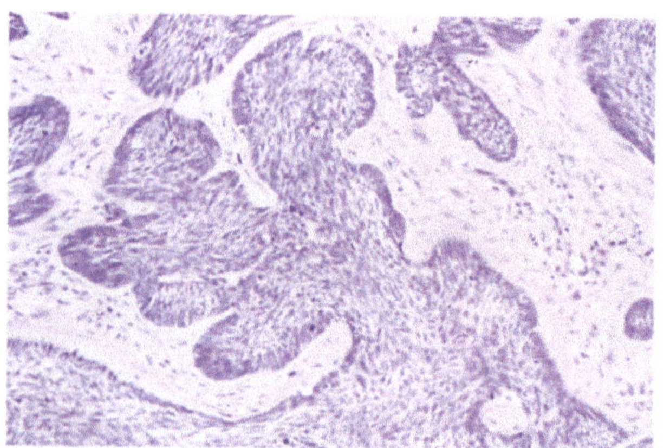

Figure 15.21 Basal cell carcinoma. The cells at the margins of the clumps of basophilic cells are arranged vertically, giving a palisaded appearance. H & E (B)

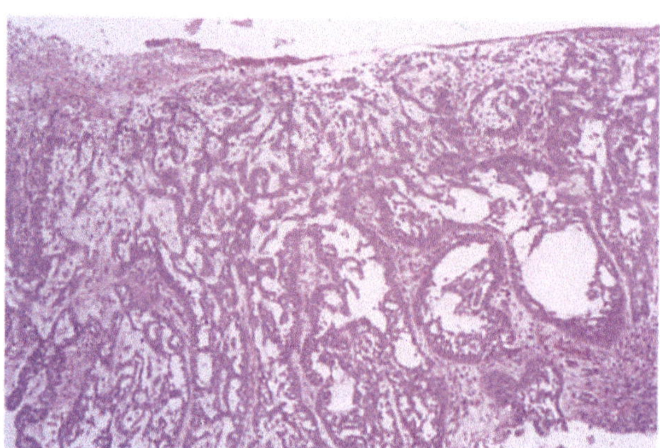

Figure 15.22 Basal cell carcinoma showing a pseudoglandular arrangement. H & E (A)

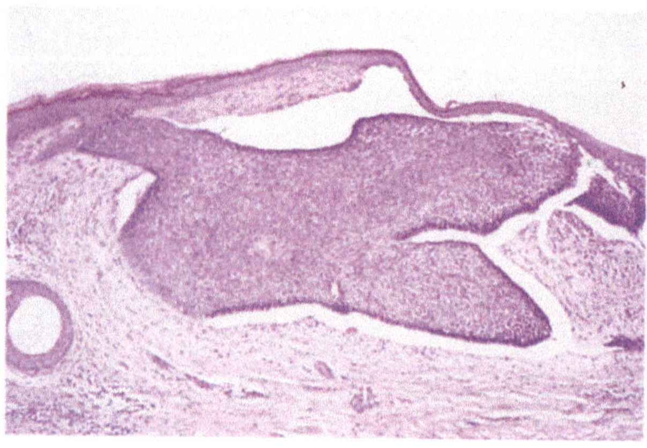

Figure 15.23a Small lobule of basal cell carcinoma showing gap between lobule and dermis due to mucoid degeneration of stroma. H & E (A)

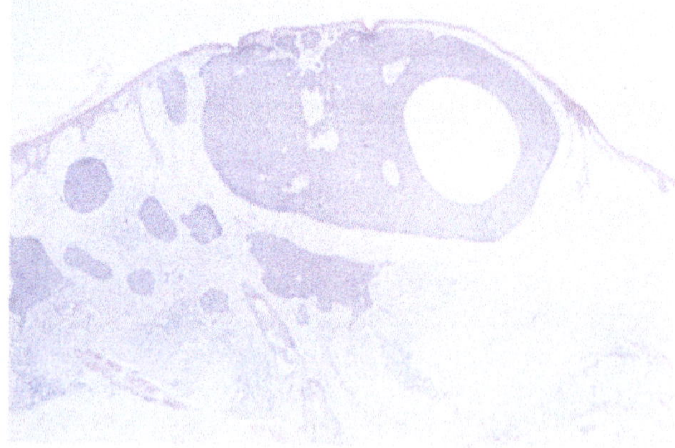

Figure 15.23b Lobule of basal cell carcinoma showing mucoid degeneration within the mass of cells. H & E (A)

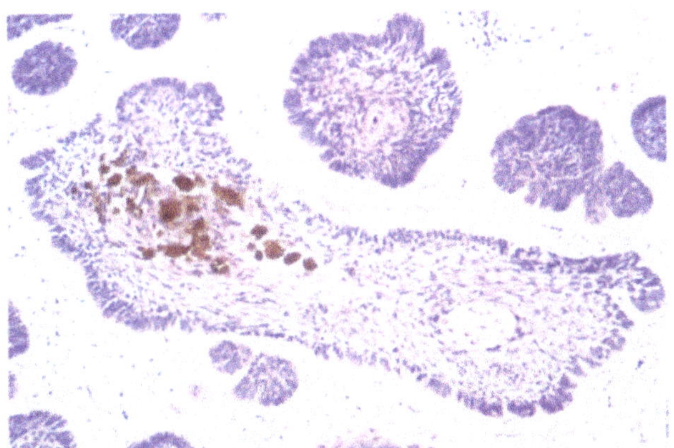

Figure 15.24 Lobule of basal cell carcinoma showing palisading and pigment within the tumour mass.   H & E (C)

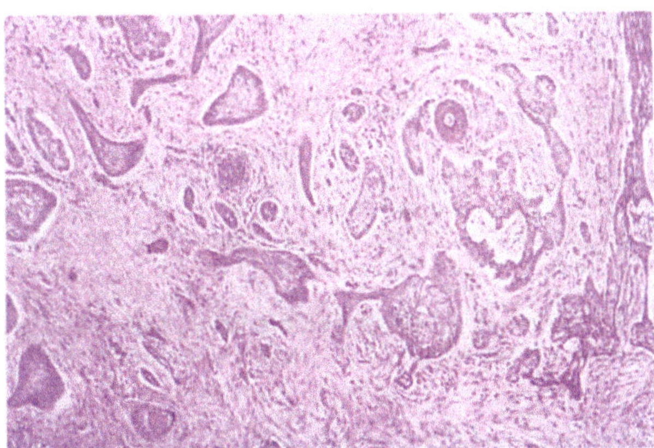

Figure 15.25 Sclerosing (morphoeic) basal cell carcinoma. Irregular strands and masses of basal cell carcinoma tissue embedded in a fibrous stroma.   H & E (B)

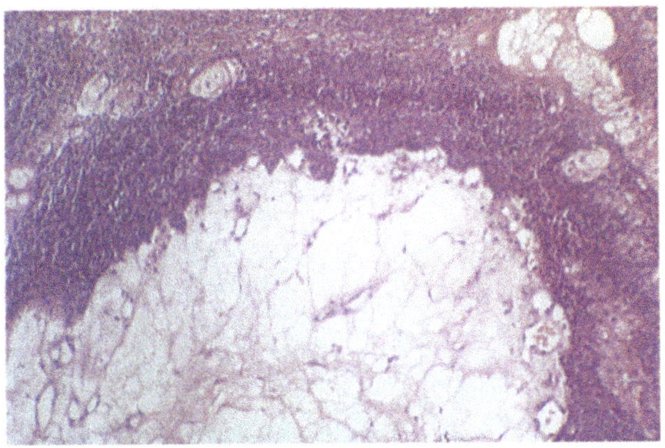

Figure 15.26a Sebaceous gland carcinoma. There is a mass of abnormal basophilic epithelial cells showing abnormal differentiation and irregular sebaceous gland cell formation.   H & E (B)

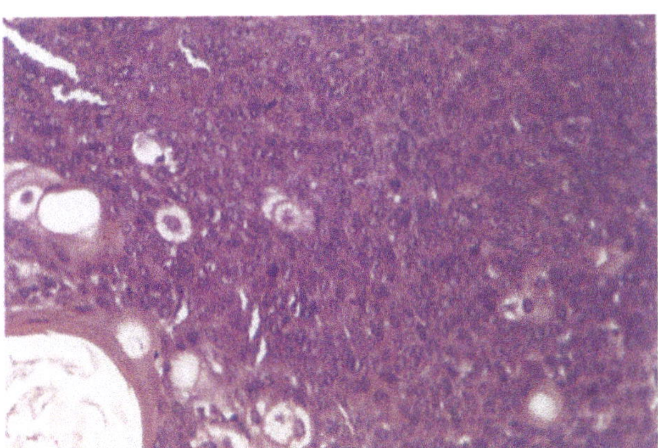

Figure 15.26b Detail of Figure 15.26a.   H & E (D)

Sebaceous Gland Carcinoma[9]

This is a rare tumour of sebaceous gland tissue usually presenting as a rapidly growing single nodule on the face or scalp. The lobular structure of the sebaceous gland and the sebaceous nature of the cell differentiation is usually retained although there may be considerable cytological abnormality (Figure 15.26). They may have a rather worse prognosis than do ordinary squamous cell carcinoma especially when located around the eyes.

Carcinoma of the Eccrine Sweat Gland

Malignant epithelial lesions deriving from sweat glands are quite rare. They may have a variety of patterns depending on from which part of the sweat apparatus they arise. Mehregan and colleagues[10] recognized four varieties eccrine porocarcinoma, syringoid eccrine carcinoma, mucinous eccrine carcinoma and clear cell eccrine carcinoma. These lesions are locally destructive and tend to local recurrence. Metastases have been noted with the eccrine porocarcinoma type.

References

1. Pinkus, H. (1967). The borderline between cancer and non-cancer. In *Year Book of Dermatology* 1966–1967, pp. 5-34 (London: Year Book)

2. Pearse, A. D. and Marks, R. (1977). Actinic keratoses and the epidermis on which they arise. *Br. J. Dermatol.*, **66**, 45

3. Tan, C. Y. and Marks, R. (1982). Lichenoid solar keratosis. Prevalence and immunologic findings. *J. Invest. Dermatol.*, **79**, 365

4. Gross, G., Hagedorn, M., Kenberg, H., Rufli, T., Dahlet, C., Grosshans, E. and Gissman, L. (1985). Bowenoid papulosis, presence of human papillomavirus (HPV). Structural antigens and of HPV-related DNA sequences. *Arch. Dermatol.*, **121**, 858

5. Paone, J. F. and Baker, R. R. (1981). Pathogenesis and treatment of Paget's disease of the breast. *Cancer*, **48**, 825

6. Jones, R. E., Austin, C. and Ackerman, A. B. (1979). Extramammary Paget's disease. A critical re-examination. *Am. J. Dermatopathol.*, **1**, 101

7. Rook, A. and Whimster, I. (1979). Keratoacanthoma – a thirty year retrospect. *Brit. J. Dermatol.*, **100**, 41

8. Ferguson-Smith, J. (1934). A case of multiple primary squamous celled carcinomata of the skin in a young man with spontaneous healing. *Br. J. Dermatol.*, **46**, 267

9. Rulon, D. B. and Heling, E. B. (1974). Cutaneous sebaceous neoplasms. *Cancer*, **33**, 82

10. Mehregan, A. H., Hashimoto, K. and Rahbam, H. (1983). Eccrine adenocarcinoma. A clinicopathologic study of 35 cases. *Arch. Dermatol.*, **119**, 104

The dermis is composed of connective tissue including collagen and elastic tissue, muscle, vessels, nerves and fat extending from the subcutis. All of these elements may give rise to tumours, either true neoplasms or congenital malformations.

Histiocytic and Fibroblastic Tumours

Dermatofibroma

These tumours are usually small and occur as red or reddish-brown papules chiefly on the extremities. They may occasionally reach a size of up to 3 cm. It is suggested by most authors that they are true neoplasms of histiocytic origin[1].

Histologically, dermatofibromas show a varying combination of vascularity, fibrosis and iron pigmentation within an area of fibroblastic and histiocytic proliferation[2] (Figure 16.1). Depending on the predominant feature the names of sclerosing haemangioma, benign fibrous histiocytoma (Figure 16.2) and dermatofibroma (Figure 16.3) have been applied to what appears to be essentially variants of the same lesion. The more fibrous lesions are composed of whorls of plump, spindle-shaped fibroblastic cells interspersed by many capillaries. A rather characteristic feature of these whorls is the way the spindle-shaped cells spiral outwards from the apparent centre of the cell bundle. This pattern has been termed storiform and is most typically seen in dermatofibroma and dermatofibrosarcoma protuberans. Between the spindle cells there is newly formed collagen. The edge of the lesion is characteristically indistinct, with prominent capillary blood vessels and spindle-shaped lesional cells infiltrating the surrounding collagen. The base of the lesion only rarely extends beyond the confines of the dermal collagen, but some small amount of penetration of the fat is occasionally observed. The epidermis overlying a dermatofibroma is usually acanthotic with prominent basal melanocytes and is separated from the lesion by a narrow band of fine collagen fibrils. Sometimes there is a distinctive irregular, basaloid type of hyperplasia in which the lower part of the thickened epidermis may simulate follicular structures (Figures 16.4 – 16.6). In some cases, the lesional tissue comes right up to the overlying epidermis, but even in these cases ulceration is extremely rare.

Fibrous histiocytomas are usually more cellular than dermatofibromas. They are composed of plumper, better outlined cells with the appearance of histiocytes. Lipid and haemosiderin are much more commonly demonstrable in such lesions than in dermatofibromas. Occasional Touton giant cells may be seen in such lesions.

Atypical Fibroxanthoma

Atypical fibroxanthomas are raised, and sometimes ulcerated nodules which occur predominantly on sun-exposed skin[3]. They are usually no more than 2 cm in diameter and are most common in old age.

Histologically, the lesions are composed of cells with histiocytic features including vacuolated or foamy cytoplasm (Figure 16.7). Nuclear pleomorphism is a constant feature and may be alarming in degree (Figure 16.8); mitoses are commonplace and may also be atypical (Figure 16.9). Characteristically, the lesion is confined to the dermis. If there is extensive infiltration of the subcutaneous tissues then the possibility of a soft-tissue malignant fibrous histiocytoma involving overlying skin must be considered[4]. Despite the alarming appearances, atypical fibroxanthomas rarely metastasize and, because of their small size, local excision is usually curative.

Dermatofibrosarcoma Protuberans

The characteristic shape of dermatofibrosarcoma protuberans is of a dermal plaque with nodules protruding from the surface. The nodules are shaded dark red or mauve in colour. Detecting the margins of the neoplasm can be almost impossible (Figure 16.10) and recurrence is common after local excision. Nonetheless, metastases are rare[5].

The characteristic cell of dermatofibrosarcoma protuberans is spindle-shaped, fibrous and arranged in a clearly storiform pattern[6] (Figure 16.11). This radiating arrangement of cells contrasts with the sheet-like, interlacing 'herring-bone' pattern more typical of fibrosarcoma. The edge of the tumour is particularly poorly defined; it extends as cords and trabeculae into surrounding fat and collagen. The overlying epidermis is usually thinned and may be ulcerated. Unlike dermatofibromas, the cells of dermatofibrosarcoma protuberans commonly form a shelf-like infiltrate beneath the epidermis which extends well beyond the nodular areas. Mitotic figures are unusual and nuclear pleomorphism is typically slight in degree.

Some recurrent cases of dermatofibrosarcoma protuberans show myxoid changes. Much rarer is the prominent presence of melanin pigment. The occurrence of pigmented dermatofibrosarcoma protuberans is difficult to reconcile with a fibrohistiocytic derivation of these tumours. There is some ultrastructural evidence which suggests that dermatofibrosarcoma protuberans may have features of schwannian differentiation.

Keloid and Hypertrophic Scar

Keloid is the name given to an abnormal reaction of dermal collagen to injury, resulting in the formation of coarse, glistening, red or pearly white firm, fibrous tissue. The essential difference between hypertrophic scar and keloid is that while the former gradually atrophies, the latter slowly increases and becomes larger than the site of original trauma[7]. It may be very difficult

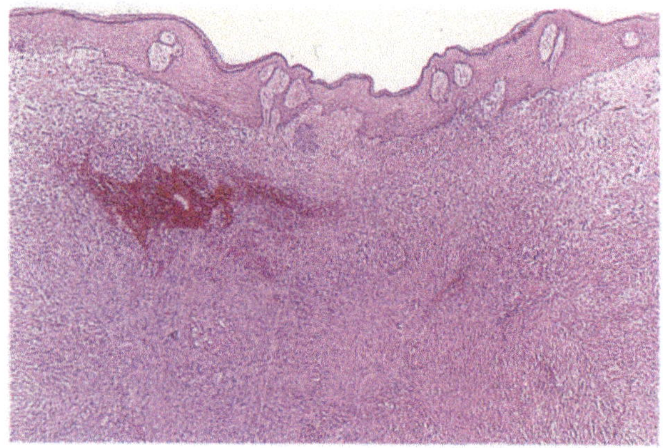

Figure 16.1 Fibrous histiocytoma. The lesion shows typical acanthosis of the overlying epidermis.   H & E (A)

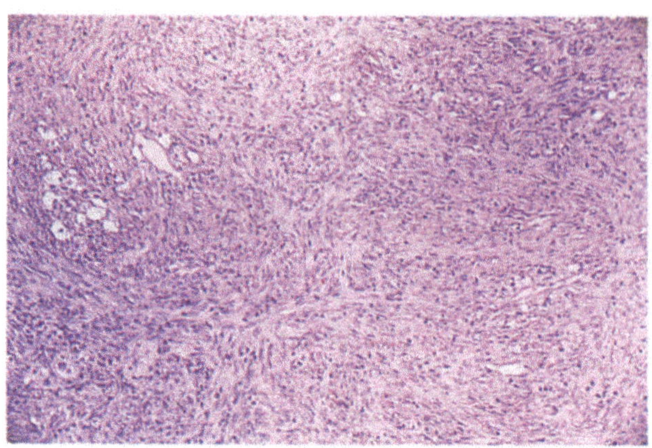

Figure 16.2 Fibrous histiocytoma. Scattered foamy macrophages with clear cytoplasm can be seen. This should not be confused with xanthogranuloma.   H & E (B)

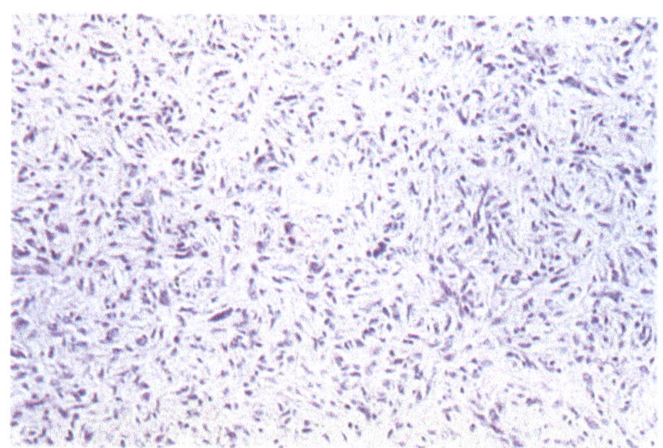

Figure 16.3 Dermatofibroma. Spindle-shaped histiocytic and fibroblastic cells are arranged in a storiform (cartwheel) pattern.   H & E (B)

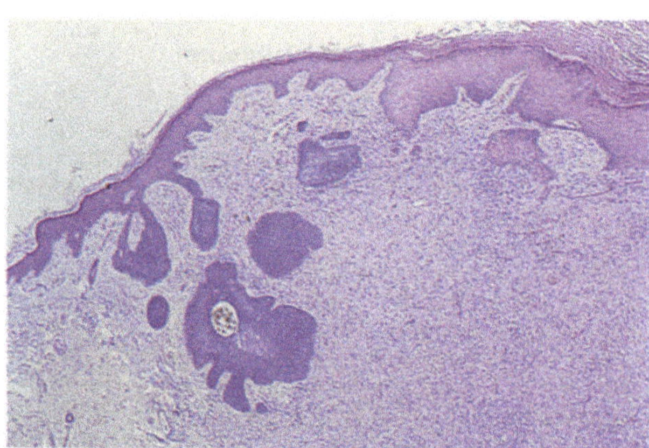

Figure 16.4 Dermatofibroma. There is basaloid hyperplasia of the overlying epithelium. Compare this with the rare co-incident basal-cell carcinoma and dermatofibroma shown in Figure 16.5.   H & E (A)

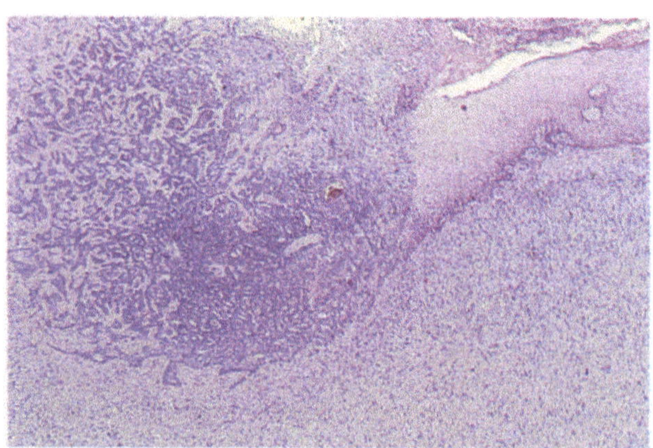

Figure 16.5 Dermatofibroma and basal-cell carcinoma.   H & E (A)

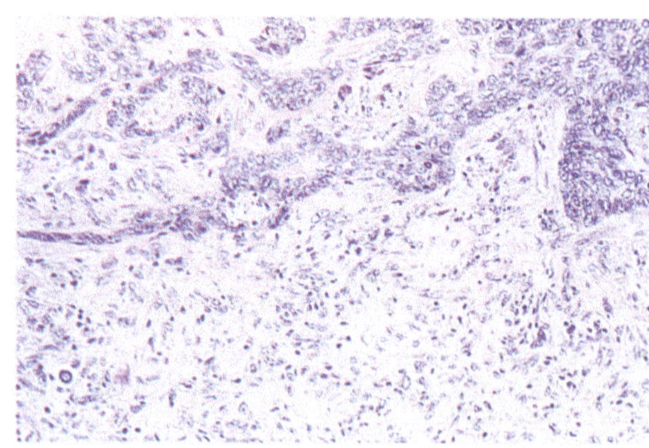

Figure 16.6 Basal-cell carcinoma invading storiform dermatofibroma in this rare collision tumour.   H & E (B)

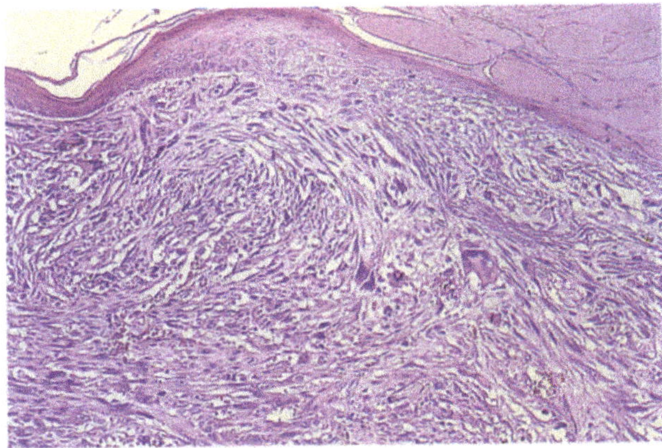

Figure 16.7 Atypical fibroxanthoma. This lesion is often ulcerated on the surface.   H & E (B)

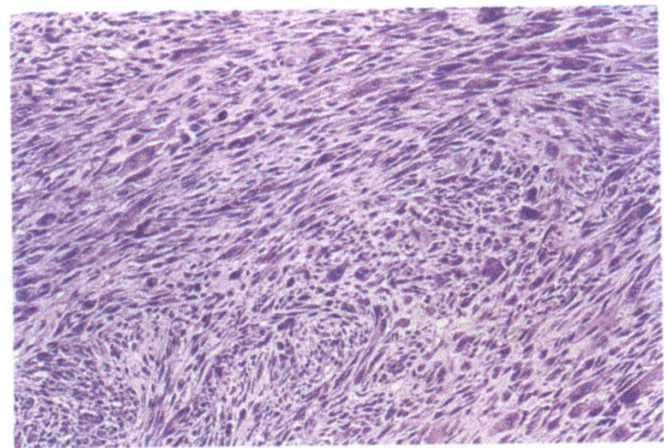

Figure 16.8 Atypical fibroxanthoma. The well-marked nuclear pleomorphism is typical of this condition.   H & E (B)

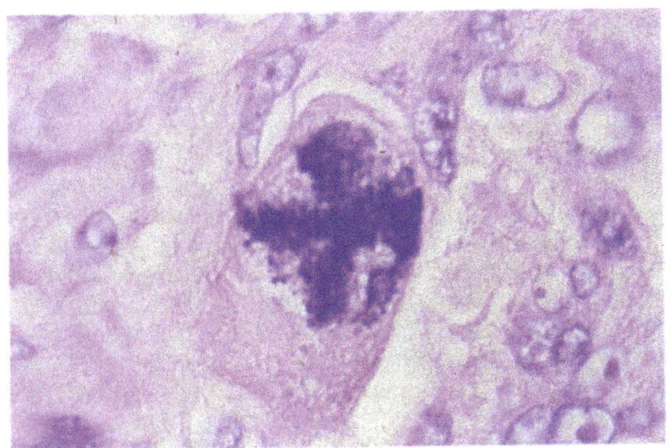

Figure 16.9 Atypical fibroxanthoma. Quadripolar mitosis.   H & E (C)

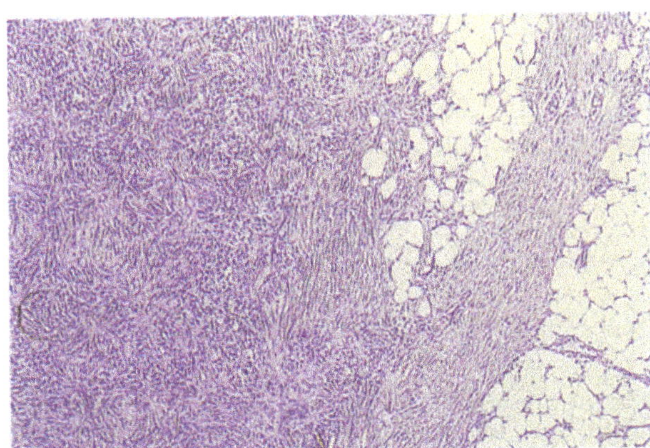

Figure 16.10 Dermatofibrosarcoma protuberans. Infiltrating bands of spindle cells are seen encroaching on subcutaneous fat.   H & E (A)

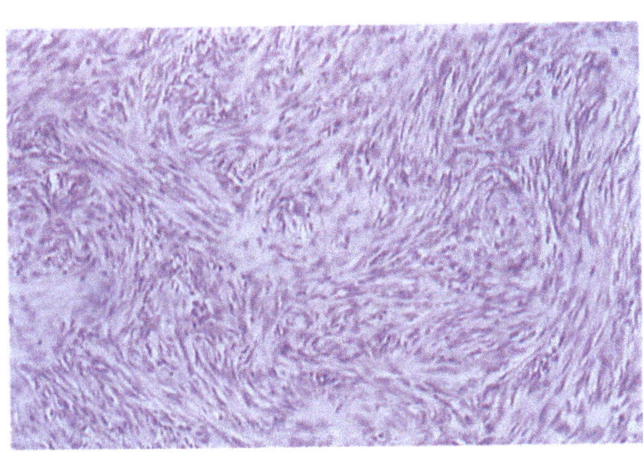

Figure 16.11 Dermatofibrosarcoma protuberans. The storiform pattern in this condition is usually more pronounced than in dermatofibroma.   H & E (B)

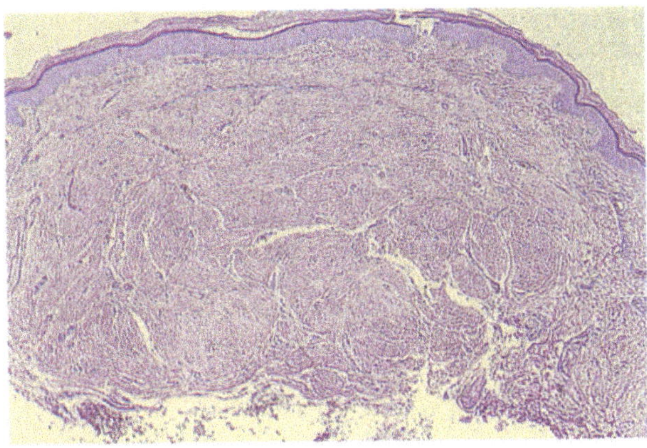

Figure 16.12 Hypertrophic scar. Whorls of hypertrophic bands of collagen are seen in the reticular dermis.   H & E (A)

to distinguish between the two on purely histological grounds.

Both keloids and scars show loss of adnexal structures and atrophy of the epidermis. The hypertrophic collagen in both conditions is devoid of elastic fibres and is arranged haphazardly in nodules (Figure 16.12). Particularly characteristic of keloid as opposed to scar is the presence of grossly thickened collagen bundles (Figure 16.13). As scars mature the collagen tends to become arranged parallel to the skin surface.

Nodular Fasciitis

This is a not uncommon lesion which is principally seen in young adults[8]. Nodular fasciitis is a lesion which is rapidly developing and has a cellular histological appearance that can easily be mistakenly diagnosed as sarcoma. Its importance lies in appreciating its benign nature. The nodule is subcutaneous and small, rarely measuring more than 2 cm in diameter. If incompletely excised the lesion normally regresses spontaneously within a few months.

Although basically composed of clumps of fibroblastic cells (Figure 16.14), the histological appearances of nodular fasciitis are very variable[9]. There are certain features which are helpful in coming to a correct diagnosis:

(1) Small numbers of extravasated erythrocytes lying free amongst the spindle-cells of the lesion.
(2) Mucoid change in the interstitium.
(3) Clefts between the fibroblastic cells.
(4) Whorling of the fibroblasts into rather long fascicles which interlace with one another in gentle curves.
(5) A scanty lymphocytic infiltrate at the periphery.

Mitotic activity is the rule in nodular fasciitis, although none of the mitoses are atypical. Although the lesion is cellular and the fibroblasts are plump, there is no nuclear pleomorphism. Giant cells may be seen, particularly in the more myxoid variants of nodular fasciitis.

Fibromatosis

These lesions are benign and self-limiting but infiltrate surrounding structures including the dermis to such a degree that they may be mistaken for fibrosarcoma[10]. This is particularly true of plantar lesions which may be much larger, more tender and more rapidly growing than the typical palmar fibromatosis resulting in Dupuytren's contracture.

The nodules of both plantar and palmar fibromatosis are initially composed of plump, mitotically active fibroblasts arranged in vascular clumps. No cytological atypia is seen but the edge of the lesion is indistinct and infiltrates the surrounding connective tissue. There is, however, no invasion of skeletal muscle as is seen in the more deep-seated desmoid type fibromatosis. As the lesions mature they become more hyaline and less cellular. A particularly hyaline form of fibromatosis is seen in infancy and childhood[11] (Figure 16.15).

Infantile Digital Fibroma

These uncommon lesions develop during the first year of life and may be present at birth[12]. They appear as small fibrous nodules on the toes or fingers. In sections, nodules are seen to be composed of bundles of fibroblasts which extend into the subcutis. A rather constant feature is the presence of eosinophilic spherical inclusion bodies some 5 μm in diameter within the cytoplasm of the fibroblasts.

Tumours of Muscle

Leiomyoma

Smooth muscle tumours of the skin may be single or multiple and derived from the arrectores pilorum or single and derived from the muscular wall of blood vessels[13]. Both types may be tender or painful.

Piloleiomyoma. These are typically intradermal nodules. They are less than 2 cm in diameter and are composed of intertwining bundles of collagen and smooth muscle with an indistinct margin somewhat reminiscent of dermatofibroma (Figure 16.16). However, the bundles of cells in piloleiomyoma are not storiform but run in straight fascicles and sheets (Figure 16.17). The cells possess a nucleus which is typically elongated but with blunted ends.

Angioleiomyoma. Smooth muscle tumours derived from blood vessels are subcutaneous and have a smooth, encapsulated margin. There is typically less collagen than in piloleiomyoma and the lesion contains multiple, medium-sized venous channels, the thickened walls of which merge with the surrounding tumour cells (Figure 16.18).

Leiomyosarcoma

These lesions appear to be derived from the walls of blood vessels. Even after lymph nodal metastasis, which is rare, truly cutaneous leiomyosarcomas are seldom if ever fatal. Subcutaneous leiomyosarcomas, on the other hand, may demonstrate haematogenous spread[14]. Histologically, the general features are those of a spindle-cell sarcoma, with bizarre mitoses and nuclear pleomorphism. More characteristic features are the presence of blunt-ended, elongated nuclei and the demonstration of myofibrils by phosphotungstic acid–haematoxylin staining.

Epithelioid Sarcoma

These malignant neoplasms usually occur in the skin of the hands and feet but they can be found in other sites, and in deeper, subcutaneous tissues. They are thought to be synovial or myofibroblastic in origin[15,16], and may metastasize to the regional lymph nodes; blood-borne spread to the lungs usually only occurs in advanced stages of the disease. The principal complication of epithelioid sarcoma is local recurrence. This is particularly true in the hands, where excision may be difficult.

Nuclear atypia is the principal diagnostic feature of epithelioid sarcoma. The tumour cells are usually admixed with plentiful lymphocytes and may superficially resemble a histiocytic inflammatory process (Figure 16.19). Even when the atypia is recognized, it is sometimes difficult to exclude a carcinoma from the differential diagnosis. Helpful features indicating a diagnosis of epithelioid sarcoma are the nodular growth pattern and the gradual admixture of tumour cells with the surrounding collagen.

Tumours of Vessels

Although true neoplasms of blood and lymph vessels do occur, many of the benign tumours of vessels are thought to be hamartomas or naevi rather than true neoplasms[17].

Capillary Haemangioma

These lesions appear in infants and young children as lobulated bright red tumours. Under the microscope, sections of capillary haemangiomas reveal multiple, thin-walled vascular channels. Young lesions show few lumina, and are chiefly composed of cords and strands of plump endothelial cells. Maturation of the lesion leads to the formation of capillary channels and results in increasing fibrosis within the lesion (Figure 16.20). Eventually, most capillary haemangiomas become completely replaced by fibrous tissue.

Cavernous Haemangioma

Being deeper within the dermis or subcutis than capillary haemangiomas, cavernous lesions are typically purple in colour and are less compressible. They are composed of thick-walled dilated vascular channels resembling veins, set in a loose collagenous stroma (Figure 16.21). Cavernous haemangiomas may be associated with systemic syndromes (e.g. osteochondromas of Maffucci) and may co-exist with capillary haemangiomas.

Lymphangioma

Lymphangiomas may be difficult to distinguish from similar tumours of blood vessels[18] (Figure 16.22). Generally the vascular spaces contain only eosinophilic hyaline material but haemorrhage into the spaces at the time of biopsy may cause a lymphangioma to be filled with blood cells. Superficial and deep types occur. Both are composed of thin-walled dilated even cystic spaces, and the two types may occur in combination. The superficial type is found at the junction of dermis and epidermis, which may show acanthosis (Figure 16.23). This type is called lymphangioma circumscriptum[19]. The deeper type (cavernous lymphangioma) is subcutaneous and is composed of multiple cystic spaces which may cause pressure atrophy of nearby muscle.

Angiokeratoma

This is a superficial form of angioma, with dilated blood spaces presenting as small, slightly warty red papules or nodules. The lesion consists of distended capillary spaces immediately beneath the epidermis and located principally in the papillary dermis. The overlying epidermis shows a greater or lesser degree of acanthosis and hyperkeratosis.

Various types of angiokeratoma occur. The solitary type (angiokeratoma circumscriptum) tends to be the largest, measuring usually a few centimetres in diameter (Figure 16.24). Multiple angiokeratomas (angiokeratoma corporis diffusum) measuring only 1–3 mm in diameter are seen in alpha-galactosidase deficiency (Fabry's disease). Although the effect of Fabry's disease is the accumulation of ceramide glycolipid throughout the body, the amount deposited in the skin is so small that it can only be detected in specially stained (Sudan black) frozen sections. Also multiple but confined to the digits are the angiokeratomas of Mibelli, which are usually less than 5 mm in diameter and occur like the other forms of angiokeratoma in childhood or early adulthood.

Pyogenic Granuloma

These lesions are rapidly growing ulcerating and bleeding lesions which develop into pedunculated nodules about 1 cm in diameter. The commoner sites include face, fingers and oral mucosa. Histological appearances are often distinctive. There is a well-circumscribed, almost spherical, exophytic, pedunculated and lobulated nodule of capillary blood vessels and cords of endothelial cells with a characteristic loose mucoid connective tissue stroma (Figures 16.25 and 16.26). Mitotic figures may be seen. When ulcerated, the nodule may

show extensive acute and chronic inflammatory changes. The rapidly expansile growth of the nodule of capillary blood vessels distorts the adjacent epidermis and adnexal structures to produce a characteristic epidermal collarette around the lesion. The overall appearances are well in accord with the recently suggested synonym of eruptive haemangioma for what has traditionally been known as granuloma pyogenicum. In rare cases, satellite lesions develop after excision of pyogenic granuloma[20]. Some involve without treatment, the remainder persist unless locally re-excised but, in either case, this occurrence does not indicate malignancy.

Angiolymphoid Hyperplasia with Eosinophilia

These lesions occur principally around the head and neck region as multiple cutaneous or subcutaneous nodules less than 1 cm in diameter[21]. Histologically, the nodules are composed of irregular capillaries surrounded by a dense inflammatory infiltrate which includes lymphocytes and histocytes but is most remarkable for the large number of eosinophils (Figure 16.27). These lesions tend to occur in young adults in contrast to angiosarcomas which are found almost exclusively on the scalp and face of the elderly.

Pseudopyogenic granuloma

There are some features of similarity between pseudopyogenic granuloma and angiolymphoid hyperplasia with eosinophilia. However, pseudopyogenic granuloma is more superficial and although the atypical capillary buds of angiolymphoid hyperplasia are seen, there is less inflammatory infiltration[22]. Some authors have suggested that these and other similar vascular proliferations are variants of a single entity – so-called Kimura's disease[23].

Glomus Tumour

Solitary glomus-cell tumours are purple nodules less than 1 cm in diameter, found on the extremities and characterized by surprising tenderness. The multiple type may be inherited and may extend to be a few centimetres in diameter[24]. They may be painful, but this is not such a common or prominent feature as it is in solitary glomus lesions. In some instances multiple glomus tumours appear to be inherited as a dominant characteristic.

Histologically, the two types of glomus-cell tumours are also somewhat different. The solitary lesion is densely cellular, contains a few vascular channels and is encapsulated (Figure 16.28). The cells have large, rounded nuclei, the cytoplasm is pale and eosinophilic and there is usually a clearly defined cell margin (Figure 16.29). Nerve fibres may be demonstrable in the capsule. Multiple glomus tumours contain prominent, dilated vascular channels (Figure 16.30). The glomus cells may be so insignificant that they are overlooked and an inadequately sampled lesion may be mistaken for a cavernous haemangioma. The thin layer of glomus cells (which are similar to those of solitary glomus tumours) are covered by the endothelial lining of the vascular space (Figure 16.31). Such tumours are often referred to as glomangiomas.

Haemangiopericytoma

These lesions are normally deep-seated, in contrast to the dermal location of glomus tumours[25]. However, occasional cases do occur in the immediately subcutaneous tissues where they form painless masses which

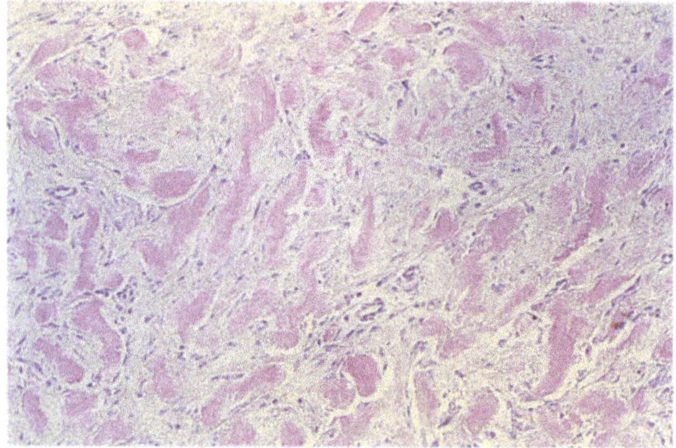

Figure 16.13   Keloid. Coarse bundles of collagen are typical of this condition, but may also be seen in hypertrophic scars.   H & E (B)

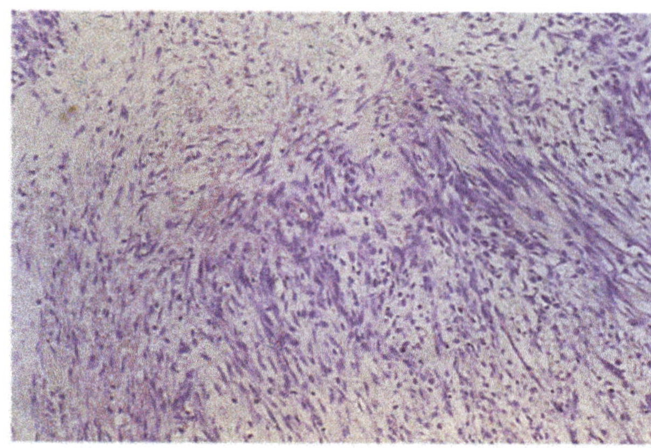

Figure 16.14   Nodular fasciitis, showing bundles of fibroblastic cells in a richly vascular mucoid stroma.   H & E (B)

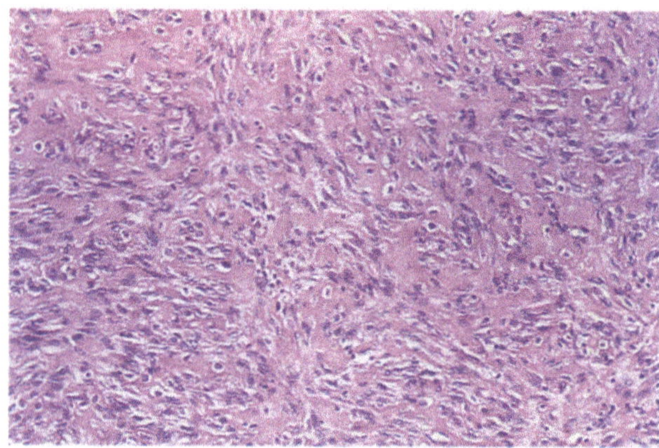

Figure 16.15   Juvenile hyaline fibromatosis. Cords of spindle cells are embedded in a hyaline eosinophilic ground substance.   H & E (B)

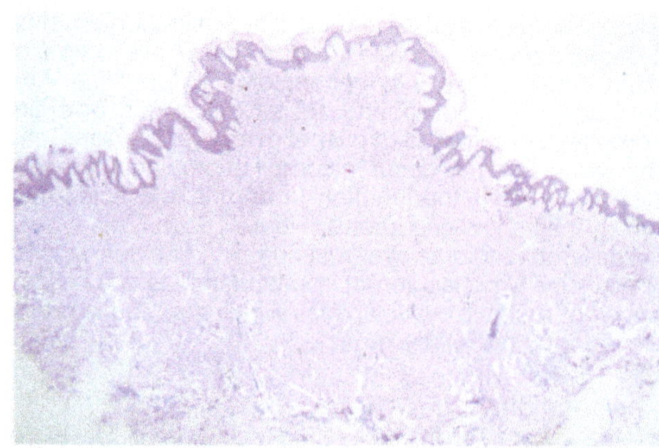

Figure 16.16   Piloleiomyoma. The lesion is typically superficial and poorly delineated.   H & E (A)

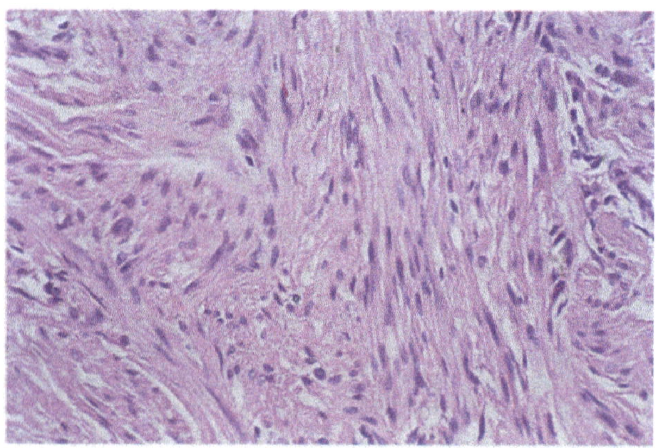

Figure 16.17   Piloleiomyoma, showing straight, intersecting fascicles of smooth-muscle cells.   H & E (C)

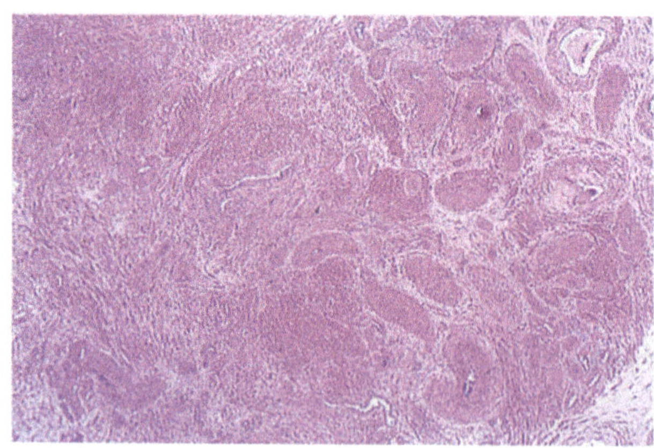

Figure 16.18   Angioleiomyoma. Thick-walled vessels merge imperceptibly with the surrounding tumour cells.   H & E (A)

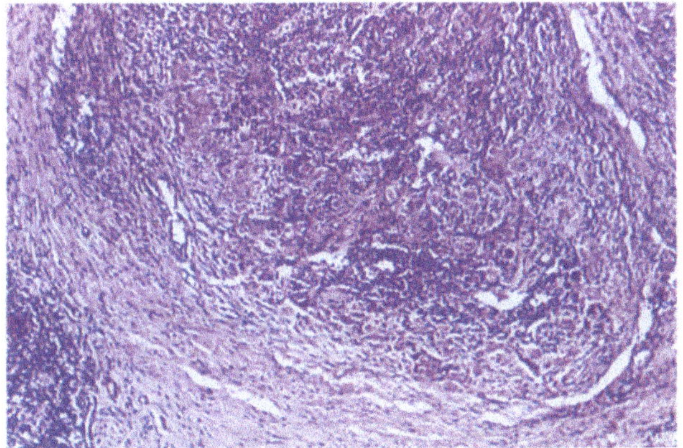

Figure 16.19 Epithelioid sarcoma. A nodule of atypical cells is partly obscured by a dense lymphocytic infiltrate.   H & E (B)

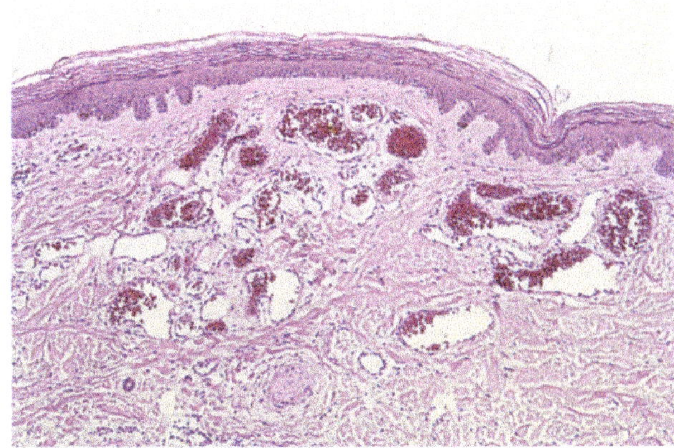

Figure 16.20 Capillary haemangioma. Small blood-filled capillary vessels are located in the superficial reticular dermis.   H & E (A)

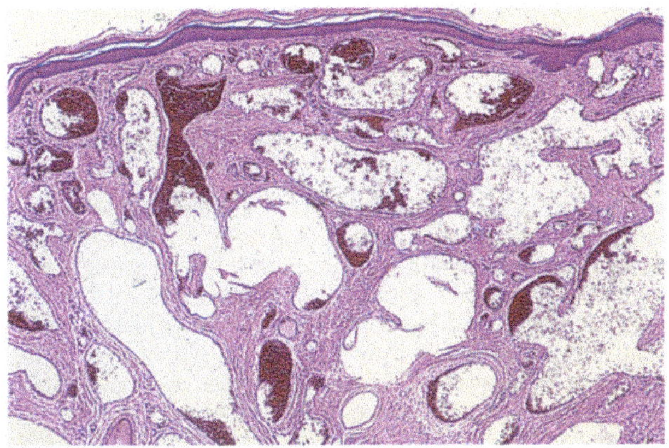

Figure 16.21 Cavernous haemangioma. As compared with capillary haemangioma, the vessels are typically larger and deeper seated.   H & E (A)

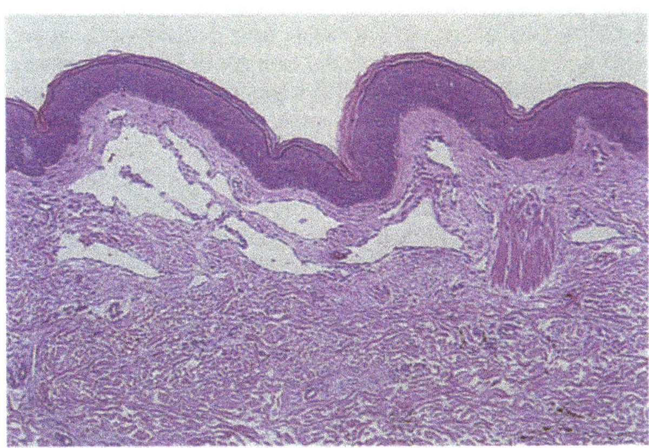

Figure 16.22 Lymphangioma. Small thin-walled channels show a typically empty appearance.   H & E (B)

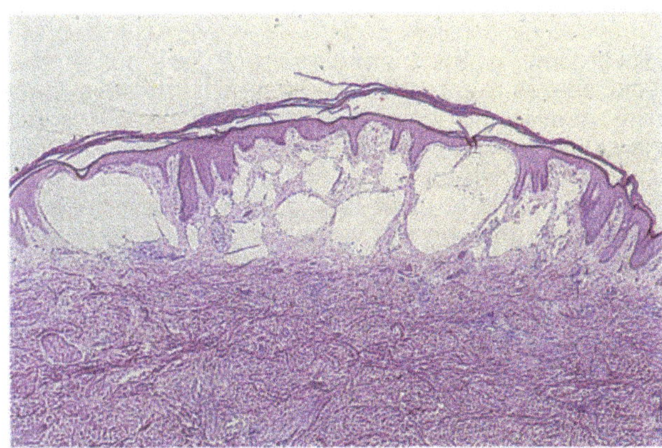

Figure 16.23 Lymphangioma circumscriptum. This type of lymphangioma may be combined with a larger, deeper cavernous type of lymphangioma in the subcutis.   H & E (A)

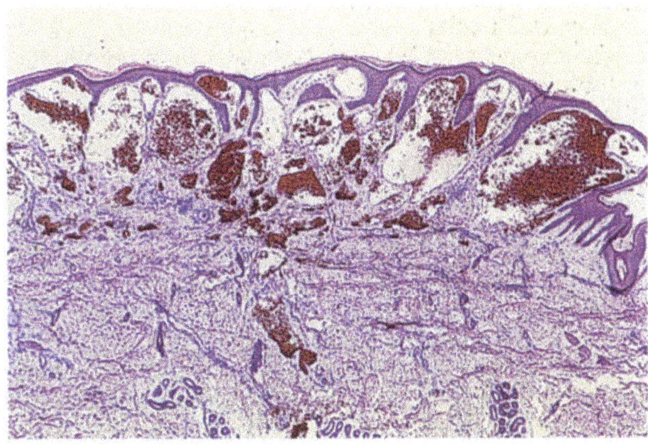

Figure 16.24 Angiokeratoma circumscriptum. Superficial blood-filled vascular spaces occupy the papillary dermis and are associated with acanthosis of the rete ridges of the overlying epithelium.   H & E (A)

sometimes reach a considerable size. In histological sections, the tumour consists of large numbers of capillary vessels surrounded by clumps and sheets of small spindle-shaped 'pericyte-like' cells. The vascularity of the tumour is best revealed by special staining for reticulin fibres which circle the vessels and then radiate out between the tumour cells. The pattern of reticulin is often particularly helpful in establishing the diagnosis.

Haemangiopericytomas may metastasize. Increased mitotic activity, cellular or nuclear pleomorphism and lack of characteristic spindle shape in the tumour pericytes have all been noted to indicate a metastatic potential.

Kaposi's Sarcoma

This rare cutaneous sarcoma presents in the classical form as plaques or nodules, purple or brown in colour and particulary situated on the lower part of the legs in elderly men of Italian or Jewish origin. Untreated, the plaques and nodules gradually enlarge, ulcerate and cause lymphoedema. This tumour is distinguished by its various patterns of association. Outside Africa, until recently Kaposi's sarcoma has been a rarity. It usually remained localized to the skin and progressed slowly with spontaneous remissions being noted occasionally. Although eventually fatal the classical form progresses so slowly that the patient often outlives the tumour. There was, however, an increased risk of the development of lymphoma in patients with Kaposi's sarcoma. In Equatorial and Southern Africa, the disease is more common, more rapidly progressive and often progresses to involvement of the gastrointestinal tract, liver, lungs and heart[26]. More recently, North American and European cases of Kaposi's sarcoma have been described in patients suffering from immune deficiency, either as a result of immunosuppression following organ transplant or as part of the acquired immunodeficiency syndrome (AIDS)[27].

In histological sections, the earliest pathological changes in Kaposi's sarcoma are quite insignificant. The appearances are quite similar to granulation tissue, the lesion being composed of thin-walled capillary channels[28]. Little atypia is seen, but the endothelial cells do tend to bulge into the lumina of the vascular channels, which characteristically contain few erythrocytes. Nodular change in the lesions is associated with the development of plump spindle-shaped cells around the vascular spaces (Figure 16.32). These cells show a moderate degree of nuclear atypia and pleomorphism, and occasional mitotic figures. The vascular spaces are reduced to narrow slits. Haemorrhage into these nodular lesions is common, and haemosiderin becomes deposited amongst the tumour cells (Figure 16.33). Appearances within a given nodular tumour may vary considerably from an almost fibrosarcomatous appearance at one extreme to an almost angiosarcomatous appearance at the other. However, the vascular slits are usually present throughout the lesion. When Kaposi's sarcoma becomes disseminated, the various tumours can also have rather different histological appearances. The pattern of 'spread' in most disseminated cases is more in keeping with multifocal origin rather than metastasis from a single primary site.

Angiosarcoma[29]

Angiosarcomas may be derived from blood or lymph vessels. They are rare in the skin and are generally confined to two distinct clinical situations[30]. Thus, the tumour may occur in persistent chronic lymphoedema (usually following radical lymph node dissection) or alternatively angiosarcomas may arise spontaneously in the elderly where they tend to affect the face and scalp. The tumours grow by gradual infiltration of the surrounding skin and deep subcutaneous tissue or even bone. Metastasis tends to be a relatively late phenomenon, but when it occurs the cervical lymph nodes and lungs are principally involved.

Under the microscope, cutaneous angiosarcoma shows areas of varying differentiation. The best differentiated areas may be indistinguishable from pyogenic granuloma or granulation tissue but adequate sampling will usually reveal the more typical dilated channels lined by atypical endothelial cells which protrude into the vascular space (Figure 16.34). In poorly differentiated areas, the malignant endothelial cells may form solid cords and nests of cells. Mitoses are seen, but are not conclusive proof of malignancy, in that they may be quite common in the benign angiomas in children. Fortunately, primary angiomas in the skin in infants are virtually always benign. There may also be confusion between Masson's intravascular papillary endothelial hyperplasia and true cutaneous angiosarcoma. The papillary structure, lack of severe atypia of the endothelial cells, and the intravascular location are the most useful distinguishing features of Masson's pseudoangiosarcoma.

Intravascular Papillary Endothelial Hyperplasia (Masson)

First described by Masson and subsequently named after him, this tumour is not a true neoplasm. It is thought to be a distinctive pattern of endothelial proliferation within a thrombus and its importance lies in the ease with which it can be confused with angiosarcoma[31,32]. Clinically, the lesion may vary from a few millimetres to 5 cm in diameter. The smaller the lesion the more superficial it tends to be. Angiosarcomas of the skin usually appear first as haemorrhagic plaques whereas Masson's tumour is often not obviously vascular on clinical examination, but appears as a non-specific nodule.

In histological sections, on the other hand, Masson's tumour is clearly vascular. The lesion consists of papillary, collagenous and rather acellular stalks covered by a single layer of plump endothelial cells (Figure 16.35). Many of the stalks are at right angles to the plane of sectioning and appear as islands floating free in a pool of erythrocytes. This pattern is useful in distinguishing intravascular papillary endothelial hyperplasia from angiosarcoma, where the predominant pattern is of sinusoid spaces surrounded by atypical endothelial cells. The intravascular location of Masson's tumour is very helpful in coming to the correct diagnosis. Accordingly, sections stained for elastic fibres are very useful, but it must be borne in mind that in many cases the lesion may erode through the vessel wall. Although most of these tumours arise within a normal vein, they have also been described within vascular malformations and benign neoplasms, further complicating the histological appearances.

Tumours Derived from Neural Tissues

Traumatic Neuroma

Similar histological appearances are seen in neuromas due to severing of a nerve (amputation neuromas) or as part of a supernumerary digit[33]. The lesions consist of well-delineated bundles of nerve fibres embedded in dense fibrous tissue (Figure 16.36). Although amputation neuromas are frequently tender, supernumerary digits are asymptotmatic and are found characteristically on the lateral margin of the fifth finger.

Granular-cell Tumour

These neoplasms (so-called granular-cell myoblastomas) present as spherical nodules in the skin[34], mucous membranes and other organs, including pituitary, gastrointestinal tract, breast and lung. Cutaneous granular-cell tumours are up to 4 cm in diameter, but most measure about 1 cm. Occasional tumours are tender.

The histological appearances are usually specific (Figure 16.37). The tumour cells are large, with plentiful cytoplasm and a small, central, almost spherical nucleus (Figure 16.38). Mitoses are rare and the nuclei show little pleomorphism. The cytoplasm contains pale, indistinct granules which are easily overlooked but are usually readily demonstrated by the period acid-Schiff stain even after diastase pretreatment (Figure 16.39). The overlying epidermis characteristically shows pseudoepitheliomatous hyperplasia. This may be of so marked a degree that a superficial biopsy may be misinterpreted as squamous-cell carcinoma. The margins of the tumour show an infiltrative pattern with clusters of tumour cells apparently surrounded by normal dermal connective tissue.

It is of interest that granular-cell tumours are positively stained in immunocytochemical procedures designed to demonstrate myelin basic protein. This finding, together with the ultrastructural appearances of granular-cell tumours, has led many authors to consider that, despite their superficial resemblance to muscle cells, these lesions are of Schwann cell origin[35,36].

Neurilemmoma (Schwannoma, Neurilemoma)

This neoplasm is derived from nerve-sheath cells and is uncommon in the skin[37]. Histological appearances are characteristic in most instances. The lesion is encapsulated and the neoplastic cells are spindle shaped with elongated cigar-shaped nuclei (Figure 16.40). In some areas of the tumour the nuclei are arranged in parallel rows (Antoni A arrangement). In other areas the stroma becomes rather myxoid and the nuclei are arranged at random (Antoni B arrangement). When the Antoni A arrangement includes palisading nuclei surrounding an acellular fibrous area the structure is termed a Verocay body. Nerves may be demonstrable in the capsule of the lesion, but there are few within the Antoni A or B areas. Mast cells are plentiful. Malignant change in neurilemmomas is rare. Nuclear pleomorphism may be readily found in degenerate neurilemmomas, but does not infer a malignant potential.

Neurofibroma

Neurofibromas are solitary and sporadic or multiple and associated with von Recklinghausen's disease[38]: a familial syndrome which is autosomal dominant in its mode of inheritance although many cases of von Recklinghausen's disease are considered to be spontaneous mutations. Besides being multiple, the neurifibromas in the familial disease occur at an earlier age than solitary, spontaneous lesions and are associated with café-au-lait pigmented macules. Whether sporadic or familial, most neurofibromas occur as soft almost spherical cutaneous or subcutaneous nodules. Plexiform neurofibromas, which are large ill-defined masses of nerves and neurofibroma tissue, are mainly seen in the familial form of the disease.

Histological examination of neurofibromas reveals a quite well delineated but unencapsulated nodule composed of elongated spindle-shaped cells (Figure 16.41).

The margins of the tumour are not always distinct. The characteristic feature of these cells is that they show a wavy appearance which is so short in its periodicity that it affects the nuclei, so that they too show a corrugated appearance. Nerve fibres may be demonstrated within the tumour (Figure 16.42). Most neurofibromas show focal myxoid change, but in some lesions the myxoid change may be so well-marked as to obscure the true nature of the lesion. There are often large numbers of mast cells scattered throughout the tumour.

Neurofibrosarcoma (Malignant Schwannoma)

Malignant change in a neurofibroma virtually only occurs in the familial tumours of von Recklinghausen's disease[39] and then it is a rare complication. Furthermore, when malignancy occurs in neurofibromatosis it only very rarely arises in cutaneous lesions. The skin may be involved in a neurofibrosarcoma arising from a larger subcutaneous nerve trunk.

Malignancy is principally indicated by the presence of mitotic figures as benign neurofibromas are typically devoid of mitoses. Mitotic activity may be the only indicator of neurofibrosarcoma in well-differentiated lesions, but poorly differentiated lesions may show such extensive pleomorphism that, without the history of neurofibromatosis, categorization of the tumour may be impossible.

Tumours of Adipose Tissue

Lipoma

These are common tumours of the subcutaneous tissues (Figure 16.43). They have a thin capsule and may contain broad fibrous bands, but otherwise have the appearance of normal mature adipose tissue.

Angiolipoma

Angiolipomas are often multiple and tender. Accordingly, they often present at a smaller size than the more common lipoma. They resemble lipomas except in that there are multiple capillary blood vessels (Figure 16.44) at the periphery of the lesion[40]. The capillaries are usually filled with erythrocytes and may be thrombosed (Figure 16.45).

Atypical Lipomas

Ordinary lipomas are commonplace lesions. Rarer forms of benign fatty tumours occur which are clinically similar to ordinary lipoma, but have a quite different histological appearance. Their importance is in realizing their benign nature, despite their sometimes bizarre histological appearance. It is noteworthy that virtually all superficial, subcutaneous fatty lesions are benign, whereas deep-seated tumours with adipose differentiation must be regarded with suspicion.

Hibernoma. Most commonly found in a subcutaneous situation on the back, hibernomas may reach up to 10 cm in diameter. They are occasionally rather tender[41]. Histologically, these lesions consist of clumps of large cells with a finely vacuolated cytoplasm and a small, often centrally placed nucleus. The number of vacuoles may vary greatly and some cells similar to those in an ordinary lipoma are usually seen.

Spindle-cell Lipoma. These tumours are usually found in the subcutis of the back of elderly men[42]. Under the microscope, the lesion is seen to consist of mature fat separated by plump fibroblastic cells with a myxoid stroma (Figure 16.46). When a large proportion of mature

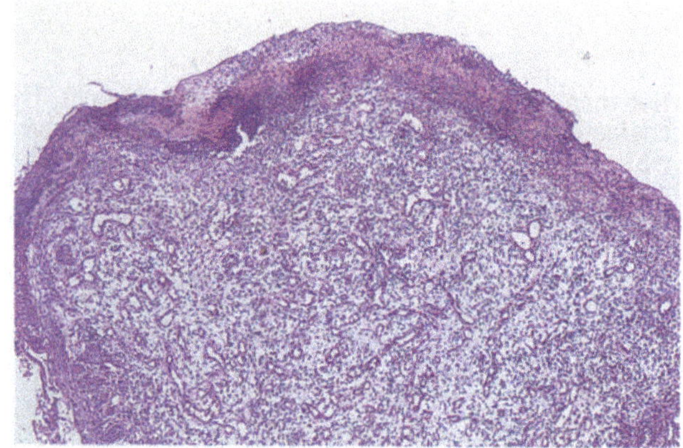

Figure 16.25 Pyogenic granuloma. Composed of granulation tissue, pyogenic granulomas are often ulcerated on the surface.   H & E (A)

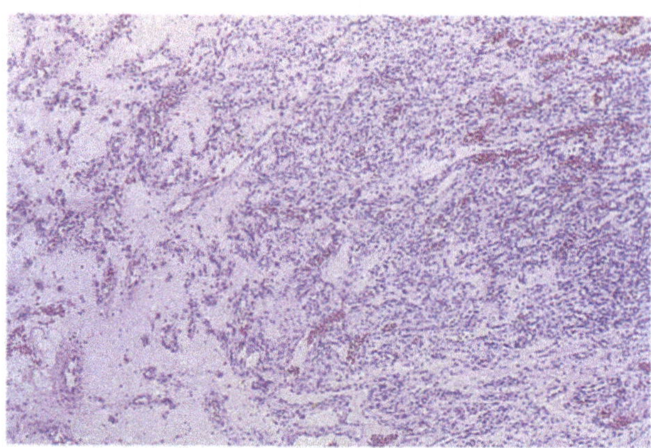

Figure 16.26 Pyogenic granuloma, showing the typical hyaline, mucoid stroma commonly seen at the base of the lesion.   H & E (A)

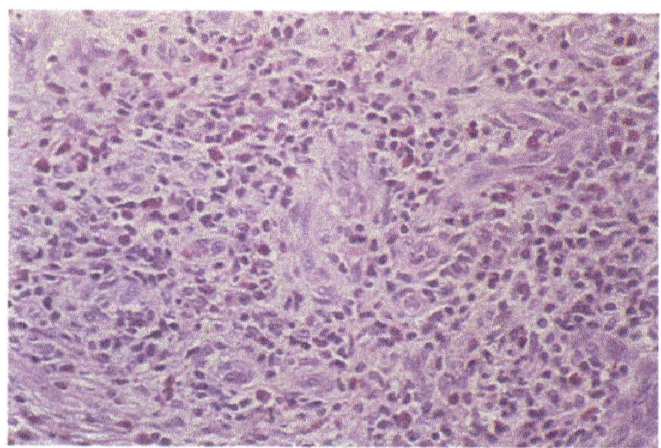

Figure 16.27 Angiolymphoid hyperplasia with eosinophilia. Although there are plump endothelial cells in the capillary vessels, the accompanying mixture of inflammatory cells and particularly eosinophils allows differentiation from pyogenic granuloma or angiosarcoma.   H & E (B)

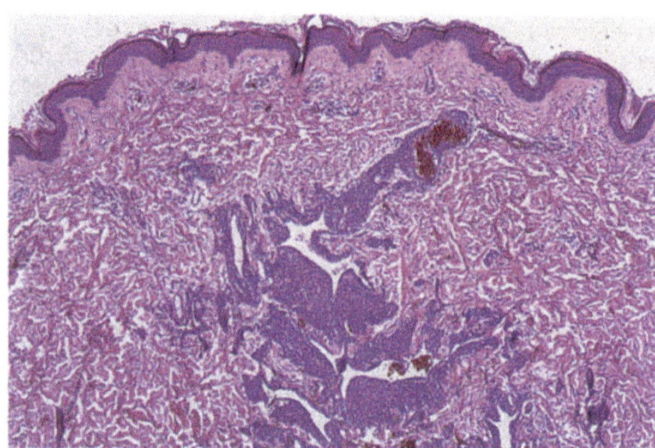

Figure 16.28 Glomus tumour. At low magnification, ill-defined clusters of basaloid cells and vascular spaces can be seen.   H & E (A)

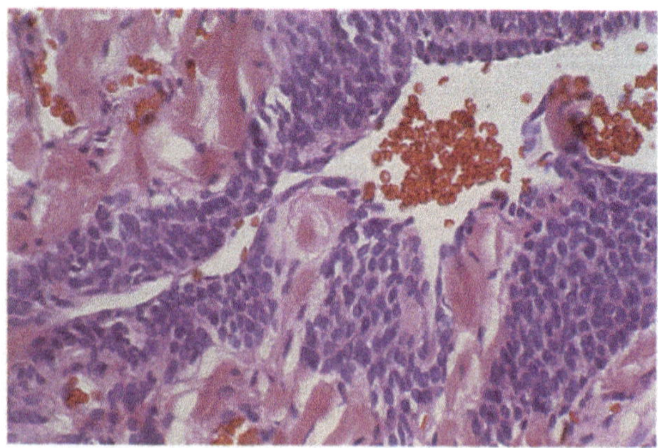

Figure 16.29 Glomus tumour. At this higher magnification the characteristic cells of the glomus tumour can be seen to be lining the sinusoidal vascular spaces.   H & E (C)

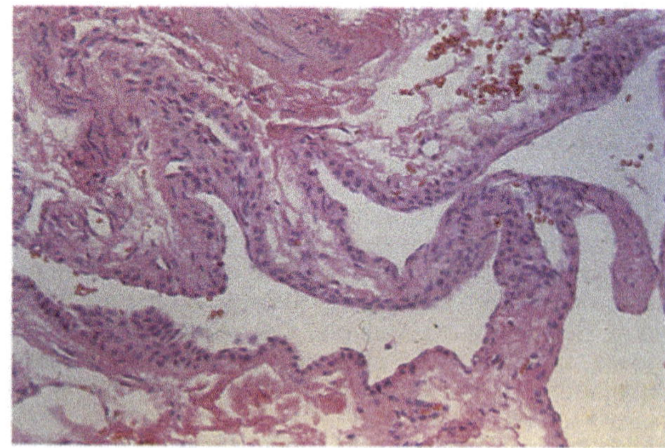

Figure 16.30 Glomus tumour (glomangioma). In these tumours the lining of glomus cells may be so scanty that first impressions are of a cavernous haemangioma.   H & E (B)

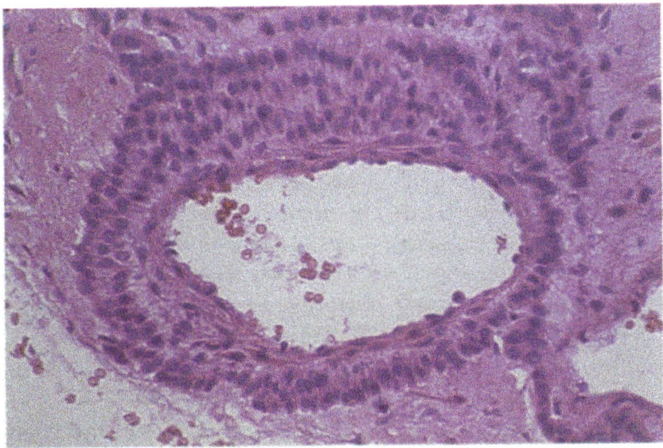

Figure 16.31 Glomus tumour (glomangioma). In places, it is usually possible to identify the characteristic small basophilic cells around vascular spaces. The cells may be arranged in double layers.   H & E (C)

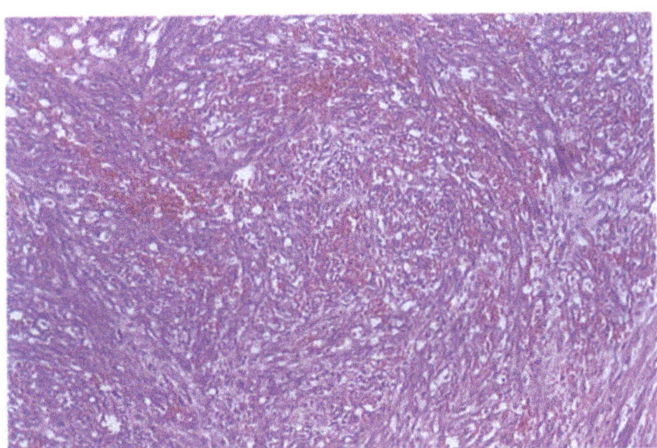

Figure 16.32 Kaposi's sarcoma, nodular phase. At low magnification, the lesion is composed of collided fascicles of plump spindle cells containing areas of apparent haemorrhage.   H & E (B)

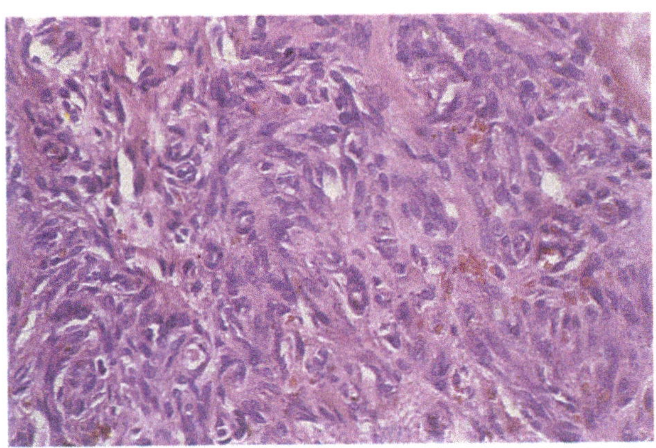

Figure 16.33 Kaposi's sarcoma. Plump spindle cells contain slit-like vascular spaces and areas of haemorrhage.   H & E (C)

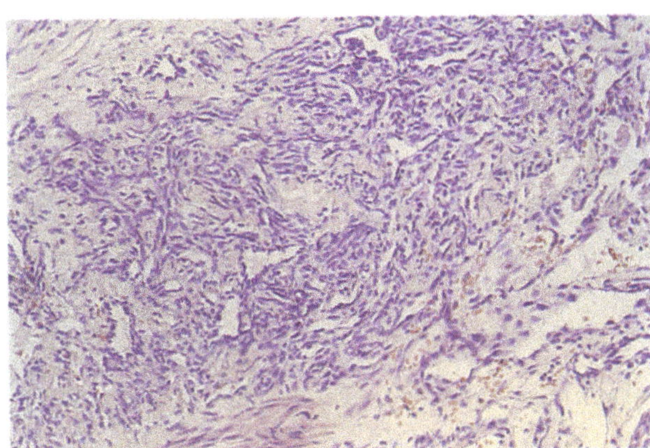

Figure 16.34 Angiosarcoma. Sinusoidal vascular spaces are lined by plump, atypical endothelial cells.   H & E (B)

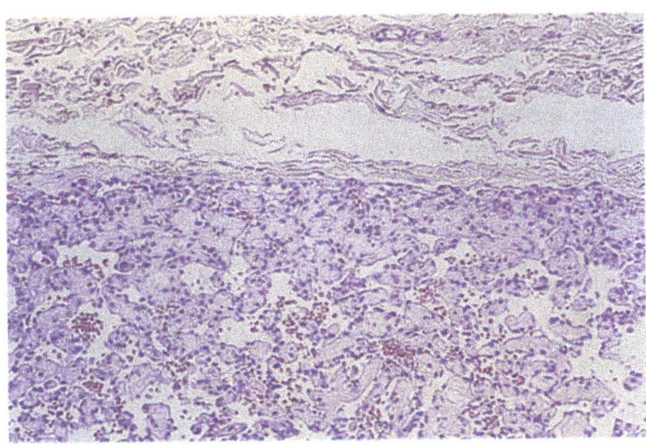

Figure 16.35 Intravascular papillary endothelial hyperplasia. (Masson's tumour). The papillary pattern of growth contrasts with the sinusoidal structure of angiosarcoma (Figure 16.34).   H & E (B)

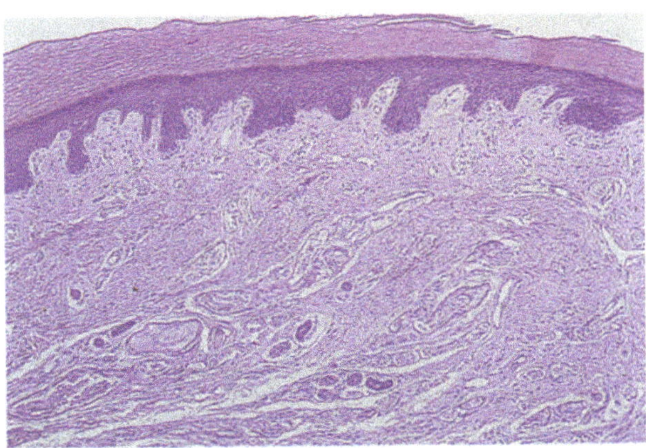

Figure 16.36 Amputation neuroma. This section was taken from an accessory digit. Nerves are surrounded by laminated coarse fibrous tissue. The appearances of traumatic amputation neuroma are the same.   H & E (A)

fat-cells are seen the diagnosis is usually straightforward. However, some samples of these tumours often consist only of the myxoid spindle cells.

Pleomorphic lipoma. Similar in clinical appearance to spindle-cell lipomas, these lesions consist of a mixture of mature fat and other cells which have pleomorphic nuclei (Figure 16.47) and may appear very similar in appearance to the lipoblasts of liposarcoma[43]. However, mitoses are rare and the tumour is well delineated from the surrounding stroma. Giant cells are frequently present. They have their many nuclei arranged overlapping at the margin of the cytoplasm of the cell. The arrangement of nuclei has been likened to the petals of a flower. Occasionally, benign lipomatous lesions are encountered which have an appearance with features of both spindle-cell and pleomorphic lipomas.

Liposarcoma

Malignant tumours of adipose tissue arise only extremely rarely from subcutaneous fat. Their origin is normally from within the deeper muscles and fascia and they involve the skin only by superficial infiltration from a lesion of considerable size[44]. The typical clinical appearance of a liposarcoma involving skin is of a large, infiltrative nodular mass.

Histologically, liposarcomas can be well-differentiated, myxoid, or pleomorphic in type. The more helpful diagnostic features of liposarcoma include the presence of mitoses (some atypical), a rich vascularity of the tumour with frequent arborizing branches of capillary blood vessels and the presence of atypical lipoblasts (Figure 16.48). Frozen sections stained to demonstrate fat may be helpful in establishing the adipose differentiation of the tumour, but it must be borne in mind that many cells contain fine lipid droplets without being lipoblasts.

References

1. Niemi, K. M. (1970). The benign fibrohistiocytic tumours of the skin. *Acta Dermatol. Venereol. (Stockh)*, **50**, Suppl. 63, 1

2. Vilanova, J. R. and Flint, A. (1974). The morphological variations of fibrous histiocytoma. *J. Cutan. Pathol.*, **1**, 155

3. Soares, H. L., Silveira, J. G., Fantini, A. and Soares, M. E. (1981). Atypical fibroxanthoma. *J. Dermatol. Surg. Oncol.*, **7**, 915

4. Enzinger, F. M. (1979). Atypical fibroxanthoma and malignant fibrous histiocytoma. *Am. J. Dermatopathol.*, **1**, 185

5. Bendix-Hansen, K., Myhre-Jensen, O. and Kaae, S. (1983). Dermatofibrosarcoma protuberans. A clinico-pathological study of nineteen cases and review of world literature. *Scand. J. Plast. Reconstr. Surg.*, **17**, 247

6. Hashimoto, K., Brownstein, M. H. and Jakobiec, F. A. (1974). Dermatofibrosarcoma protuberans. *Arch. Dermatol.*, **110**, 874

7. Linares, H. A. and Larson, D. L. (1974). Early differential diagnosis between hypertrophic and nonhypertrophic healing. *J. Invest. Dermatol.*, **62**, 514

8. Mehregan, A. H. (1966). Nodular fasciitis. *Arch. Dermatol.*, **93**, 204

9. Bernstein, K. E. and Lattes, R. (1982). Nodular (pseudosarcomatous) fasciitis, a non-recurrent lesion. *Cancer*, **49**, 1668

10. Gonatas, N. K. (1961). Extra-abdominal desmoid tumours. *Arch. Pathol.*, **71**, 214

11. Kitano, Y. (1976). Juvenile hyalin fibromatosis. *Arch. Dermatol.*, **112**, 86

12. Bhawan, J., Bacchetta, C., Joris, I. and Majno, G. (1979). A myofibroblastic tumour. Infantile digital fibroma (recurrent digital fibroma of childhood). *Am. J. Pathol.*, **94**, 19

13. Fisher, W. C. and Helwig, E. B. (1963). Leiomyomas of the skin. *Arch. Dermatol.*, **88**, 510

14. Jegasothy, B. V., Gligor, R. S. and Hull, M. (1981). Leiomyosarcoma of the skin and subcutaneous tissue. *Arch. Dermatol.*, **117**, 478

15. Enzinger, F. M. (1970). Epithelioid sarcoma. A sarcoma simulating a granuloma or a carcinoma. *Cancer*, **26**, 1029

16. Blewitt, R. W., Aparicio, S. G. and Bird, C. C. (1983). Epithelioid sarcoma: a tumour of myofibroblasts. *Histopathology*, **7**, 573

17. Johnson, W. C. (1976). Pathology of cutaneous vascular tumors. *Int. J. Dermatol.*, **15**, 239

18. Peachey, R. D. G., Lim, C. C. and Whimster, I. W. (1970). Lymphangioma of the skin. *Br. J. Dermatol.*, **83**, 519

19. Bauer, B. S., Kernahan, D. A. and Hugo, N. E. (1981). Lymphangioma circumscriptum – a clinicopathological review. *Ann. Plast. Surg.*, **7**, 318

20. Zaynoun, S. T., Juljulian, H. H. and Kurban, A. K. (1974). Pyogenic granuloma with multiple satellites. *Arch. Dermatol.*, **109**, 689

21. Wells, G. C. and Whimster, I. W. (1969). Angiolymphoid hyperplasia with eosinophilia. *Br. J. Dermatol.*, **81**, 1

22. Wilson-Jones, E. and Bleehan, S. S. (1969). Inflammatory angiomatous nodules with abnormal blood vessels occurring about the ears and scalp (pseudo or atypical pyogenic granuloma). *Br. J. Dermatol.*, **81**, 804

23. Burrall, B. A., Barr, R. J. and King, D. F. (1982). Cutaneous histiocytoid hemangioma. *Arch. Dermatol.*, **118**, 166

24. Pepper, M. C., Laubenheimer, R. and Cripps, D. J. (1977). Multiple glomus tumors. *J. Cutan. Pathol.*, **4**, 244

25. Angervall, L., Kindblom, L.-G., Nielsen, J. M., Stener, B. and Svendsen, P. (1978). Hemangiopericytoma. A clinicopathologic, angiographic and microangiographic study. *Cancer*, **42**, 2412

26. O'Connell, K. M. (1977). Kaposi's sarcoma. Histopathological study of 159 cases from Malawi. *J. Clin. Pathol.*, **30**, 687

27. Hymes, K. B., Cheung, T., Greene, J. B., Prose, N. S., Marcus, A., Ballard, H., William, D. C. and Laubenstein, L. J. (1981). Kaposi's sarcoma in homosexual men – a report of eight cases. *Lancet*, **ii**, 598

28. Ackerman, A. B. (1979). Subtle clues to diagnosis by conventional microscopy. The patch stage of Kaposi's sarcoma. *Am. J. Dermatopathol.*, **1**, 165

29. Girard, C., Johnson, W. C. and Graham, J. H. (1970). Cutaneous angiosarcoma. *Cancer*, **26**, 868

30. Maddox, J. C. and Evans, H. L. (1981). Angiosarcoma of skin and soft tissue: a study of forty-four cases. *Cancer*, **48**, 1907

31. Clearkin, K. P. and Enzinger, F. M. (1976). Intravascular papillary endothelial hyperplasia. *Arch. Pathol.*, **100**, 441

32. Salyer, W. R. and Salyer, D. C. (1979). Intravascular angiomatosis: development and distinction from angiosarcoma. *Cancer*, **36**, 995

33. Reed, R. J., Fine, R. M. and Mettzer, H. D. (1972). Palisaded, encapsulated neuromas of the skin. *Arch. Dermatol.*, **106**, 865

34. Goette, D. K. and Olsen, E. G. (1982). Multiple cutaneous granular cell tumors. *Int. J. Dermatol.*, **21**, 271

35. Armin, A., Connelly, E. M. and Rowden, G. (1983). An immunoperoxidase investigation of S-100 protein in granular-cell myoblastomas: evidence for Schwann cell derivation. *Am. J. Clin. Pathol.*, **79**, 37

36. Seo, I. S., Azzarelli, B., Warner, T. F., Goheen, M. P. and Senteney, G. E. (1984). Multiple visceral and cutaneous granular cell tumors. Ultrastructural and immunocytochemical evidence of Schwann cell origin. *Cancer*, **53**, 2104

37. Das Guptas, T. K., Brasfield, R. D., Strong, E. W. and Haiju, S. I. (1969). Benign solitary schwannoma (neurilemmoma). *Cancer*, **24**, 355

38. Foot, H. C. (1940). Histology of tumors of the peripheral nerves. *Arch. Pathol.*, **30**, 772

39. Knight, W. A. III, Murphy, W. K. and Gottlieb, J. A. (1973). Neurofibromatosis associated with malignant neurofibromas. *Arch. Dermatol.*, **107**, 747

40. Dixon, A. Y., McGregor, D. H. and Lee, S. H. (1981). Angio-

lipomas: An ultrastructural and clinicopathological study. *Hum. Pathol.*, **12**, 737

41. Dardick, I. (1978). Hibernoma: A possible model of brown fat histogenesis. *Hum. Pathol.*, **9**, 321

42. Brody, H. J., Meltzer, H. D. and Someren, A. (1978). Spindle cell lipoma. *Arch. Dermatol.*, **114**, 1065

43. Shmookler, B. M. and Enzinger, F. M. (1981). Pleomorphic lipoma. A benign tumor simulating liposarcoma. *Cancer*, **47**, 126

44. Enterline, H. J., Culberson, J. D., Rochlin, D. B. and Brady, L. W. (1960). Liposarcoma. A clinical and pathological study of 53 cases. *Cancer*, **13**, 932

Figures 16.37–16.48 will be found overleaf.

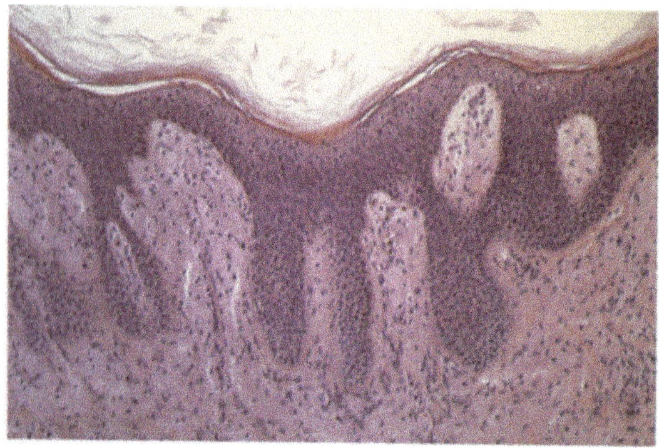

Figure 16.37   Granular cell tumour. There is typical pseudoepitheliomatous hyperplasia of the epithelium overlying the lesion.   H & E (A)

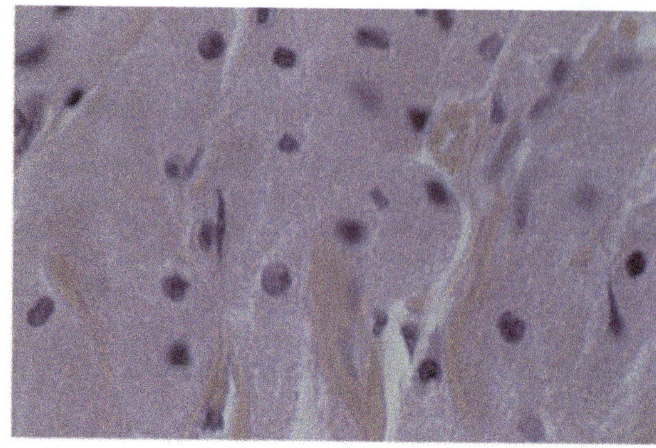

Figure 16.38   Granular-cell tumour, with large tumour cells which have a centrally placed nucleus and plentiful granular cytoplasm.   H & E (C)

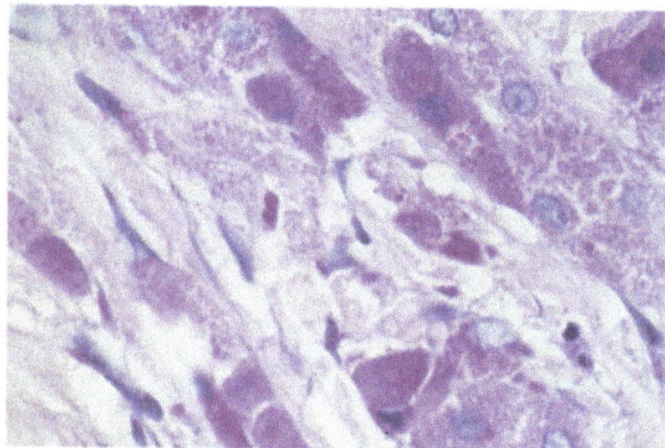

Figure 16.39   Granular-cell tumour, showing the positive staining of the cytoplasmic granules with PAS reagents.   PAS (C)

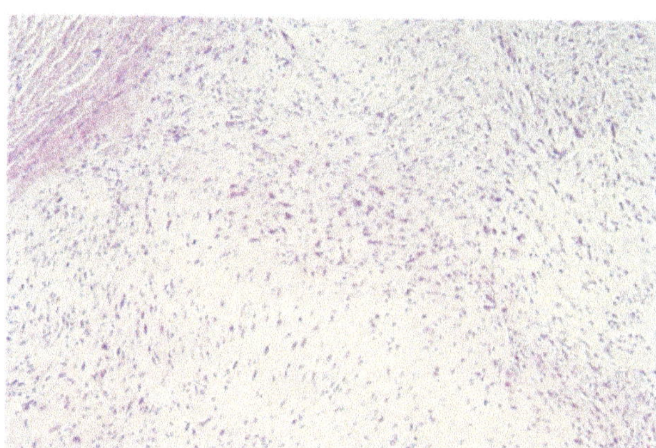

Figure 16.40   Neurilemmoma. Spindle-shaped cells are arranged in a pale stroma. Areas of pallisading are apparent in the lower part of the photomicrograph.   H & E (B)

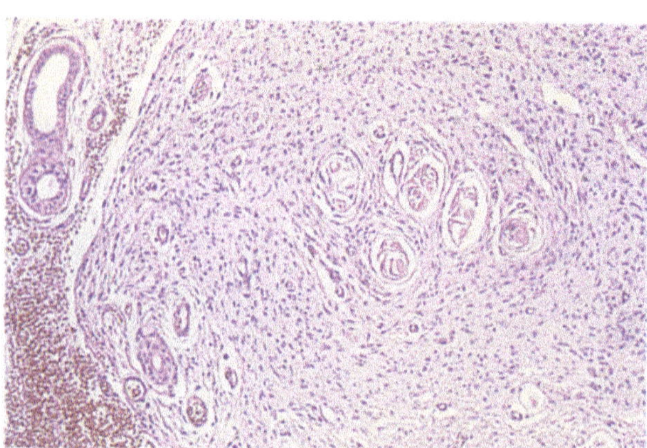

Figure 16.41   Neurofibroma, enveloping nerve bundles. The tumour cells contain typical nuclei with a wavy contour.   H & E (B)

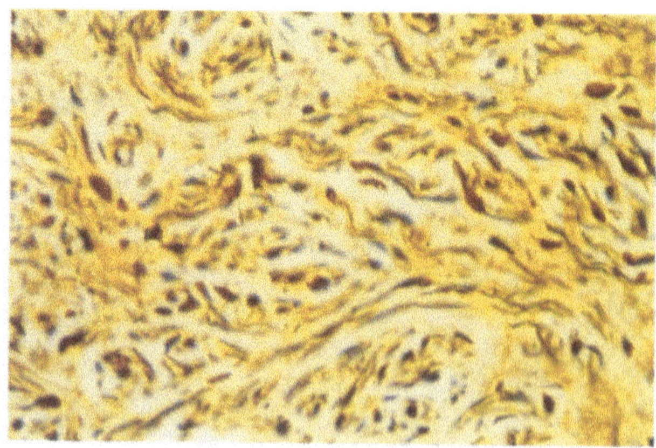

Figure 16.42   Neurofibroma. Special staining reveals nerve axons within the fibrous stroma. Palmgren's stain   (C)

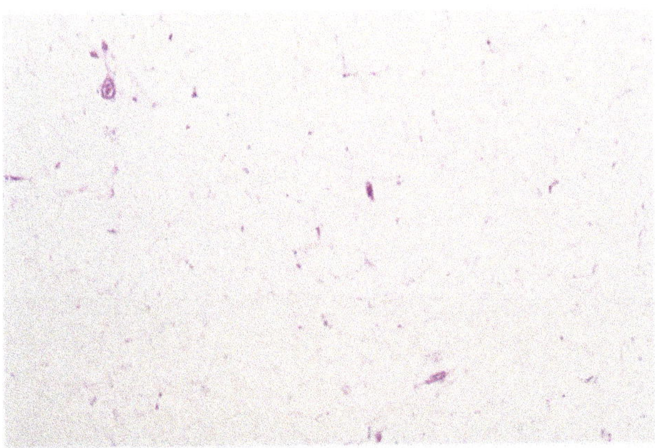

Figure 16.43 Lipoma. The appearances are identical with normal mature adipose tissue. H & E (A)

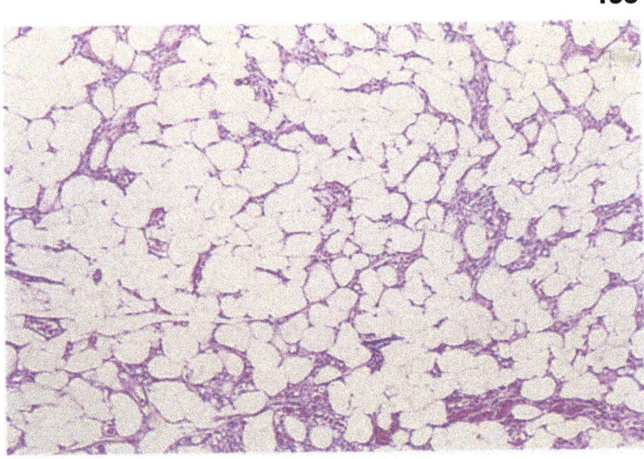

Figure 16.44 Angiolipoma. Compare the degree of vascularity with that of a typical lipoma. H & E (A)

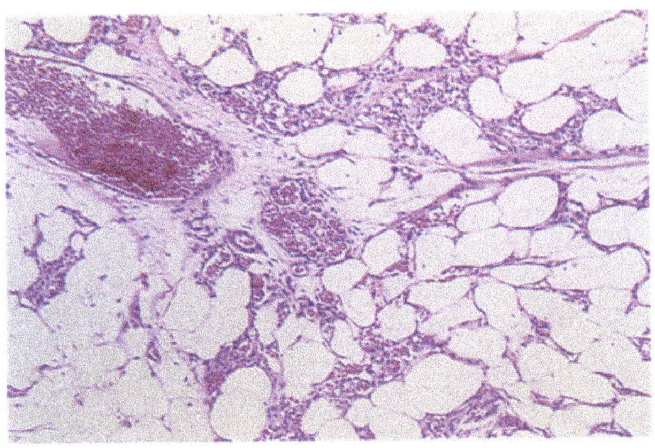

Figure 16.45 Angiolipoma. Higher magnification demonstrates the rich capillary network of angiolipoma. H & E (A)

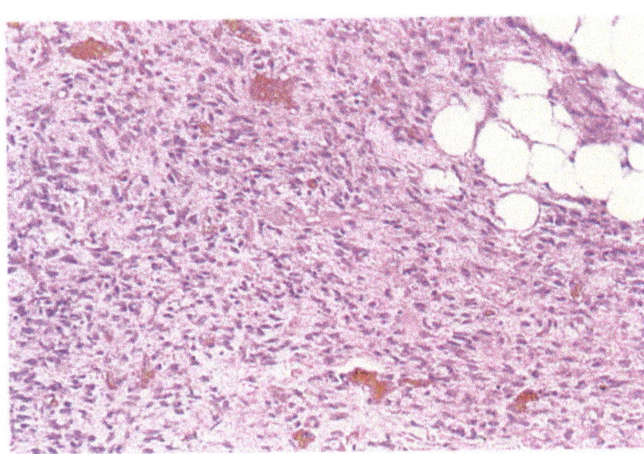

Figure 16.46 Spindle-cell lipoma. Spindle cells are set in a mucoid stroma and intermingle with normal mature fat-cells. H & E (B)

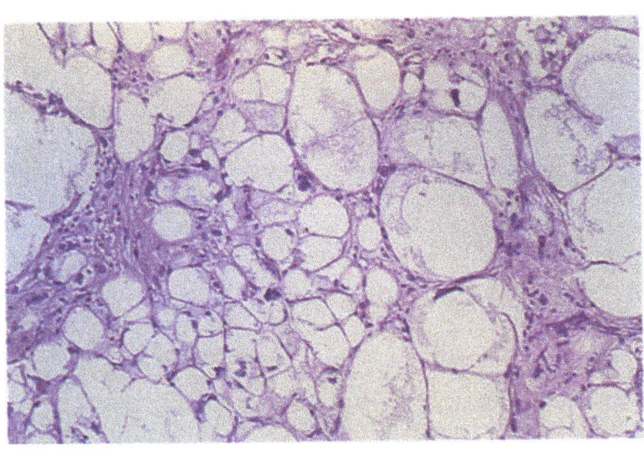

Figure 16.47 Pleomorphic lipoma. There is well-marked nuclear pleomorphism, but the absence of a typical vascular pattern or lipoblasts serve to distinguish this lesion from liposarcoma. H & E (B)

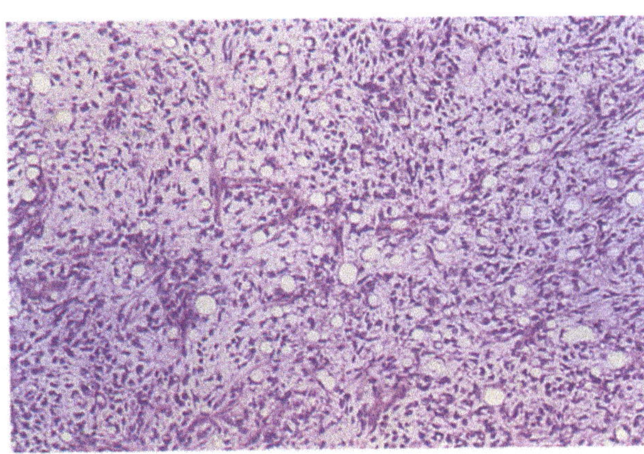

Figure 16.48 Myxoid liposarcoma, showing typical arborizing capillary blood vessels and lipoblasts in a mucoid stroma. H & E (A)

Lymphocytic, Mast-cell and Atypical Histiocytic Skin Tumours and Dermal Leukaemia

Among the diagnostic problems of skin biopsy, lymphocytic and histiocytic proliferations may prove the most bewildering[1]. This difficulty stems from the fact that chronic inflammatory infiltrates are commonplace in the skin and can be so prolific and histologically bizarre that an erroneous impression of lymphoid neoplasia can be created. On the other hand, in the early stages of mycosis fungoides (a T-cell lymphocytic neoplasm) the changes may be so minor that appearances vary little from inflammatory dermatoses. There are also conditions like histiocytosis X, neither certainly neoplastic nor certainly reactive, which affect the skin and may cause diagnostic difficulty. Unfortunately, no general rules apply to assist histological diagnosis in this field (save the golden rule of caution), but there are some features of lymphoid infiltrates which should raise a suspicion of

Table 17.1 General features of dermal lymphoma and reactive lymphocytic infiltration

	Lymphoma	Reactive lymphocytic infiltration
Site	–Reticular dermis and subcutaneous fat	–Papillary and reticular dermis
	–Epidermis and Grenz zone spared except in mycosis fungoides	–Epidermis may be involved
Structure	–Tightly packed, monomorphic infiltrate	–Oedematous, polymorphic infiltrate
	–Germinal centres absent	–Germinal centres may be present
	–Obliterates adnexal structures	–Infiltrates adnexal structures as single cells
	–Single-file invasion of collagen by strands of cells	–Single-cell diffuse infiltration of collagen
Cytology	–General nuclear atypia may be present	–Nuclear atypia only focal, if present
	–Mitotic activity variable but may include atypical forms	–Mitotic activity not uncommon, but *no* atypical forms seen

a neoplastic process (Table 17.1). Nodular lymphomas or leukaemic infiltrates tend to occupy the reticular rather than the papillary dermis and tend to extend into subcutaneous fat. The infiltrate tends to obliterate adnexal structures, rather than surrounding them as does an inflammatory lymphoid proliferation. A neoplastic lymphoid infiltrate tends to be densely cellular with little associated dermal oedema and tends to be composed of one cell type (monomorphism). Features which tend

to be of little help in differential diagnosis (and may raise a false suspicion of malignancy) include ulceration of the lesion, mitotic activity within the infiltrate (unless many of the mitoses are clearly atypical) and cellular pleomorphism. Cytologic atypia is a useful feature in the assessment of mycosis fungoides but it is also seen in other non-neoplastic lymphoid infiltrates. Finally, even though the skin may be easily accessible for biopsy in cases of lymphoma, leukaemia or myeloma in which there is cutaneous involvement, it is usually the lymph node or bone-marrow biopsy which will provide the reliable histological diagnosis.

Histiocytosis X

Histiocytosis X is the general name given to a group of mysterious conditions occurring in children and young adults and in which there is uncontrolled proliferation of histiocytes[2]. Three types of histiocytosis X are described: Letterer–Siwe and Hand–Schüller–Christian diseases, and eosinophilic granuloma. Cutaneous lesions are most common in Letterer–Siwe disease which is also the type of histiocytosis X which affects the youngest infants and is the most generalized and rapidly progressive. About 30 per cent of cases of Hand–Schüller–Christian disease have skin involvement but skin deposits are unusual in eosinophilic granuloma. Some cases of Hand–Schüller–Christian disease and most cases of Letterer–Siwe disease present as a crusting, papular dermatitis. Other cases of Hand–Schüller–Christian disease appear as erythematous, destructive plaques which tend to ulcerate.

Histological sections of skin affected by histiocytosis X show a dense infiltration of the upper dermis by a mixture of cells which include eosinophils, neutrophils, plasma cells and lymphocytes but are predominantly histiocytic in type (Figures 17.1–17.3). Many histiocytes are cytologically atypical with a prominent reniform nucleus. The cytoplasm of these cells may be deeply eosinophilic or may show xanthomatous change. The infiltrate is usually centred on the superficial dermis and involves the overlying epidermis. Electron microscopy of the histiocytic cells shows that their cytoplasm contains the granules seen in normal Langerhans cells of the skin[3]. This finding is a useful confirmatory test in that normal histiocytes do not contain these granules.

The various forms of histiocytosis X show a somewhat different histological appearance; variants of the above general description. As would be expected from its relatively benign clinical course, skin lesions in eosinophilic granuloma show little cytological atypia and may include histiocytic giant cells. Eosinophils are numerous and appear in clumps. The most aggressive form, Letterer–Siwe disease, is characterized by epidermal invasion by histiocytic cells showing nuclear atypia and

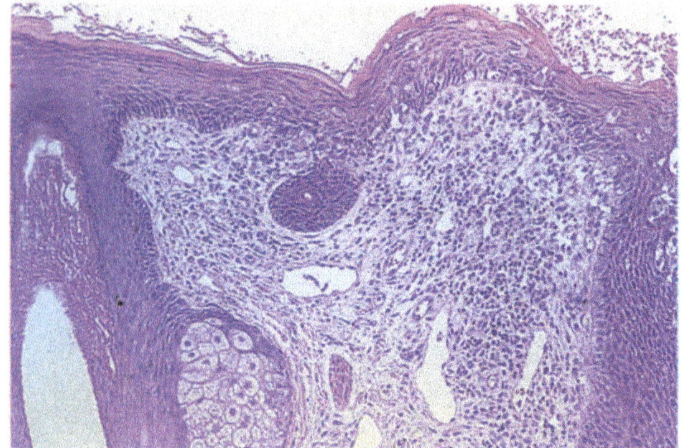

Figure 17.1 Histiocytosis X. At low magnification, the infiltrate is seen to be primarily located in the papillary dermis. Epidermotropism (infiltration of the epidermis by atypical cells) is typical of histiocytosis X.   H & E (A)

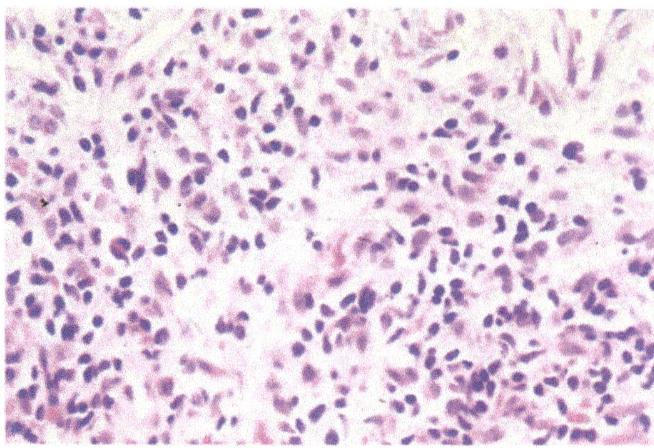

Figure 17.2 Histiocytosis X. The infiltrate is polymorphic, consisting of histiocyte-like cells, lymphocytes and eosinophils.   H & E (B)

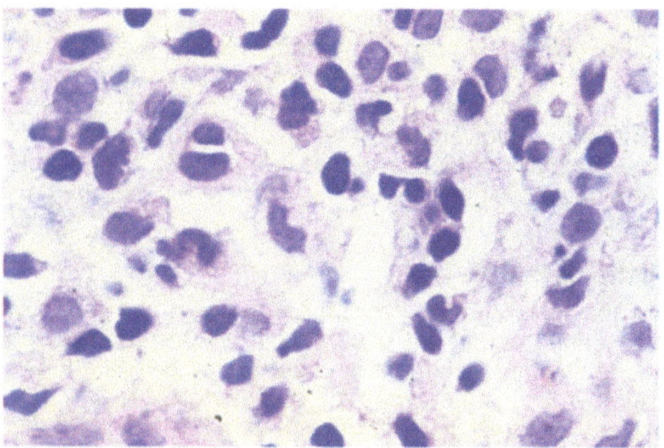

Figure 17.3 Histiocytosis X. At high magnification, the nuclei are seen to be atypical, with reniform nuclei being apparent.   H & E (C)

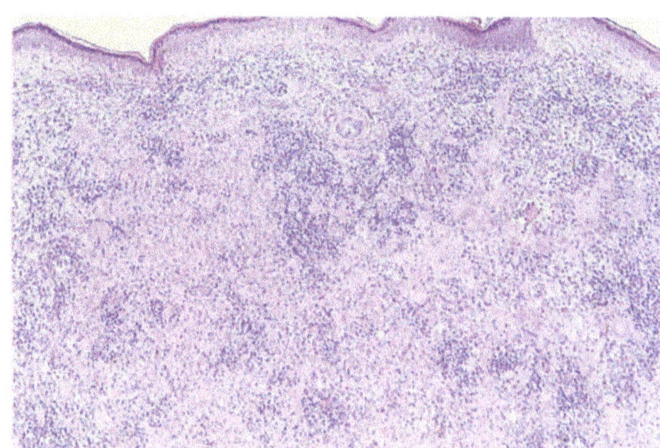

Figure 17.4 Juvenile xanthogranuloma. At low magnification, the dermis is expanded by an infiltrate composed of large eosinophilic cells, interspersed by clumps of lymphocytes.   H & E (A)

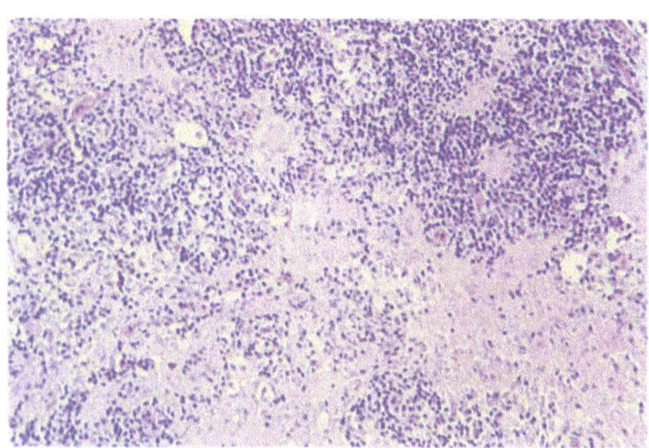

Figure 17.5 Juvenile xanthogranuloma. The inflammatory infiltrate includes foamy histiocytes, scanty lymphocytes and some eosinophils.   H & E (B)

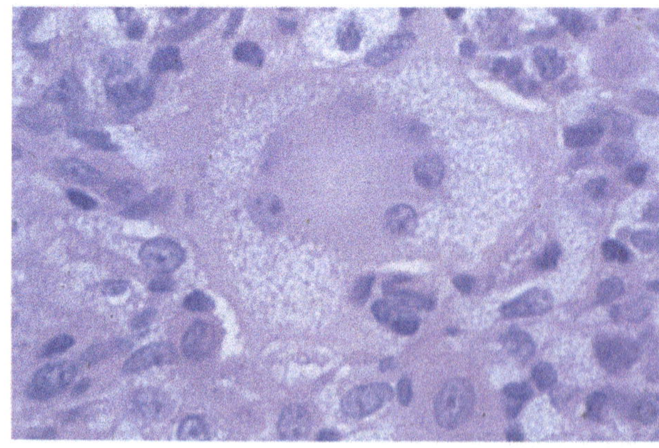

Figure 17.6 Juvenile xanthogranuloma. Touton giant cell.   H & E (C)

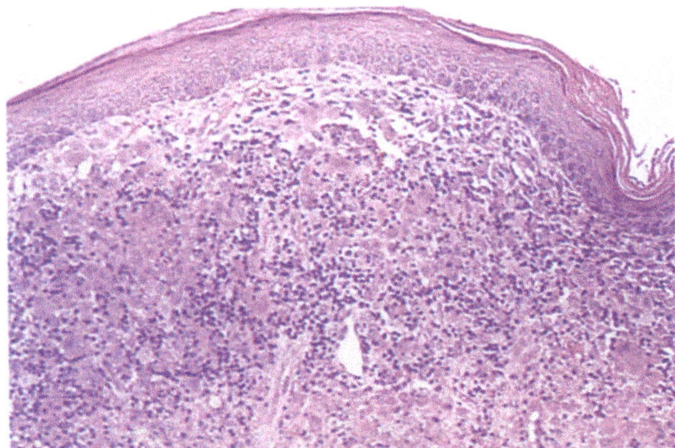

Figure 17.7 Reticulohistiocytic granuloma. Appearances are similar to those of juvenile xanthogranuloma, but Touton giant cells are scarce. H & E (B)

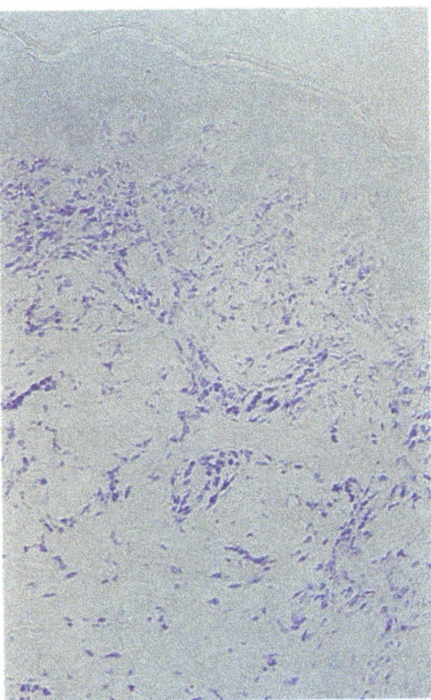

Figure 17.8 Mastocytosis. Special staining with toluidine blue demonstrates large numbers of mast cells around superficial dermal capillaries. Toluidine blue (B)

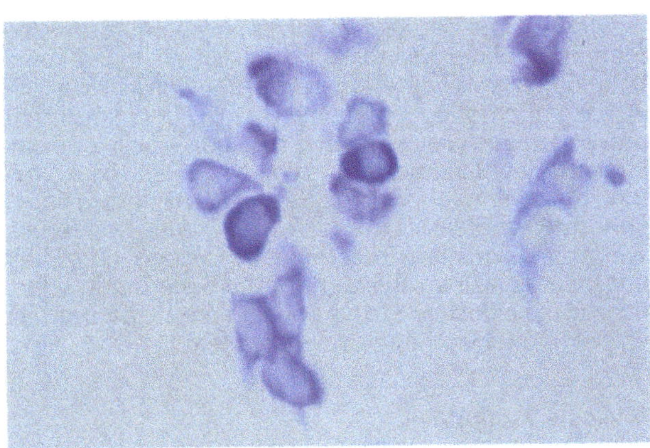

Figure 17.9 Mastocytosis. Mast cells are readily demonstrated by toluidine blue staining. (C)

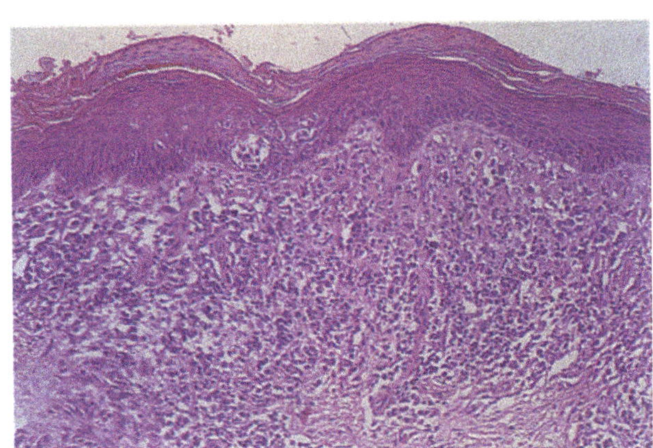

Figure 17.10 Mycosis fungoides, erythematous stage. A Pautrier microabscess can be identified in the epidermis. H & E (B)

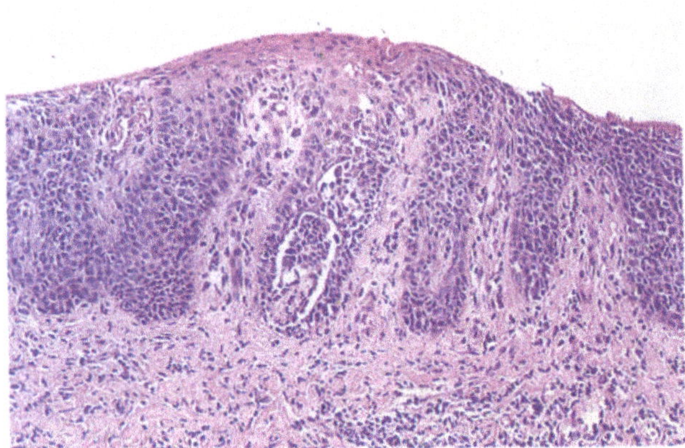

Figure 17.11 Mycosis fungoides, erythematous stage. Psoriasiform hyperplasia of the epidermis. H & E (B)

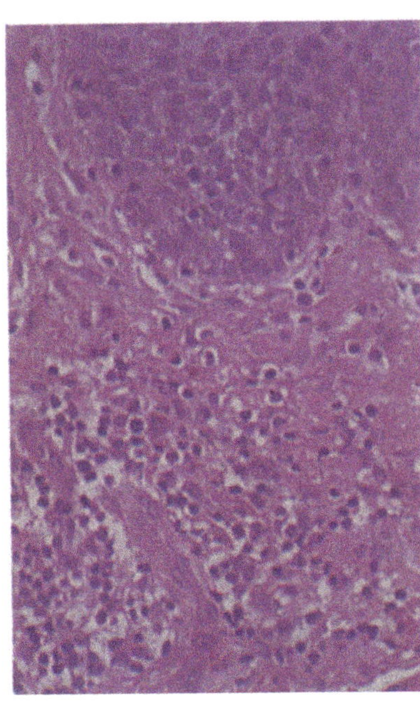

Figure 17.12 Mycosis fungoides, erythematous stage. Cellular infiltrate. H & E (C)

scanty eosinophilic cytoplasm. Most cases of Hand–Schüller–Christian disease are intermediate between these extremes, but in some cases the histiocytes are almost entirely xanthomatous. Unfortunately, in such cases Langerhans granules may be difficult to demonstrate by ultrastructural examination of the foamy histiocytic cytoplasm. These cases can be difficult to distinguish from lipidized fibrous histiocytomas or juvenile xanthogranuloma. The characteristic features of xanthomatous Hand–Schüller–Christian disease are a relative paucity of Touton-type giant cells and the mixed nature of the inflammatory infiltrate, with prominent eosinophilic polymorphonuclear leukocytes.

Juvenile Xanthogranuloma

Juvenile xanthogranuloma (naevoxanthogranuloma[4]) shows many histological features of similarity with histocytosis X, and there has undoubtedly been some confusion between the two entities. Ultrastructural studies, however, suggest that the two conditions are separate, for no Langerhans granules have been demonstrated in cases of juvenile xanthogranuloma[5], whereas they are regularly demonstrable in all forms of histiocytosis X except for some cases of the most xanthomatous variant. The lesions are usually solitary or few in number, occur early in life and are red or yellowish nodules, usually about 1 cm in diameter. Although normally confined to the skin, there may be haemorrhagic nodular lesions of the iris and rare cases of infiltration of other organs have been described.

Lipidization is a common feature of juvenile xanthogranuloma, even in early lesions (Figures 17.4 and 17.5). In older nodules, the inflammatory infiltrate includes histiocytes (many lipidized), lymphocytes and some eosinophils. A characteristic feature is the presence of prominent foreign-body type and Touton giant cells (Figure 17.6). Finally, regressing lesions may show significant fibrosis. Touton giant cells are not unique to juvenile xanthogranuloma; small numbers are seen in some cases of histiocytosis X or lipid-laden dermatofibromas.

Reticulohistiocytic Granuloma and Multicentric Reticulohistiocytosis

In many ways, reticulohistiocytosis is the adult and old age counterpart of juvenile xanthogranuloma[6]. The two types of reticulohistiocytosis have the same histological appearance. Reticulohistiocytic granulomas occur singly or as one or two nodules up to 2 cm diameter and almost exclusively on the head and neck. The multicentric variant of reticulohistiocytosis has multiple nodules on the face and hands together with an arthritis, again most severe in the hands, in many patients.

The characteristic cell of reticulohistiocytosis is a pale, swollen histiocyte with pale mauve homogeneous cytoplasm with the appearance of ground glass (Figure 17.7). Aging of the lesion is associated with the fusing of these histiocytes into large giant cells. The nuclei are randomly distributed and Touton forms are rare. In most cases the granular cytoplasm can be demonstrated to be PAS-positive even after diastase pretreatment. In between the histiocytic cells is a prominent lymphocytic infiltrate, particularly in early lesions. Fibrosis may be a prominent feature in later lesions demonstrating large numbers of giant cells.

Mast-cell Proliferations

Mast cells are easily demonstrated in sections of skin by staining of their metachromatic cytoplasmic granules by such stains as toluidine blue or Giemsa's reagents (Figures 17.8 and 17.9). Increased numbers of mast cells are seen as a non-specific feature in granuloma annulare and scleromyxoedema where they appear to be a response to connective tissue mucins. They are seen in large numbers in many tumours such as basal-cell carcinoma or neurofibroma. Although mast cells play an essential role in the development of urticaria through the release of histamine, in histological sections of urticarial lesions the inflammatory infiltrate is usually not intense. Accordingly, the total numbers of mast cells are not grossly increased although they form a relatively high proportion of the inflammatory infiltrate. Dense mast-cell infiltration of the skin indicates a diagnosis of either urticaria pigmentosa or systemic mastocytosis[7]. The infiltrate is principally located around the capillary blood vessels of the superficial dermis. In places the aggregates of mast cells become frank tumours and may extend from the dermis into the subcutaneous fat. It is most unusual for there to be epidermal infiltration by mast cells in either urticaria pigmentosa or systemic mastocytosis.

Although the histological appearances of urticaria pigmentosa and mastocytosis are similar, the clinical presentation is very different. Urticaria pigmentosa is a disease of childhood, presenting as multiple small light-brown papules which become red and swollen on being stroked. Spontaneous regression of the lesions is common at the time of puberty. Systemic mastocytosis is a very rare progressive disease which occurs in adults. The skin lesions may resemble those seen in children, but there is also involvement of the bone marrow (producing radiolucency of the bones) and of the liver and spleen producing hepatosplenomegaly.

Mycosis Fungoides

Mycosis fungoides is a form of lymphoma peculiar to the skin[8,9]. It has a prolonged course which may last over many years but is inexorably progressive without treatment, passing through erythematous, plaque and tumourous stages until there is dissemination into the lymph nodes and internal viscera. The eczematous, erythematous phase may be very varied in its distribution and extent. A particularly localized variant described by Woringer and Kolopp[10] is characterized by a focus of acanthosis and papillomatosis with an epidermotropic infiltrate of atypical mononuclear cells. Local excision is usually curative. At the other extreme is the Sézary syndrome, a combination of exfoliative dermatitis or generalized erythroderma and the appearance in the peripheral blood of atypical mononuclear (so-called Sézary) cells.

The principal feature of mycosis fungoides in its early erythematous stage is the presence of an epidermotropic infiltrate of atypical mononuclear cells (Figures 17.10 – 17.12). The abnormal cells are somewhat larger than usual and have large irregular basophilic, reniform or cerebriform nuclei. The infiltrate is often arranged in a band-like pattern. The particular characteristic of the epidermotropism is that, unlike epidermal inflammatory infiltrates in inflammatory dermatoses, there is little or no associated spongiosis. In places, the epidermotropic cells form small clumps of 10 or 20 cells. These so-called Pautrier 'microabscesses' are highly suggestive of mycosis fungoides, particularly when the surrounding epidermis shows no evidence of reactive spongiosis. Sometimes there is regular epidermal hyperplasia and parakeratosis with a superficial resemblance to psoriasis. When spongiosis co-exists with Pautrier-like microabscesses, even when there is some hyperchromasia and atypia of the nuclei in the inflammatory cells, appearances must be interpreted with caution because such changes have been described in inflammatory dermatosis.

Histological diagnosis of mycosis fungoides may be very difficult in the early erythematous stage. Recent advance has been made with the application of monoclonal antibodies to leukocyte surface markers to frozen sections of skin[11]. In some cases, the monotypical T–cell nature of the infiltrate can be demonstrated using such antibodies in immunocytochemical procedures. Monotypicality is a good indicator that the infiltrate is neoplastic rather than inflammatory. In other cases, when there is a well-marked inflammatory reaction to the neoplastic infiltrate, the polyclonal nature of these inflammatory cells reduces the value of immunocytochemistry in diagnosis.

Once the plaque stage has developed, histological diagnosis is much more straightforward (Figures 17.13 – 17.17). Many more atypical mononuclear cells are seen and are diffusely distributed throughout the dermis. The nuclei of the cells tend to have an irregular shape and are hyperchromatic, rather than being enlarged. As the plaque stage progresses the nuclear irregularity becomes more marked and enlarged, clearly malignant nuclei are seen. Epidermotropism and Pautrier abscess formation are the rule in the plaque stage of mycosis fungoides, but ulceration of the epidermis is unusual. An occasional non-specific feature is the presence of follicular mucinosis in hair follicles involved in the plaques. Immunocytochemical studies are usually able to demonstrate the monoclonal nature of the overwhelming majority of the cells in plaque-stage mycosis fungoides.

The tumour stage is clearly malignant. Large nodules of pleomorphic, hyperchromatic cells fill the dermis and infiltrate the subcutaneous fat and epidermis producing ulceration of the skin. When the tumour becomes disseminated it affects many organs, but the clinical symptoms of systemic involvement are often slight and death is usually due to intercurrent infection. Early lymph nodal involvement can be difficult to detect in histological sections but as the disease progresses there is disruption of the nodal architecture in a manner very similar in appearance to Hodgkin's disease. The infiltrating cell has a rather histiocytic appearance but can be shown by use of immunocytochemical procedures to be a monotypical T-cell proliferation.

Cutaneous Involvement by Lymphoma and Leukaemia

Hodgkin's Disease

Direct involvement of the skin in Hodgkin's disease by infiltration from an affected nearby lymph node is uncommon, primary involvement of the skin is extremely rare[12]. The histological appearances of tumour-stage mycosis fungoides and Hodgkin's disease may be very similar. Immunocytochemical studies may help in differentiating between those conditions. In mycosis, the infiltrate shows evidence of T-lymphocyte surface markers. The crucial diagnostic feature of Hodgkin's disease is the presence of multinucleate Reed–Sternberg giant cells. The cells have a pale eosinophilic cytoplasm which tends to shrink away from the surrounding tissue during preparation of the sections. There are typically two nuclei in direct contact with one another. Each nucleus has a pale, open chromatin pattern and contains a prominent, angular, eosinophilic nucleolus. Less common forms have multiple nuclei. Similar mononuclear, so-called 'lacunar' cells are more common but less specific in histological diagnosis. The nuclei of the cellular infiltrate in tumour-stage mycosis fungoides may be similar to those in Hodgkin's disease, but they tend to be more hyperchromatic and have less prominent nucleoli which are also less eosinophilic in their staining reactions.

Non-Hodgkin's Lymphoma

Non-Hodgkin's lymphoma, a tumour most commonly of B-lymphocytes, usually arises in the lymph nodes and bone marrow. However, primary cutaneous lymphoma does occur and frequently presents problems in histological diagnosis[13]. These problems tend to fall into two categories. Either the biopsy shows an infiltrate which is obviously malignant because of its degree of cytological atypia and mitotic activity but is not obviously lymphoid in origin or alternatively the biopsy contains an infiltrate which is clearly of well-differentiated lymphocytes but is not obviously malignant. In well-differentiated lymphoid infiltrates of the skin, features suggestive of malignancy are: (1) monomorphic infiltrate – the cells appear to be all of one type and do not include many neutrophil leukocytes; (2) lack of oedema in the reticular dermis or spongiosis or basal vacuolation in the overlying epidermis; (3) densely packed lymphocytes; (4) lack of germinal centres; and (5) sharp delineation of individual nodules of the infiltrate, with invasion of the surrounding collagen by rows of cells rather than randomly distributed lymphocytes (Figures 17.18–17.20). Unfortunately, none of these features is pathognomonic of lymphoma and it may not be possible to make a diagnosis in all skin biopsies. In poorly differentiated lymphocytic infiltrates it is usually necessary to use immunocytochemical techniques (on frozen sections) to determine whether the neoplasm is B- or T-cell in type. Immunocytochemistry may also be useful in showing that a poorly differentiated tumour is lymphoid rather than a primary or metastatic carcinoma or sarcoma.

Multiple Myeloma

Myeloma is a neoplasm of plasma cells and it arises in the bone marrow. The plasma cells often produce a monoclonal immunoglobulin which can be detected in the serum and which may be associated with amyloidosis. Metastasis to the skin is rare but can precede the systemic manifestations of the disease. In ordinarily stained sections, the infiltrate appears monomorphic and is composed of densely packed atypical plasma cells. Antibodies to λ- and ϰ-light chains and IgG, IgM and IgA immunoglobulin can be used on paraffin sections to demonstrate that the infiltrate is monoclonal.

Leukaemia Cutis

Leukaemia arises in the bone marrow, but it is a systemic disease and skin involvement is not uncommon. The histological appearances depend on the type of leukaemia. In chronic lymphatic leukaemia the infiltrate is identical to that in well-differentiated non-Hodgkin's lymphocytic lymphoma. Infiltration of the skin in acute lymphocytic leukaemia is very rare. The cells may demonstrate T-cell markers. Cutaneous involvement is also uncommon in granulocytic leukaemia, but may be the first sign of disease in both acute granulocytic and in myelomonocytic leukaemia. The cellular infiltrate is atypical and may be almost entirely monomorphic, falsely suggesting a diagnosis of lymphoma. In paraffin-embedded sections, it is usually possible to demonstrate

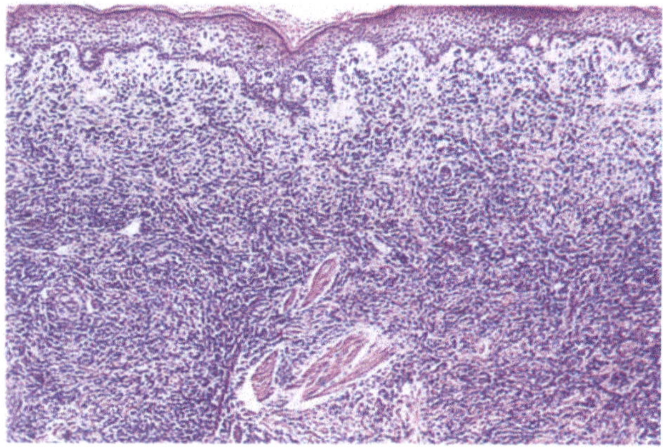

Figure 17.13 Mycosis fungoides, plaque stage. A dense, diffuse, atypical lymphocytic infiltrate fills the reticular dermis.   H & E (A)

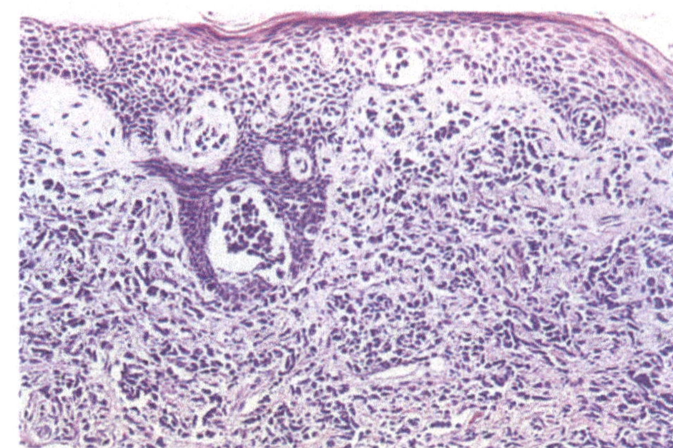

Figure 17.14 Mycosis fungoides, plaque stage. Multiple Pautrier microabscesses are seen in the epidermis.   H & E (B)

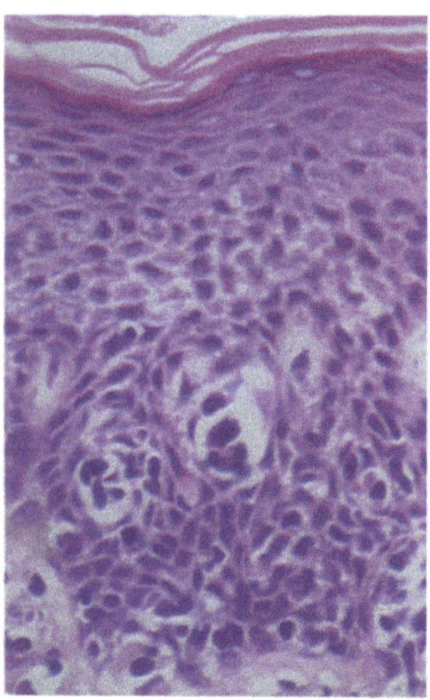

Figure 17.15 Mycosis fungoides, plaque stage. Pautrier microabscess. H & E (C)

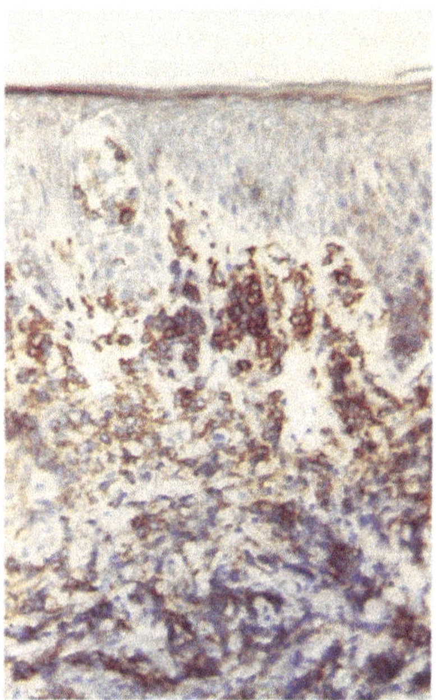

Figure 17.16 Mycosis fungoides, plaque stage. Immunocytochemistry can provide useful confirmation that the atypical lymphocytic infiltrate is monotypic. Virtually all the lymphocytes seen in this frozen section stain positively with antibody to T-helper subset surface markers (compare with Figure 17.17). Leu 3a immunostain   (B)

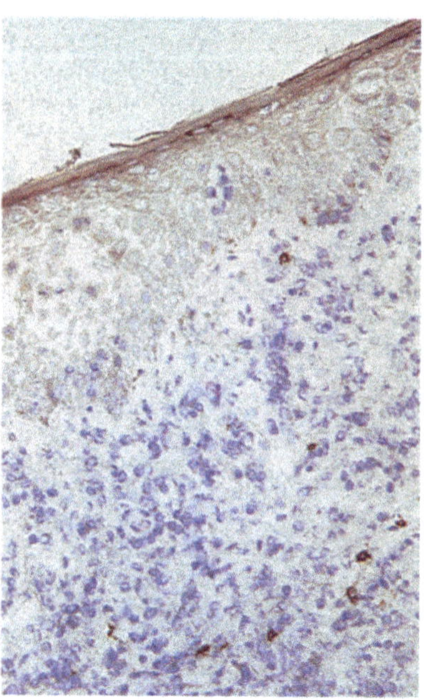

Figure 17.17 Mycosis fungoides, plaque stage. Only scanty, reactive T-suppressor lymphocytes are seen in this immunocytochemical staining of serial section from the specimen shown in Figure 17.16.   OKT-8 immunostain   (B)

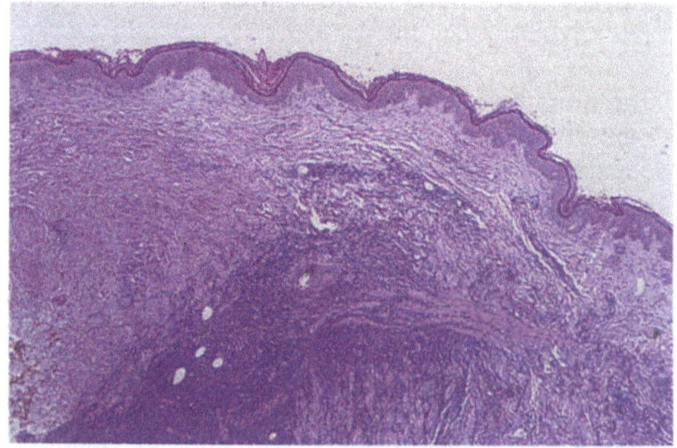

Figure 17.18 Non-Hodgkin's lymphoma. A dense infiltrate is seen to be separating bands of dermal collagen.   H & E (A)

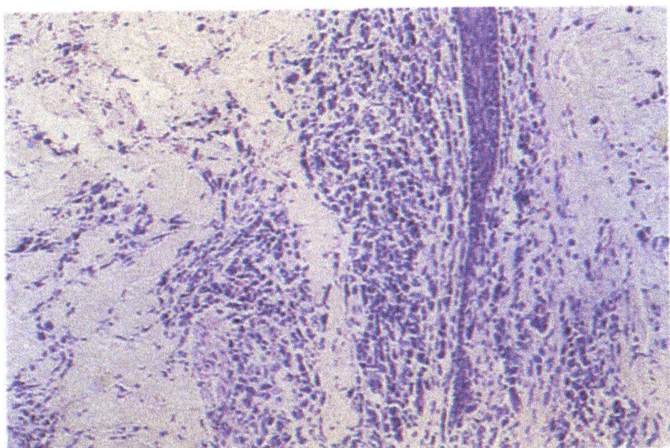

Figure 17.19 Non-Hodgkin's lymphoma, showing infiltration by cords of neoplastic lymphocytes around a hair follicle.   H & E (B)

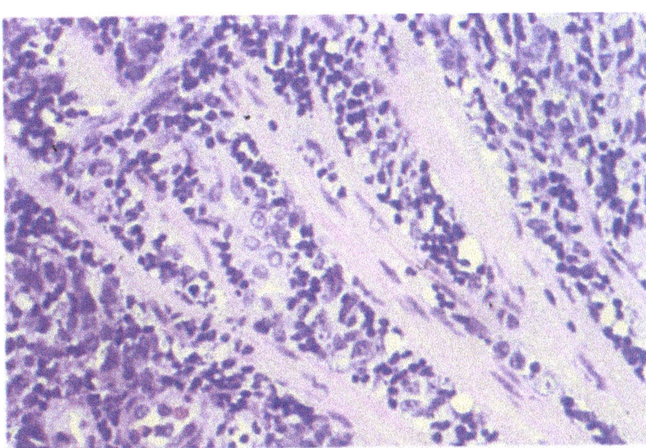

Figure 17.20 Non-Hodgkin's lymphoma. The collagen of the reticular dermis is being infiltrated by cords of lymphocytes which show nuclear atypia.   H & E (C)

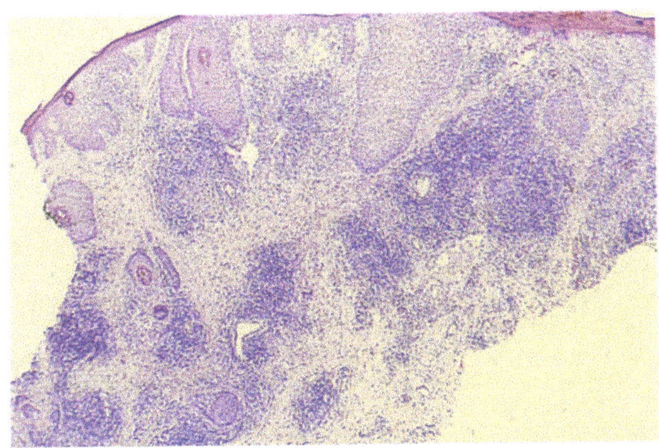

Figure 17.21 Reactive lymphocytic infiltration of the skin. The infiltrate is loosely packed, perivascular in distribution and the nodules of lymphocytes are ill-defined.   H & E (A)

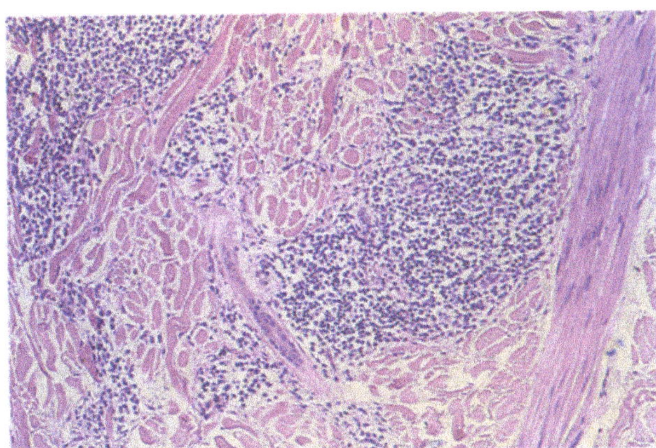

Figure 17.22 Reactive lymphocytic infiltration of the skin. A single-cell infiltrating pattern, lack of nuclear pleomorphism, perivascular distribution and associated oedema of dermal collagen are indicative of a reactive process.   H & E (B)

chloroacetate esterase activity in a proportion of the cells and thus confirm their myelocytic nature. Nonetheless, marrow trephine biopsy is mandatory to establish the diagnosis.

Lymphocytoma Cutis (Pseudolymphoma of Spiegler–Fendt)

The general term 'pseudolymphoma' is applied to all situations where there is such a dense lymphocytic infiltration of the skin that a spurious diagnosis of lymphoma may be made. Such conditions include insect bites[14], actinic reticuloid and Jessner's lymphocytic infiltration. In addition to these conditions there are others which may progress to lymphoma after many years or heal spontaneously, including lymphomatoid papulosis[15] (see page 64), angiolymphoid hyperplasia with eosinophilia (see page 125), angioimmunoblastic lymphadenopathy and lymphomatoid granulomatosis. These are systemic diseases with cutaneous manifestations, but have a similar histological appearance to the isolated skin condition lymphocytoma cutis.

Lymphocytoma usually occurs as a solitary or, more rarely multiple lesions which may occur at any site but are more frequently encountered on the face. They are fleshy red or violaceous papules which tend to heal spontaneously but which may recur and rarely progress to lymphoma.

The histological picture is of a massive lymphoid infiltrate extending into the subcutaneous fat (Figures 17.21 and 17.22). The infiltrate is a mixture of lymphocytes and histiocytes and has a rather nodular appearance. Mitotic activity may be well-marked, but the follicular pattern usually serves to distinguish the appearance from that of lymphoma which also shows significant atypia when it is of the mixed lymphocytic–histiocytic type. It is also important to sample the lesion of a suspected case of lymphocytoma with care to eliminate the possibility of a reaction to an arthropod sting or persistent scabies.

References

1. Clarke, W. H., Mihm, M. C. Jr, Reed, R. J. and Ainsworth, A. M. (1974). The lymphocytic infiltrates of the skin. *Hum. Pathol.*, **5**, 25

2. Mihm, M. C. Jr, Clarke, W. H. and Reed, R. J. (1974). The histiocytic infiltrates of the skin. *Hum. Pathol.*, **5**, 45

3. Gianotti, F. and Caputo, R. (1969). Skin ultrastructure in Hand–Schüller–Christian disease. *Arch. Dermatol.*, **100**, 342

4. Helwig, E. B. and Hackney, V. C. (1954). Juvenile xanthogranuloma (nevoxantho-endothelioma). *Am. J. Pathol.*, **30**, 625

5. Gonzales-Crussi, F. and Campbell, R. (1970). Juvenile xanthogranuloma. Ultrastructural study. *Arch. Pathol.*, **89**, 65

6. Goltz, R. W. and Layman, C. W. (1954). Multicentric reticulohistiocytosis of the skin and synovia. *Arch. Dermatol. Syphilol.*, **69**, 717

7. Moheit, G. D., Murad, T. and Conrad, M. (1979). Systemic mastocytosis and the mastocytosis syndrome. *J. Cutan. Pathol.*, **6**, 42

8. Winkelmann, R. K. and Caro, W. A. (1977). Current problems in mycosis fungoides and Sézary syndrome. *Ann. Rev. Med.*, **28**, 251

9. Brehmer-Anderrson, E. (1976). Mycosis fungoides and its relation to Sézary's syndrome, lymphomatoid papulosis, and primary cutaneous Hodgkin's disease. *Acta. Derm. Venereol. (Stockh.)*, **75**, (Suppl.56), 9

10. Deneau, D. G., Wood, G. S. Beckstead, J., Hoppe, R. T. and Price, N. (1984). Woringer-Kolopp disease (pagetoid reticulosis). Four cases with histopathologic, ultrastructural, and immunohistologic observations. *Arch. Dermatol.*, **120**, 1045

11. Chu, A.C., Fergin, P.E. and MacDonald, D.M. (1982). *In-situ* T lymphocyte identification in cutaneous tissue sections of benign and malignant dermatoses. *Histopathology*, **6**, 25

12. Smith, J. L. and Butler, J. J. (1980). Skin involvement in Hodgkin's disease. *Cancer*, **45**, 345

13. Evans, H. L., Winkelmann, R. K. and Banks, P. M. (1979). Differential diagnosis of malignant and benign cutaneous lymphoid infiltrates. *Cancer*, **44**, 699

14. Thomson, J., Cochran, T., Cochran, R. and McQueen, A. (1974). Histology simulating reticulosis in persistent nodular scabies. *Br. J. Dermatol.*, **90**, 421

15. Sanchez, N. P., Pittelkow, M. R., Muller, S. A., Banks, P. M. and Winkelmann, R. K. (1983). The clinicopathologic spectrum of lymphomatoid papulosis: study of 31 cases. *J. Am. Acad. Dermatol.*, **8**, 81

Index

Italic references are to figure numbers. Those which start with *I* refer to figures in the introduction.

GPSR Compliance
The European Union's (EU) General Product Safety Regulation (GPSR) is a set
of rules that requires consumer products to be safe and our obligations to
ensure this.

If you have any concerns about our products, you can contact us on

ProductSafety@springernature.com

In case Publisher is established outside the EU, the EU authorized
representative is:

Springer Nature Customer Service Center GmbH
Europaplatz 3
69115 Heidelberg, Germany

www.ingramcontent.com/pod-product-compliance
Ingram Content Group UK Ltd.
Pitfield, Milton Keynes, MK11 3LW, UK
UKHW050740080726
473059UK00008B/2360